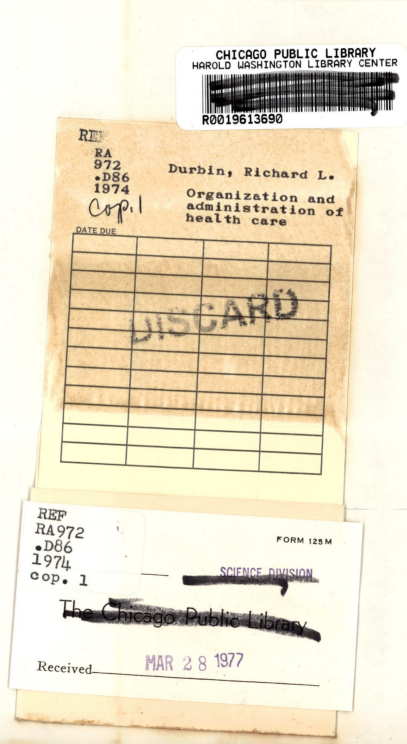

ORGANIZATION
AND
ADMINISTRATION
OF HEALTH CARE

ORGANIZATION AND ADMINISTRATION OF HEALTH CARE

THEORY, PRACTICE, ENVIRONMENT

RICHARD L. DURBIN, A.B., M.B.A., M.P.A.

Vice President for Planning and Development,
College of Medicine and Dentistry of New Jersey;
Interim Project Director,
Newark Comprehensive Health Service Plan;
Assistant Professor, Preventive Medicine,
New Jersey Medical School,
Newark, New Jersey

W. HERBERT SPRINGALL, A.B., M.P.H.

Director of HMO Development,
Philadelphia Health Management Corporation;
Adjunct Associate Professor of Health Care Management,
Temple University College of Allied Health Professions,
Philadelphia, Pennsylvania

SECOND EDITION

with 59 *illustrations*

THE C. V. MOSBY COMPANY

Saint Louis 1974

Second edition

Copyright © 1974 by The C. V. Mosby Company

All rights reserved. No part of this book may be reproduced in any manner without written permission of the publisher.

Previous edition copyrighted 1969

Printed in the United States of America

Distributed in Great Britain by Henry Kimpton, London

Library of Congress Cataloging in Publication Data

Durbin, Richard L
    Organization and administration of health care.

    Bibliography: p.
    1. Hospitals—Administration. 2. Public health
administration. I. Springall, W. Herbert, joint
author. II. Title. [DNLM: 1. Hospital administration—U. S. WX150 D953o 1974]
RA972.D86 1974   658'.91'36211   74-1114
ISBN 0-8016-1472-4

CB/CB/B 9 8 7 6 5 4 3 2 1

For

**those who explore the boundaries
of organizational reality**

and
our wives

Carolyn and Helen

FOREWORD

Two surpassingly important features of the current American scene are affecting both theory and practice in the administration and management of organizations.

The first is the growing recognition—again in both theory and application—that there is a great core of necessary lore common to all employing institutions, whether they be strictly governmental, strictly private, or anywhere in between.

The reasons for this emerging perception lie in the growth in size and complexity of these organizations and in the accelerated blending, especially in post–World War II America, of private and public functions. In fact, such institutions as universities, health care organizations, ports of authority, foundations, COMSATS and like corporations, and privately organized manpower training efforts endowed with public funds have experienced a greater rate of growth during the past quarter century than any other form of enterprise.

The result has been an intensified effort to understand the factors affecting the problems of how to manage, how to organize, how to administer—in a world where old forms and formats and compartmentalized systems have had to give way to the burst of change that emphasized innovation and the need to interact with large sectors of the environment that could previously be ignored.

The second important feature is the growing recognition of the need to define organizational goals, objectives, aims, and aspirations in overt and measurable terms; to construct corresponding organizational forms responsive to those goals; and to set up, simultaneously, systems for providing the necessary intelligence that permits an evaluation of how good that correspondence is.

The reasons for this emerging perception lie in the great growth of technology and its generation of upending change and in the growing scarcity of the prime factor of production: manpower. If for no other reason, the sheer shortage of the hands, skills, and talents needed to consummate organizational goals has put an enormous emphasis on ensuring the most clear-cut avowed institutional aims and the most responsive pathways for getting them achieved.

All of this is in the context of an outlook for the immediate years ahead, which juxtaposes, for example, a 1 million reduction in the number of workers in such a critical age cohort as the 35 to 45 year olds and an urgently increasing demand for experienced personnel to carry out an equally urgent demand for a growing range of services.

Cutting across these two forces has been the emergence of a new national stance in terms of public policy. Just within this decade we have witnessed the emergence of a new economic policy that seeks to mitigate, if not prevent, fluctuations in business activity by the intervention of fiscal and monetary measures. At the same time there has emerged a new manpower policy that seeks to mitigate, if not prevent, the educational disabilities related to the job market by the intervention of publicly financed training and retraining efforts. Simultaneously, we have adopted a national incomes policy that seeks to mitigate, if not prevent, the syndromes of those at the bottom of the earnings ladder by the intervention of a series of programs against poverty.

Every organization, public or private, has been affected by the avalanche of programs mounted to give effect to these policies, and every organization now seeks organizational formats that can deliver in the most responsive manner the substance required by these developments.

In very few, if any, other arenas are these occurrences more relevant than in the field of health care. Its growing complexity, its technologic change, and its role in the mainstream of the new public policy have no rivals.

This book goes to the heart of these matters in two ways. It confronts the prob-

lem of administration and management, and, from the spectrum of efforts in this field, puts before the house the essence of a viable system and a viable process of organization. And it meets the challenge of that confrontation by setting forth a concrete and specific system applicable to hospital administration. In doing so, the authors are both innovative and responsive to a great need in an enormously important sector of our national effort.

No foreword should review or anticipate the volume to which it is prefatory. But as the reader moves on to the book itself he will want to look forward to finding and following the authors' reasoning that "an organizational theory is a conceptual point of reference that prepares us to better understand an organization."

And the reader will want to see how the authors' definition of a hospital as "an administrative organization—a process within a structure—that is a social system contributing to a larger social system" so clearly meshes with the social, economic, and political requirements of the United States in the last third of the twentieth century.

Seymour L. Wolfbein, Dean

School of Business
Temple University

PREFACE

In the 1960s America became vividly aware of needs for change because of the stirring from the core of her social conscience. In an era marked by a strong government-industrial partnership and famed for scientific and economic growth, the people of our country began to actively voice dissatisfaction with the national approach to solving deepening social and human problems. Revealing self-examination brought on by Vietnam first and Watergate later flowed through the 1960s into the 1970s, and now, in the 1970s, a large segment of the resulting change in social views focuses on health, the struggle to define its parameters, and the search for effective organization.

These changes are happening in an environment somewhat more receptive to change, but, at the same time, an environment that has so far offered little in the way of workable solutions. The source of the problem lies primarily in the fact that the base reality of American social, economic, and government organization has been framed in a competitive, bureaucratic mode. Such a base, founded on technologic efficiency, has shaped self-serving cultural patterns that induce people to work together for material gain through threat, fear, punishment, or promise of reward.

At the same time, science and technology have expanded to a point of almost unfathomable complexity, which requires entirely new types of organizations based on more genuine cooperation. Thus an environment in which people are motivated to cooperate for material gain is fast reaching its limits. The complexity of future organizations will require people who have a feeling of human commonality that will enable them to work together easily and happily without bureaucratic restrictions or competitive one-upmanship.

These people who work for the fun of being and doing together, which is genuine cooperation, and the synergistic organizations that will coordinate their efforts are at a great distance in the future, but not at such a great distance that they can be ignored, because current change is moving in just that direction, albeit largely unconsciously. We must recognize this in our efforts to define and deliver health services. While writing and revising this book, we have tried to bring this recognition into play and combine it with a look at the past and future that is usable now. This approach is valid, we believe, if it serves only to stretch the mind a bit. But, beyond that, it has current value for all phases of education and practice in health care organization and administration.

The second edition adds an evaluation of the organizational approach taken at Case Hospital. This material could have been added in small segments to several of the chapters or, as was our decision, kept intact as the concluding chapter of Part Four. It was handled in this way to retain the integrity of the original manuscript so that the reader would find an unaltered picture of the original ideas, plans, and actions as he progressed through the book. No doubt he will have a multitude of reactions and questions by the time he reaches Chapter 12, where he will find an evaluation that can be compared, intact, to the preceding story.

We are indebted to many people for help in this undertaking. We wish especially to express our thanks to Shaw Livermore and to countless other educators, physicians, and administrators who provided their advice and critique during the formation and revision of the book. Appreciation is also extended to John C. Aird, who made significant contributions to the section on "Structure and Spectrum of Ability, Behavior, and Values," to Paula Weinstein and Roberta Zengerle, who prepared the original manuscript, and to Jackie Denning, who managed the revision.

A special word of thanks must go to **Bob Bucher**; Robert Edgecumb, executive vice president of the Commission for Administrative Services in Hospitals; and Edward C. Butterbaugh, partner in the consulting firm of Ernst & Ernst, for permission to use their work as examples of industrial engineering applied to hospitals.

Material from a prior book* and articles published in *Hospital Management*† and *Hospital Administration*‡ have been used in this book. We are indebted to James A. Connelly, Clissold Publications, and the American College of Hospital Administrators for permitting their use.

Richard L. Durbin
W. Herbert Springall

*Durbin, R. L., Connelly, J. A., and Springall, W. H.: Ivory tower to workshop, Tucson, Ariz., 1964, Tucson Medical Center Press.

†Durbin, R. L., and Springall, W. H.: Systems organization for a hospital, Hosp. Manage. 104:36, Sept. 1967; **104:**57, Oct. 1967; **104:**38, Nov. 1967.

‡Springall, W. H.: Group practice in the university teaching environment, Hosp. Admin., Spring, 1971.

CONTENTS

PART ONE
SPECTRUM OF ADMINISTRATION

The spectrum of administration discusses the formal schools of theory about organizations and their administration, the experiences of operations in practice, and the environment in which theory and practice occur and by which they are influenced.

chapter one
THE SPECTRUM

The most frequently cited characteristics of an organization are its shortcomings. Many of these shortcomings are real, the result of piecemeal means or solutions to problems that have been latched onto as panaceas in an inflexible framework. Not only have they been taken as panaceas when they were not but they have often become ends in themselves, thus diverting attention from the original ends. Such individual means are drawn from a spectrum of theory, practice, and environment, including such subjects as definition, rationality, human physiology, psychology, decisions, authority, organizational structure, and administrative process. This broad spectrum is seen in depth as being made up of a host of smaller spectrums.

In considering the spectrum it should be noted that the concepts found there have been strongly influenced by changes in religious, social, political, and economic circumstances that gained momentum in the eighteenth century and went hand in hand with the Industrial Revolution. These circumstances impinge upon and are a part of today's organizations. They have been built in and, although sometimes obsolete, are hard to dislodge from the ruts they have carved.

The spectrum includes theory about organizations and administration, experience of operations in practice, and information about the environment in which theory and practice occur and which influences them. In using the spectrum, formal schools of theory, experiences of many organizations, and the historical and present environment in which they occur may be drawn upon. The different types of organizational structure into which concepts from the spectrum are drawn serve as a point of graphic reference.

Presented graphically, the spectrum ranges from an organization represented by a straight vertical line to an organization represented by a straight horizontal line. The type of organization found most often between these two occurs near the vertical extreme and is portrayed as a pyramid. This pyramidal organization is the one upon which schools of theory often focus and after which businesses and organizations have most frequently fashioned their operations (Fig. 1-1).

In the pyramidal organization a hierarchy of jobs forms a pyramid in which there is a heavy reliance on monistic authority. Toward the other extreme, in the horizontal organization, jobs are arranged in a flat plane and authority arises from collaboration. Between the two extremes lies a variety of organizational structures drawing concepts from the spectrum. The concepts emerge in the form of organizational structure and administrative pro-

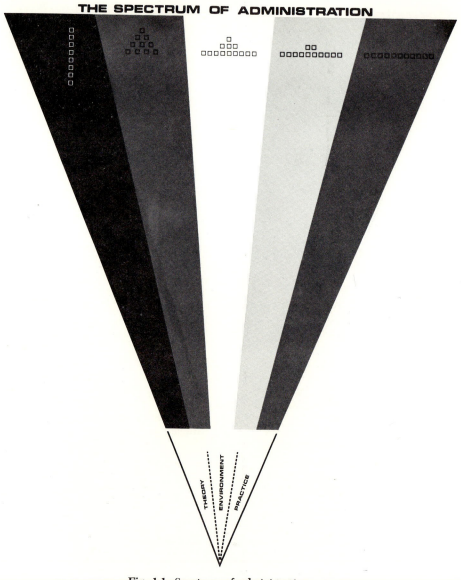

Fig. 1-1. Spectrum of administration.

cess. In tandem the two determine the graphic shape and functional process of an administrative organization. This spectrum is the organizing concept of this book. It is the spectrum of administration.

Organizations approximating the pyramid are of three types: (1) those in which leadership and authority depend on charisma—a magical orientation; (2) those in which leadership and authority depend on traditionalism—an organization oriented toward "traditional ways"; and (3) those in which leadership and authority depend on routinized specialization and the offices of a director—a bureaucratic orientation.[1] Descriptively, all three may be seen as a pyramid in which there is a heavy reliance on a monistic leader. They evolved from a period when a single leader could effectively control the entire organization through application of personal qualities, force, and knowledge. As organizations began more and more to follow the spirit of technology in insisting on scientific methodology and as workers began more and more to specialize in order to gain the depth of knowledge necessary to work in a technologic setting, the monistic leader lost the ability to possess sufficient knowledge to be a director, but retained the right.

The fashionable structure of American organizations has centered on a pyramidal orientation. A strong organization of this type is an efficient organization for applying scientific methodology and technology since unskilled workers and technical specialists use stable routines for efficient performance. Technical specialization requires departmentalization, the division of the overall organization into many specialized parts that are all tied together in pyramidal fashion. It also requires the division of goals and information into subgoal and subinformation categories that correspond to departmentalization. This requires that workers in departments internalize subgoals and work with fragmented information without necessarily recognizing their interrelationships to the larger whole. It requires that subgoals be met and fragmented information be used in a routine and predictable way.

Technologic emphasis, however, has led in the direction of seeking a *hard* science of organizations. In order to have a hard science of organizations, there must be a hard science of man—as long as man remains a part of organizations. Judging from the state of the science of man, we are a long way from a hard science of organizations. The trap into which this leads is one of accepting that anything which cannot be analyzed and understood in terms of hard science is bad for the organization and should be eliminated.

In the fiercely competitive business world the goal was to produce the same product at a lower cost through routinization. Some industries found that they could only reach a lower cost by not including costs for depreciation, research, and development. Therefore the fierce competition theory did not allow for replacement of plant machinery or for research and development in product areas. Corporate bodies then looked for ways of getting an edge on the market either by control of raw materials or by patent advantages. The federal government, through the Sherman Anti-Trust laws, acted to disallow this type of practice. At this point, competition was not productive, and the monopoly was illegal. American ingenuity, being what it is, gave rise to oligopolies.

The McGraw-Hill Dictionary of Modern Economics gives the following definition of oligopoly:

[Oligopoly is] a type of market structure in which a small number of firms supply the major portion of an industry's output. The best known examples in the U. S. economy are the automobile industry in which three firms account for 92% of the output of passenger cars; the gypsum industry in which four firms supply 90% of the industry's output; and the aluminum industry in which three firms provide nearly all the supply of aluminum ingots.*

Competition is defined as follows:

Prices in oligopolistic industries generally fluctuate less widely than those in more competitive industries; each seller hesitates to lower prices because he knows that his few competitors will immediately match the cuts, leaving him with essentially the same share of the total market and lower profits. Nevertheless, other forms of competition, such as styling, quality, new features, marketing and advertising may be very keen.*

In the last sentences comes the focus on the role of the new, innovative specialist who creates change and makes product innovation. Modern organizations must seek out these specialists, attract them to the

---

*Greenwald, D., and associates: The McGraw-Hill dictionary of modern economics: a handbook of terms and organizations, New York, 1965, McGraw-Hill Book Co., pp. 357-358.

organization, and keep them actively interested in their specialization.

The technical and innovative specialists, particularly in the health industry, have at times been forced to leave their specialty and go into management's hierarchal chain of command in order to be recognized statuswise and salarywise and to have their ideas accepted. The form of management today has not changed from the old hierarchal system where charisma and the right to decision making persists. There appears to be a large and ever increasing distance between the manager's right to decide, which is defined by Fayol and others as authority, and the ability to decide, which is a specialized or judgmental ability. The distance between authority to decide and ability to decide is growing. It probably is caused by increasing technologic advances that result in specialization. This increased knowledge expansion is occurring at a much faster rate than changes in the cultural definition of hierarchal roles.

Pyramidal organizations are not conducive to creativity, innovation, or professional judgment. They are often diametrically opposed to the needs of the innovative specialist and the professional. Organizations approximating the horizontal extreme of the spectrum allow freedom of action and flexibility that support and encourage judgment and innovation. In this type of organization, broad goals often are not subdivided and information is not fragmented. There is indeed a heavy dependency upon judgment and innovation, and hence they are legitimate. In this sense the organization is less hard-science oriented in its structure and administrative process. Its environment supports improvision for new sets of circumstances. Although all situations will have some similarities, it is only to the similarities, and among these the ones that occur most often, that routine may be applied with predictability. It is to accommodate dissimilarities that the horizontal organization is needed, based on influence among innovators and professionals in collaboration rather than in subordination.

Increasing necessity to incorporate innovative specialists and professionals into their structure has made pyramids obsolete as the overall organizational framework; it has also outmoded the motivational practice of punishment and reward often associated with it. Twentieth-century organizations must accommodate a much wider variety of practices and abilities. They are experiencing increasing pressure to innovate at the same time that they are carrying out day-to-day operations. They cannot rely upon a vertical or a horizontal application alone; they cannot depend on a single motivational strategy. A broader framework is required, one into which many concepts may be drawn from the spectrum and interrelated in a flexible and fluid matrix. Such a framework is synergistic in nature.

Health care organizations exemplify the need for incorporating unskilled and semiskilled workers, technical specialists, innovative specialists, and professionals into a synergistic framework. It is with this need in mind that the spectrum of administration is applied to Case Hospital.

While concentrating on the application, it is paramount not to lose sight of the framework that has been drawn from the spectrum and into which many of the concepts found there have been fitted. The particular means that were chosen to fill out the framework are the ones that were believed applicable in the situation under consideration. Others could have been chosen and arranged and applied in a different manner. Whatever the means, it is the flexible, synergistic framework and broad use of the spectrum that is crucial.

REFERENCE

1. Gouldner, A. W.: Studies in leadership: leadership and democratic action, New York, 1950, Harper & Brothers, p. 645.

chapter two

THEORY, DEFINITION, AND RATIONALITY

THEORY

An organizational theory is a conceptual point of reference that prepares us to better understand an organization. It is not limited to the tight, logical meaning it carries in the hard sciences but rather takes on a more generalized and flexible meaning of what the basics are and how they apply.

In this context, theory should be used as a platform for creativity and as a means of gaining a deeper understanding of what goes on in an organization. Experience alone does not allow depth of insight into what goes on and therefore does not provide sound foundations for systematic evaluation. An academic mind must be at play, using both science and experience. The spectrum holds a wealth of information that must be used in this way if the chasm that has developed between academics and practice is to be bridged. An intermixing of the two, with academicians participating in practice and practitioners participating in academics, will go a long way toward this.

As administration becomes more and more a profession, we will find that its professionals draw more heavily upon science and the experience of their colleagues and less heavily upon personal experience. As

this takes place, theory will become a tool that sensitizes people to processes and relationships instead of experienced techniques alone. Professionals will seek a systematic approach to administration, and thus an organization theory. As a result, the transition from theory to practice will become a great concern.

The theorist can maintain his state of intellectual purity as long as he remains in the theoretical. Once he moves into the practical and attempts to apply his theory, he comes face-to-face with the world as it is. At this point he must either retreat to the theoretical or make concessions to practicality. The nature of these concessions measures his metamorphosis.

The theorist becomes a practitioner when he accepts the responsibility for successful application of theory. If the success of the operation is identified by the environment with the individual, then, once committed to the theory and its application, the negative aspects become equally important with the positive. The theorist works on the causes of success; the practical man works on the removal of the causes of failure.

If theory has the potential of being applied, the transition from theoretical to practical may not be so noticeable. Here the theoretical has some common area with the practical. The practitioner, who believes in theory and is dedicated to its practice, attempts to broaden this common area. He succeeds or fails according to his acceptance or rejection by the world in which he finds himself.

If the theory is good, one means of testing its validity is to expand the size and select the population to which it will be applied. The theory applied must have unity and must be specific, compact, and singular in purpose. These aspects will reduce the theoretical area to its smallest possible size. This creates an artificial atmosphere, a greenhouse in which theory can be cross-bred with practicability. The creation of this semi-artificial environment gives the factors of success a chance to grow and at the same time inhibits the causes of failure. Here this theory-practice resultant has the opportunity to be observed, sifted, encouraged, and strengthened to withstand the adverse elements in the total population.

Health care organization needs to develop the use of this middle ground rather than to continue to use its present methodology of scattering theoretical seeds on any soil in any kind of weather. The transition from theory to practice in health care is becoming evermore frequently the responsibility of the health care administrator; it is through intelligent use of theory, research, and implementation in the middle ground that it will most often succeed. The use of theory in administration is difficult, requiring familiarization with theory, reasonable value judgments, and a rigor of application that is exhausting and often unrewarded.

Organization and administration, as an area of theory in their own right, have come about in response to the industrialized society that grew out of the Industrial Revolution. In the United States the growing complexity of government and industry has led to new administrative concepts and theories in schools of business administra-

tion, psychology, sociology, anthropology, political science, and public administration, to name a few. Consequently, emphasis has developed according to enclaves of interest reflecting the particular views of given schools. Emphasis has shifted from machine to man to organization to social institution. There is no single, complete theory, but the entire spectrum of theory may be drawn upon in organizational practice provided there exists a flexible framework for their understanding and use. Among the theories that may be drawn into this framework are the schools of thought known as scientific management, human relations, and structuralism.

Scientific management, for instance, is the most frequently used in organizations as we see them today. Its physiologic considerations, time and motion applications, engineered work standards, and methods improvement techniques are of great value in hospital organizations when used in proper perspective. If accepted as absolutes or as panaceas, however, they may create extreme conflict with psychologic and environmental factors.

The school of human relations has contributed important understandings and tools related to the psychologic aspect of organizations. The findings of the Hawthorne Studies, for instance, are a significant contribution. Here again, we do not have a complete theory in and of itself. Many organizations have fallen into the trap of attempting to make the organization a completely happy and conflict-free situation. Organizations, by their very nature of having more limited boundaries than does general society, will inevitably have some unhappiness and conflict. One should attempt to view unhappiness and conflict with objectivity.

The structuralists have acknowledged scientific management and human relations as usable tools but have established a broader frame of reference for considering structural and functional processes. This approach is demonstrated by the work of Max Weber in his treatment of bureaucracies. The bureaucracy, however, has too often been accepted as an inevitable form of organization.

Scientific management

Frederick Winslow Taylor is commonly accepted as the father of scientific management. Taylor developed his ideas during the late 1800s and early 1900s. In an effort to systematize a group of procedures, a set of underlying principles, and a fundamental philosophy, he published the book *Scientific Management* in 1911. This book, and Taylor's participation in a controversy involving his techniques, the federal government, and the railroad industry, brought scientific management national attention.

Students of the school initially set out to study the interaction between human characteristics, the machine, and the elements that make up the industrial work process. They sought basic principles for a science of management which would be the foundation of the total organization. As their work progressed, however, they limited their interests primarily to the physical characteristics of the human body in routine jobs.

The product of their efforts combines a study of worker capacity, speed, and durability with a motivational approach that views the worker as driven by fear, hunger, and the need for material reward. The underlying theme is that if work effort and money are closely related the worker will respond to the maximum of his physical capacity. This eventually led them to conclude that rather than man and machine being adaptable to one another, man was an appendage to the machine. They believed that once a worker was taught the best way to perform and his reward was tied to his performance he would perform to his maximum.

Using the principles of finding and teaching the one best way of performing each job, finding the one best man to perform each job, and creating good labor relations, scientific management developed a group of systems and procedures involving time and motion studies, foremanship, differential rates of pay, routing systems, and cost accounting. The basic philosophy was a belief that once the techniques were refined, management, labor, and the public would insist on efficiency. Cooperation between the three was seen as the essential element that would lead to a true science based on the techniques.

Considering researchers who seek a clear definition of things to be studied before proceeding and those who believe that a true definition can only be arrived at by originally bypassing it and going directly to activities that in the end will render a definition in real life operational terms, scientific management may be placed by and large with the latter group—skip the definition and dig in. This is one of the reasons why the theory produced results that were often isolated from an overall organizational approach. It resulted in a number of useful tools and principles that are of great assistance to managers, but they are not a complete organization theory. A second criticism points to the fact that only physiologic factors were considered; psychologic factors were not considered. This theme was picked up by proponents of human relations.

Among the various tools developed by scientific management, time and motion techniques and methods improvement have been developed in recent years for hospital use. Taken as tools in proper perspective to the total organizational framework, they have considerable potential.

Scientific management was the first of two schools of thought usually referred to as the classical approach to organization and administration. The second, typified by the book *Papers on the Science of Administration*, edited by Luther Gulick and L. Urwick, undertook an examination of organizational structure. Moving from a basic division of labor of the type described by Adam Smith, proponents worked out schemes for the unity of command, or scalar chain, necessary to control and administer the pyramidal organization resulting from the division of labor.

Building on the belief that each job to be performed can be divided and subdivided until it is broken into its most basic parts and that a worker can be taught depth in the skills of performing those basic parts better than the entire, broader job, this division of classicists pondered the type of supervision necessary to control workers. The organization should be built from the bottom up, they said, and in so doing each worker in each job must be organized according to the major purpose he is serving, the process he is using, the persons or things he is dealing with or serving, or the place where he renders his service. After having grouped the workers, they then considered the problem of control. Since supervisors are limited by knowledge, time, and energy, each five or six workers will require one first-line supervisor, each group of five or six first-line supervisors will require a second-line supervisor, and so on up the scalar chain to the monistic center of authority.

At the top of the pyramid, the chief executive should employ POSDCORB in conducting the administrative affairs of the organization.

POSDCORB is, of course, a made-up word designed to call attention to the various functional elements of the work of a chief executive because "administration" and "management" have lost all specific content. POSDCORB is made up of the initials and stands for the following activities:

Planning, that is working out in broad outline the things that need to be done and the methods for doing them to accomplish the purpose set for the enterprise;
Organizing, that is the establishment of the formal structure of authority through which work subdivisions are arranged, defined and co-ordinated for the defined objective;

Staffing, that is the whole personnel function of bringing in and training the staff and maintaining favorable conditions of work;
Directing, that is the continuous task of making decisions and embodying them in specific and general orders and instructions and serving as the leader of the enterprise;
Co-ordinating, that is the all-important duty of interrelating the various parts of the work;
Reporting, that is keeping those to whom the executive is responsible informed as to what is going on, which thus includes keeping himself and his subordinates informed through records, research and inspection;
Budgeting, with all that goes with budgeting in the form of fiscal planning, accounting and control.°

The problems created throughout the organization by the interrelationships between the division of labor with its psychologic side effects, the characterization by purpose, process, person or thing, and place, the implications of mathematical supervisory schemes, and POSDCORB defy one best way of organizing. Each of the elements considered by itself lends valuable insight to organization and administration, but they do not add up to a total theory.

Numerous American organizations have applied this model. In those where work could be reduced to repetitive routine it has had a fair share of success. In those that required nonroutine, nonrepetitive performance it has created untold trouble. Hospitals in this country have copied the industrial model. As will be pointed out throughout the book, the organizational and administrative needs of a hospital do not lend themselves to one center of control, to a reduction of all supervision to a singular chain of command, or to minute division of labor. Some areas of hospital

---

°Gulick, L., and Urwick, L., editors: Papers on the science of administration, New York, 1937, Institute of Public Administration, Columbia University Press, p. 13.
As Gulick notes, this idea is adapted from *Industrial and General Administration* by Henry Fayol.

organization do; some do not. Yet the prevailing hospital organizational concept has been a pyramidal structure.

The classicists were there first with theory. American industry grew hard, fast, and competitive, and these men furnished schemes and insights that worked better than "things prior." In the environment of competition they were used, ingrained, and became supporting stores of the organization. Some of these tools were and still are valid when used properly; others are not valid beyond short-run gain, and others are untrue. Many of each type have been carved deep into our organizations. Classical theory is a fact of life to be dealt with in most current modes of organization and administration.

Human relations

Human relations grew out of concern over the limited physiologic concerns of the classicists; they did not consider the psychologic factors at play in the organization. As an area of study, human relations includes psychology and sociology in studying the behavior of individuals and groups in the organization as related to organizational goals. Departing from the classical approach, human relations studied the emotional, psychologic, and social forces in the organization. As can be seen in the Hawthorne Studies, the significance of social relationships between workers and between workers and supervisors was recognized.

The founder of the movement, Elton Mayo, was not satisfied with the mechanistic, physical machine model used by Taylor. He was more interested in the psychologic implications of man's relationship with machines. The resulting approach of attempting to discover efficient methods of relating man to machines, using social as well as mechanical considerations, has become an important factor in today's organizations and their administration. This approach began with a realization of

human interaction in the organization. The main interest was in small groups because this was where interaction was most apparent.

The Hawthorne Studies, with which Mayo was deeply involved, were the first major attempt to use structured research in studying organizations. Using controlled experiments over a period of some 8 years, the Studies disclosed that adjustment of physical working conditions had little effect on productivity but that there was a relationship between social structure and increased or decreased productivity. Because of their lasting effects on the whole field of human relations, it is of benefit to dwell in some length on the Studies.

The experiments were conducted in Chicago at Western Electric's Hawthorne Works plant.[1] The Studies developed from a series of experiments conducted in cooperation with the National Research Council of the National Academy of Sciences. There were three types of studies conducted, each growing out of the preceding:

1. The *Test Room Studies* were experimental in nature. They were designed to assess the effects of single, physical variables on employee performance.
2. The *Interviewing* Studies were psychologic in nature. They were designed to find ways of improving employee attitudes and morale.
3. The *Observation Studies* were sociologic in nature. They were designed to give a greater understanding of the factors influencing the informal organization of work groups.

Test Room Studies. Collaborating with the National Research Council, the research staff designed the Test Room experiments to study the effect on performance when intensity of illumination is varied. It was expected that by increasing illumination worker production would correspondingly increase and that in the control group, where illumination was held constant, no significant change would occur. Unexpectedly, however, output rose in both groups.

Furthermore, in a second study in which the illumination was decreased similar results were obtained; output rose in the test group and the control group. The researchers were forced to conclude that either adequate control had not been effected or that illumination could be discounted as a factor that alone affected performance. Other studies in which rest periods were introduced and working hours were reduced reaffirmed that there could not be a causal relationship between any single variable and performance.

Relay Assembly Test Room Study. The Relay Assembly Test Room Study was undertaken to observe the effects of changes in the working conditions and to enact more strict experimental control. Arrangements were made to measure the temperature and humidity and the output and quality of work in a special room isolated from the rest of the plant. The room was staffed by a group of women volunteers who were considered average assemblers. They were controlled on a piecework basis, and efforts were made to keep their work attitudes consistent throughout the study. The women were given physical examinations before the experiment began and every 6 weeks thereafter to discover whether the study affected their health. An observer-supervisor, who kept records of output and other factors, was stationed in the test room to maintain a friendly atmosphere in the group through a quasi-supervisory role.

During the first 2½ years a very complicated time schedule was used to experiment with hours of work and rest periods. The changes were interrupted with periods of return to previous work arrangements so that there would not be a cumulative effect. Again there were unexpected results. Output increased during the experiment irrespective of the changes. In addition, tardiness and absenteeism decreased. When questioned, the women said that their new work experience was highly satisfying.

Relief from fatigue, relief from monotony, increased wage incentives, and the change in supervision were suggested by the researchers as reasons for the increased efficiency. After the researchers studied the data, relief from fatigue and relief from monotony were disregarded. Two more experiments with other groups were undertaken to study the effects of pay incentive and changes in working conditions as separate factors. The results seemed to indicate that both were important but were not the sole reasons for overall improvement.

One additional factor considered was the high degree of esprit de corps that developed. The observer-supervisor indicated a shift in attitude of employees in the test room as exemplified by the women's making up in output for a worker who did not feel well and by group activities that developed outside the work situation. This was attributed to the freer atmosphere, the less authoritative supervision, and the personal interest shown by top management in the employees.

Researchers felt that the security afforded the employees regarding jobs and bonuses, their participation in change, and the introduction of the observer-supervisor had profoundly altered the total social situation of the operators. They found the situation so complex that it could not be described in terms of isolated variables; it needed to be described and understood as a system of interdependent elements. At the core of the system they saw not the specific factor of supervision but the more general and vague factor of the employee's "attitude and preoccupations." From this it appeared that conditions of work (lighting, hours, rest periods, pay, and supervision) could not be viewed independently as things in themselves affecting the work of people but that these conditions take on meanings in terms of the perceptions, interpretations, and attitudes of those involved. They then proceeded to develop studies that isolated simple relationships in order to identify causes and effects brought about by changes in the environment.

Interviewing Studies. The Interviewing Studies developed out of an increasing interest in the morale of the worker. The technique, individual interviews with 21,000 people, attempted to gauge the workers' attitudes about their jobs, working conditions, and supervisors. The research staff hoped that if these attitudes could be discerned they could implement improvements in job satisfaction and motivation.

The program was only partially successful. Dissatisfaction could not be tangibly identified. Too much of the workers' dissatisfactions were based on their personal feelings and emotions, the effects of the working conditions, fair pay, and supervisory behavior toward them. These personal feelings could be traced to general life experiences at home and in the community. The conclusion was that manipulation of the environment did not necessarily provide a compatible work situation for the individual. Many of the problems believed to be connected with the work situation were actually problems of the individual. However, one thing the study did point out was that an individual could somehow better understand himself and his relationship to his job by talking things over with a good listener. This "nondirective" interviewing technique became an integral part of the employee counseling program at Western Electric.

Observation Studies (Bank Wiring Observation Study). The Observation Studies highlighted the importance of social factors in the motivation of the workers. Fourteen men and their supervisors were studied under routine operating conditions. The working hypothesis of this study was that the employees of any department constituted a social group, with established relationships, between each other, their super-

visors, and their jobs. The method selected for the study was a combination of observation and interviewing.

The Bank Wiring Observation Study, which involved the wiring of switchboards, brought a major breakthrough in the research program. When this study began, the workers were producing less than that of which they were physically capable. In spite of the fact that they could earn more (through management's piecework system) by producing the maximum they were capable of, they chose to follow a social norm of production agreed upon by their co-workers. The term *artificial restriction of output* was coined by the researchers to contrast it with the "natural" output that the management engineer determined was possible. Following Frederick Taylor's thinking that if men were enticed with money they would work as hard as they physically could and would help each other increase output, management had established a piecework payment system.

It was revealed that a norm of wiring only two complete switchboards was set and enforced by the group. In spite of the fact that Western Electric had no such practices, the group firmly believed that if they produced more their rate of pay would be reduced or some of them would be laid off and that if they produced less they would get into trouble. To reiterate, the workers firmly believed this, and this belief was influential in establishing their norm. Management did not have a given level of production that it considered adequate. Nonetheless, the group's conception of management's expectations directly influenced production.

It was evident from this study, then, that the workers constituted a social group quite different from that of the formal organization. They established their own norms and attitudes, decided how much work they would do, and determined how much communication with supervisors and contact with outsiders they would have. For instance, the standard of work output set by the group was maintained even though social pressures and wage incentives were imposed.

The important thing derived from this study seemed to be that the individual in a group considered the importance of his relationships with his fellow workers as a significant factor in his motivation. External influence from plant management and elsewhere in the company structure actually played a minor role. The worker felt that he had to defend himself from policy change. The study recognized the need to innovate new modes of communications between management and the workers and to utilize such relationships as existed to work for the benefit of the company.

•   •   •

The Hawthorne Studies had considerable impact on organizational thinking. They gave vivid relief to the fact that the *informal organization* and its effects were not well understood. Among the major findings of the Studies, the following have strongly influenced today's employee relations, industrial psychology, and management practices:

1. Scientific management assured that the foremen and supervisors formally appointed by management would provide the sole leadership for workers. The Hawthorne Studies pointed out that informal leaders who arise in a group are often much more influential than formal leaders.
2. Scientific management prescribed one-way directives, nonquestioning obedience, and monistic authority. The Hawthorne Studies revealed the importance of multidirectional communications between the ranks, group participation in decision making, and democratic leadership in a viable organizational social structure.
3. Scientific management believed that economic factors were the primary motivation forces at play among workers. The Hawthorne Studies, concluded that social forces were more important and that they largely limited the effect of economic incentives.
4. Scientific management prescribed a high degree of job fragmentation and specialization. The Hawthorne Studies showed that individual behavior is related to the group and suggested that the division of labor should not violate group solidarity.
5. Scientific management saw workers as single individuals primarily related to machines. The Hawthorne Studies saw workers as members of groups related to one another.
6. Scientific management related fluctuations in productivity to physiologic factors. The Hawthorne Studies were interpreted to mean that social norms, not physiologic capacities, determine the level of production.

The interpretation of these findings has often been in diametric opposition to scientific management. It is evident that both views have a degree of validity in practice. For instance, noneconomic factors do tend to counteract economic factors, especially when strong social norms are at play, but it is dangerous to assume that economic incentives are useless. Economic incentives are often primary factors *in spite of* social norms. It is also erroneous to assume that worker satisfaction and happiness are directly correlated to high production. Similarly, both psychologic and physiologic factors will influence productivity.

Not long after the Hawthorne Studies were concluded, the anthropologist W. Lloyd Warner undertook a study of changes in the social and economic structure of the community. His study of Newburyport, Massachusetts, drew conclusions similar to those of the Hawthorne Studies. This study concluded that social structure is important in placing the individual in a satisfying relationship with society, that the happiness of man depended on being an accepted part of a stable group. Warner found several class divisions in Newburyport, and from these he generalized a concept of class and status structure. To his way of thinking, some mobility between these classes was good, but too much would cause class structure to become meaningless and people would be lost for the lack of a stable group to relate to.

During Warner's study, there was a strike at the shoe factory. As reported in *The Social System of the Modern Factory* by Warner and J. O. Low, the cause of the strike was attributable to social rather than economic factors; control of the factory from outside the town, mechanization, and increased social mobility of workers were to blame. In earlier years there had been the stability that comes from the status of a well-developed hierarchy of skills under local ownership and management. But expansion of the firm had displaced the local citizens in favor of management from outside the town by "big city capitalism," and increased technology had downgraded the old, high-status jobs. As a result of both, plus improved education, worker social mobility had increased. Seen in this light the strike was a protest against the breakdown of their old, cohesive society.

In many ways these generalized conclusions are more trying to an organization that is committed to meeting a limited purpose more efficiently than they are to a larger society.

By way of critique, W. H. Whyte, Jr. has commented as follows:

Someday someone is going to create a stir by proposing a radical new tool for the study of people. It will be called the face-value technique. It will be based on the premise that people often do what they do for the reasons they think they do. The use of this technique would lead to many pitfalls, for it is undeniably true that people do not always act logically or say what they mean. But I wonder if it would produce finds any more unscientific than the opposite course.

That strike at Newburyport, for example. Warner

did devote a couple of sentences to the logical, economic factors, but it's clear in reading the other three hundred pages that he feels that the real cause lay in the fact that there was no longer any "hierarchy of skills" that used to give workers a sense of satisfaction and status. Well, maybe so, but most of the workers who struck didn't happen to have been around to remember the idyllic days of old described by Warner, and it is somewhat debatable if they would have liked them quite as much as Warner seems to believe they would. As far as I can gather from a careful reading of Warner's account of it, the workers acted with eminent logic. They wanted more money; the employers didn't want to give it to them; the workers banded together in strike, and the employers gave in. Is it so very naive, then, to explain this strike as very much of an economic matter? Any more naive than to attribute it to a nostalgia for ancient paternalism? Who has the nostalgia?[*]

Much of the thought of the human relations school has been repudiated, but it still remains prominently influential in present-day administration and management. One of the greatest problems with and perhaps the strongest criticism of human relations lies in that it is a kit of tools that never has been developed into a workable, usable framework that can be applied to problematic situations. And there is always that hint that *efficiency* is the goal and manipulation is the means. Too often management accepts good human relations as *the* way to organize and administer. There seems to be a "good Christian" compulsion—a literal messianic complex.

The organization will not be a completely satisfying place to work. Frustrations and conflict may be reduced. Conflict and unhappiness may be made objective. Employees may "believe in" and be "loyal to" the organization. But the organization will not be all things to all people, and seldom will it be all things to any one person. A manager who pursues organizational perfection through human relations will become as frustrated as the employees

[*]Whyte, W. H., Jr.: The organization man, New York, 1956, Simon & Schuster, Inc., p. 40.

whom he is trying to satisfy or to convince they are satisfied.

Taken with no tongue in cheek, human relations can provide endless turmoil. For instance, taken literally it would attempt to abolish conflict. Conflict provides tension that sparks innovation and creativity. Conflict makes the organization stay on its toes; it forces differences to the surface for evaluation; it provides an outlet for what might become deeply latent alienation.

Another mistake to which human relations has frequently led management is that of pretending to allow workers to participate in decision making. Workers have valuable insights and knowledge. They can make worthwhile contributions to the planning, decision-making, and implementation process. Often, however, they are asked to be a part of this process when in fact management has already decided. The effort is to make them feel a part of the process when in reality they are not. Management is presenting a façade. How long can the pretense be maintained? What happens when it is discovered?

Other criticisms have also been leveled. But the fact remains that much of its contribution is usable in proper perspective. It added the informal mate to the formal idea of the classicists. It pushed other students to consider the relationships between the two. And it provided new tools.

Structuralism

Between them, scientific management and human relations approached the two major segments of any organization: (1) its designed structure and (2) its life-giving function carried on by people. Neither of the schools paid much attention as to how the two interrelate. Max Weber and later students of bureaucracy identified and spelled out this interrelationship. Other men such as Robert K. Merton, Philip Selznick, and Peter M. Blau studied particular aspects of bureaucracy in depth. Still others, Herbert Simon, for instance, approached particular subjects such as decision making in the organization.

The German sociologist Max Weber wrote from a concern with the dehumanization of society brought about by the increasing trend toward institutionalized rationalization, culminating in what he called the bureaucracy. He identified an evolutionary graduation from charismatic to traditionalistic to bureaucratic orientation. The bureaucratic structure is found most profoundly in formal organizations but has residual effects on general society. Weber saw society as moving from primitive obedience to a charismatic leader to a highly structured system that rationally weighs means and ends. The path from charisma to bureaucracy pushed individuals into an institutional or bureaucratic role and thus changed their nature. This change in nature suppressed spontaneity, creativity, and innovation.

Weber's theory was based on a universal approach to what he believed was happening in society. The bureaucratic entity that he identified as the direction in which change was moving is characterized by the following:

offices A series of jurisdictional areas to which regular and repetitive duties and activities are assigned

hierarchy The structural arrangement of offices in pyramidal fashion, with authority assigned to vertical levels

technical quality Technical ability qualifies a person for a given office and *secures* his position in the hierarchy

impersonality A high degree of impersonality is maintained in offices as a result of the hierarchal structure and its rules and regulations

rules and regulations There is a set of rules and regulations for each office which ensures accountability and promotes impersonality

efficiency The overpowering and central goal of bureaucracy

Proceeding from this outline, Weber and other students sought insights into the need for confident, creative people and confident, sometimes creative, bureaucracies, and the value of each to society. If, for instance, formal organizations are formed to serve certain needs of society, if organizations tend to become bureaucratic, and if bureaucratic organizations tend to limit the ability of society to progress beyond its current boundaries of reality, who is servant and who is master? Which is the tool? Who has power in relation to whom? Is regimentation the essence of diminishing returns?

With Weber the study began with society at large and then focused on formal organizations. With others the study has been confined to organizations. Robert Michels explored the concentration of power in the hands of bureaucracy through a study of the diminishing voluntary participation of organizational members in the affairs of the organization. This is brought about by a conversion of means to ends— the displacement of original ends by current means—as exemplified by persons in power suppressing "comers" to protect their own welfare (or, on a larger scale, a bureaucratic organization suppressing the needs of society to protect its vested interests). Michels believed that there develops in a bureaucracy a situation in which goals become generalized as value or ethical problems and the operating organization entity as a factual problem. In this situation the orientation to the organization displaces the orientation to goals or overall values.

From this understanding comes further penetration of the problem at hand. An organization assumes an obligation to perform its function efficiently. To do so it develops the characteristics described by Weber, and in so doing and in carrying them out it uses its own discretion and decision making. As a part of its larger context, tension develops in relation to it and its clientele (society, owners, directors). Thus the question "Who is servant and who is master?" is extended to "Who is expert and who is not?" and "How do we establish effective control over bureaucracy and

yet allow it to be autonomous enough to perform its required functions?" Another question is "Who sets which goals and to what end?"

Another student, Robert Merton, pursued human relations in bureaucracy, concerning himself with the functional and dysfunctional effects of the interrelationships between people and organizational structure: Merton employed structural-functional analysis to identify the following:

Functions
Dysfunctions
Manifest functions and dysfunctions
Latent functions and dysfunctions
Intended consequences
Unintended consequences

Having developed his definitions, Merton then described the reaction of organizational members in terms of conformity, rebellion, ritualism, retreatism, and innovation; he employed the definitions to ascertain the effect on the organization.

Yet another student, Talcott Parsons, followed a broad, sociologic approach and considered the allocation and manipulation of resources in social systems.

Each study scouts the relationship of people to organizations and the relationship of organizations to society. The question remains, "Whose goals, to what end, by which means?"

Such discussion furthers the consideration of an organizational overview. In its pure sense, bureaucracy is not the answer to flexible progress linked with effective routine. Yet many of its students seem to have accepted it as an inevitable end.

DEFINITION

Inherent to the idea of theory is the idea of definition. Originally we began to describe the spectrum in terms of specific definition. This approach soon returned full circle to abstraction because of the many subtle but real relationships between concepts. Our final approach is much more abstract, allowing for a more complete inter-play with real life situations. Some defini-tive discussion is used, however, in order to solidify the text. The definition of a hos-pital, for instance, views it as an adminis-trative organization—a process within a structure—that is a social system contribut-ing to a larger social system.

A formal organization is formed delib-erately as a smaller unit in society. It is formed to perform a specific function or set of functions, and it is expected to perform these functions better than the larger so-ciety. To perform in this manner the for-mal organization must become an expert in its area of operations. In the case of health care organizations, they must be-come the experts in creating and imple-menting systems and programs for the delivery of health care; they must be given authority to do so and accept responsibility for it. Having done this, they must be recognized and respected as experts in their area of endeavor. It is the organiza-tion's responsibility to sustain its expertise.

In order to organize and administer a hospital it is necessary to establish what its responsibilities are and to formalize a con-cept for its formation and operation. A formal concept may be identified through working with those characteristics that dis-tinguish it from other organizations. Hos-pitals, with their complexity of personnel and organizational characteristics, may be seen as individual organizations in and as an integral part of society. Their goals must reflect the needs, demands, and expecta-tions of society. Seen in this way, the hos-pital is a social system that seeks to fulfill certain goals that contribute to a larger social system. An organization of this type may be defined by identifying its institu-tional value system, by identifying its goals in specific terms, and by identifying the ways it interacts with the community.

American society places high value on human life and health in and of them-selves. Illness is undesirable. Health is to

be promoted and maintained. When a per-son becomes ill, he is to be cared for and returned to his place in society. In the interest of the individual, if he cannot be returned to his place, every care must be given him. In light of these values in our culture the hospital is assigned by society the responsibility of dealing with illness. In meeting this commitment the hospital's functions may be subsumed under the labels of care, education, and research.

Care is the most singular characteristic. Although ambiguous, the term may be dis-cussed under the categories of medical, nursing, and hospital care. Medical care is the responsibility of the physician, al-though it is often initiated by nurses, and the hospital shares with the medical staff the responsibility of ensuring that safe and adequate medical care is practiced in the hospital.

Upon entering the hospital the patient must be oriented to its environment and to the role of the patient. This adjustment is socialization. In the hospital the patient is removed from the dangers of his usual environment, which often includes unsani-tary conditions, poor nutrition, and inade-quate health care and maintenance. Society may also be protected from the patient, as in the cases involving communicable disease or a mental disorder.

The hospital shares these characteristics with other organizations. However, it is the unique combination of care, socialization, and protection, with emphasis on care, that differentiates the hospital. It is upon such a concept that the following defini-tion is built.

Externally, the hospital is a formal, social or-ganization charged with the responsibility of pro-moting and maintaining health and treating illness within the community, and of functioning inter-nally to discharge this responsibility through pro-grams of care, of which socialization and protec-tion are a part.

In a university teaching setting, signifi-cant emphasis is placed on teaching and research as well as care. This emphasis makes the characteristics of a university teaching hospital somewhat different from a community general hospital. Here promotion and maintenance of health through teaching and research stand in greater relief than treatment of illness per se, and admission of patients for treatment may be governed by their teaching and research value.

In undertaking to meet its responsibility the hospital has taken on bureaucratic characteristics. The organization of a hospital has been based mostly on values arising within the hospital, and this is perhaps good in terms of ongoing operations for the hospital has been and still is in the position of choosing its own course while the public debates what the course should be. Routine efficiency is met based on internal values interpreted in terms of offices, hierarchy, technical quality, impersonality, rules and regulations, and efficiency. Much of the effectiveness that this type of organization might have, however, is negated at the point where care is rendered by professionals. The negation arises from failure to create a flexible environment in which theory and practice are organized and where routine, innovation, and professional ability can be applied equally as well.

Values in hospitals have traditionally been internal. New external values are now being pressed upon them. Many hospitals seem reluctant. They will, it seems, fight for arbitrary rights granted by a public that has now changed the basis for granting or protecting those rights. Instead of reexamining themselves and reshaping their values to remain in tune with society, these hospitals are resisting change. If hospitals were to apply their experience in devising and implementing programs of health care in a partnership with the public, then solid progress could be realized. But if instead they fight for the old way, then they will not have a chance to apply their

ability. In the end the public will get what it thinks it wants without the benefit of the people and organizations in the voluntary sector who are equipped to help them make that decision. This idea is picked up again in the discussion of the Regional Health Authority.

This approach to definition has allowed us to cut through a maze of traditionalism, opinion, and myth to a rather simple presentation of the health care organization. It has also allowed us to reduce the "hospital" from a jack-of-all-trades that attempted broad social planning, manipulated whole reserves of resources, and hoped it could control programs of patient care to a program in which reserves are coordinated and channeled into patient care. We have not reduced the requirements, but we have provided a new perspective.

This perspective, which uses definition and goal determination, will be increasingly needed as health resources and programs are coordinated into health plexuses on areawide and regional bases. The primary orientation of programs in any one health plexus may be toward care, teaching, or research, and this orientation will influence its priority on resources according to social and economic need and value.

RATIONALITY

Another set of terms found frequently in the spectrum is *rational action* based on *rationality*. The meaning of these terms varies. As used here rational action refers to activity within the boundaries of a set of values that have met the organization's pragmatic test. Rationality is the state of being in line with these accepted organizational values. Heavy organizational emphasis on the methodology of hard science has caused organizational values to parallel its approach. Rational action in this type of situation risks two difficulties: first, it tempts the organization to lose contact with its external environment and become static; second, it imposes the same risk upon people who work there. It is just this process that Max Weber identified as dehumanization and upon which W. H. Whyte, Jr. placed the responsibility for his social ethic.

It is accepted that people desire to belong. Once a member of an organization internalizes organizational values, he acquires a trained incompetence to participate fully in society. The same applies to an organization. This may be acceptable or even desirable in "caretaker" situations because over many years of repetitive operation certain "sure" and "reliable" modes have proved themselves. The values and decisions are there. They are accepted as efficient and effective according to the old standards. And the people? They can be counted on to do the predictable thing.

Rigidity is not desirable, however, when innovation and judgment are needed. And such is the case in the health care industry. Creative organizations are needed. Organizations per se are not creative. They contain creative potential—individual human beings. The potential of a group is only as great as the potential that it serves to multiply—individuals. This being the case, a flexible, elastic organization that will not suffocate creativity and initiative is necessary. Here again is a bid to combine and interweave theory and practice in the environment of operations in order to seek the actual causes of success.

Innovation often involves intuition; it is sometimes charismatic. Organizational values must allow these areas if the organization is to be an effective place for innovation to occur. The total information system, discussed in Chapter 7, furnishes reliable information for the technical specialist to carry out his job in a predictable manner. It also furnishes information that may be used for innovation. But the person pursuing innovation sometimes does not carry out his activity in a predictable manner. He must be allowed and encouraged to challenge the validity of information, to play a hunch, to fail, to dispute norms, to move freely, to be his own man, not a man pushed to be approved by others. A creative organization must have this environment where routine and innovation exist together—both accepted, both encouraged. Such an environment must ensure that every concept of reality has a chance to be evaluated. It must be broad, with a broad set of values; if it is not, too many potentially creative ideas will be judged irrational by a narrow set of organizational values and disregarded or buried as undesirable conflict.

REFERENCE

1. Heyel, C., editor: The encyclopedia of management, New York, 1963, Reinhold Publishing Corp., vol. 1, pp. 276-279.

PART TWO
ENVIRONMENT
AND
ORGANIZATION

A university teaching hospital is challenged (1) to substantiate what efficient/effective care is and to provide it that way, and (2) to innovate.

To this end a synergostructure is formed, which provides a framework for collaborative action among discrete entities so that the total effect is greater than the discrete effects taken independently.

chapter three

ENVIRONMENT AND ORGANIZATION OF A HOSPITAL

ENVIRONMENT

The extent of government involvement in medicine surprises many who have not tallied the figures. The spirited battle that the American Medical Association waged against the passage of the Medicare bill left the impression that this was government's first sizable venture into the field of medicine. Nothing could be further from the truth.

The government accounts for approximately 70% of the hospital beds in the country and 32% of the institutions, although it handles only about 24% of the admissions. The reason for the discrepancy between the number of beds and the number of admissions is that government is almost solely responsible for the treatment of tuberculosis and mental disease, two illnesses that require long-term hospitalization. The average hospital stay for tuberculosis is 3 years whereas for mental disease it is about 10 months.

The traditional role of government has been to care for special groups of people who might otherwise be left without adequate medical care. This includes individuals with the long-term illnesses already mentioned and such groups as Indians, veterans, armed service and merchant marine personnel, and now the aged. Local governments are responsible for care of the indigent to a degree. The extent and quality of care varies extensively from city to city, and it is now imminent that federal agencies and money must be used if the despair of disadvantaged groups is to be assuaged. It is very likely, then, that still more segments of our population will become the responsibility of federal government insofar as their medical care is concerned.

The government accomplishes this care in two ways. It either builds its own hospitals or buys the services from existing hospitals. The Public Health Service hospitals care for merchant seamen primarily, but certain other government personnel and their families have access to them. The Veterans Administration is an extensive network of government medicine and has vast property and personnel involvement. The Medicare program buys the services of hospitals already in existence.

The difficulties inherent in government ownership and operation of hospitals have been given wide publicity over the years. The government has been accused of giving substandard care and of featherbedding. Scandals have rocked state mental institutions and county and city hospitals again and again. They have been accused

23

of overcrowding, slovenliness, and a host of other evils.

Actually, the problems of imposing high standards of care on all the hospitals in the country have been numerous. Progress has seemed at certain times to be uncommonly slow. In a historical perspective, Veterans Administration hospitals are good examples of government-managed hospitals. They have been among the pioneers in instituting job procedures, training methods, and evaluation techniques and in securing living wages for their residents and nonprofessional personnel; they have sometimes forced their civilian counterparts to do the same. Furthermore, their sources of funds, when expansion of facilities was necessary, have been more available and reliable than many civilian hospitals have found theirs to be. It is in the realm of state and local institutions where the serious abuses of government medicine occur and, although some of the situation is the result of poor management, many of the shortcomings are the result of insufficient funds. State mental institutions are almost invariably overcrowded and understaffed. It is possible with some of the newer medications to drastically reduce the hospital stay for many of the mentally ill, but there must be some kind of follow-up system for these discharged persons. Ideally, clinics could provide excellent follow-up, but unfortunately not many do and referrals between hospitals, psychiatric clinics, and neighborhood mental health facilities remain loose and fragmented.

City and county hospitals are another story; they are large and unwieldy, with staggering numbers of patients and outpatient visits. Overworked emergency rooms are frequently understaffed. Many of these hospitals lie in the most deteriorated parts of the city, and they reflect their environment. They are resistant to change, and many of them suffer from a chronic shortage of funds. It is not uncommon for them to operate on a month-to-month basis and

to run out of money for vital medication before the month is over. Morale can be appallingly low for the staff as well as the patients.

The clinics that are operated in connection with these hospitals were, of course, started for the poor, and the stigma that outpatient departments are for the poor has remained despite the awareness that the less costly ambulatory services must be used more frequently if we are ever to provide all of the medical care that a sophisticated population wants. Medical school and university affiliations have failed to bring the hoped-for improvements in morale and management. Unfortunately, situated as they are in the decayed parts of our cities, these hospitals reflect the despair of their surroundings and therefore resist change.

Some of the more specific complaints about the clinics are the long waiting periods, overcrowded waiting rooms, lack of amenities for those who must use them, and the absence of any workable appointment system. If an appointment system is in existence, it is not always possible to make it workable because of too many missed appointments. In addition, these institutions are frequently used for political ends. Unfortunately it is not uncommon for a politician to prefer to have his name attached to a new building rather than to spend the money on consumable items. Each political rift brings a new investigation.

The role of the medical school in this has been amazingly detached. Through the years the schools sought out such institutions in the belief that large volumes of indigent patients made the best source of teaching and practice material. By remaining dedicated solely to the teaching of their students, they have managed to stay uninvolved with the community and its problems and many times have even avoided any involvement with the management of the hospital. The patient is looked on not as an end in himself but as a means toward that end—teaching. In the community hospital the same situation exists, except that the patient is seen as a means toward another end—a source of money for the physician and the hospital. Many of the problems of modern medicine are unquestionably attributable to this peculiar emphasis that persists in placing the patient and his interests last. As evidenced by budding efforts to establish comprehensive family and community care programs,* there is increasing hope that medical schools in the future will become involved in all their environments: the university, the community, and the patient.

Hill-Burton Program

At the close of World War II a shortage of hospital beds seemed to exist, although then as now there was no criteria to establish this conclusively. The government's answer was the establishment of the Hill-Burton Program, which has become known as the Hill-Harris Program. A specified sum of money is made available each year to every state on the basis of congressional appropriations and presumably the needs of the individual state. A state Hill-Burton committee then reviews the requests that have accumulated during the course of the year and decides which projects will get the money. It is a system of matching funds between the project and Hill-Burton. Hill-Burton has matched as little as one third of the funds or as much as two thirds, depending on the fiscal health of the project.

When the program first came into being, much of the construction occurred in small towns throughout the country. This was based on the theory that physicians and nurses could be attracted to those areas if a hospital were available for their use. A study[1] of certain counties in downstate Il-

linois questioned the success of this plan. The results of the study showed very strongly that the existence of a hospital did not necessarily attract the desired personnel. Many times if a physician were amenable to small-town life, his wife was not, and after a few years they left for more sophisticated surroundings. This study actually demonstrated that when a hospital was built general practitioners left the area or if they died they were not replaced. Hospitals attract specialists, a more costly method of care.

Hill-Burton has some influence on the quality of beds that are being planned, but only in planning is it able to wield any influence at all. The management and financing, once the beds have been established, are forever outside Hill-Burton's jurisdiction. It is an undisputed fact that the actual building of the instituton is the most accountable step in the venture, whereas financing it over the years is subject to every variable in the economy and can be a backbreaking thing if conditions are not right.

As in every government agency, there is always the likelihood that the funds will be disbursed on a political basis. This is more evident in some states than in others. Therefore, although current government emphasis is on larger health care centers, particularly in relation to the regional health complexes, hospitals continue to be built in small towns in sparsely populated states even after a highway system of unexcelled quality, built at enormous government expense, links these out-of-the-way places to accessible medical centers of good repute.

It is the ardent wish of many knowledgeable medical people to be spared the ordeal of an automobile accident in one of these out-of-the-way places and to be carried unconscious into one of these small hospitals that Hill-Burton sprinkles so generously throughout the land.

For some time after World War II the need for beds in areas of dense population went unsatisfied, and existing hospital

---

*See pp. 30 and 31 for more discussion of family and community care programs.

beds continued to deteriorate. This opened the way to financial speculation on the part of many operators of proprietary hospitals. These hospitals added confusion and expense to an already fuzzy health care picture. The folly of these hospitals has been regretted in many communities because of the duplication of facilities and the high cost of medical care.

Certainly the intentions of the Hill-Burton Program were admirable: to give the people financial help with costly construction, but to leave the actual practice and distribution of medicine to those who knew most about it. It was, however, a more or less artificial means of determining the location of the beds. At the same time, third-party payers were paying only for hospital admission and were completely ignoring the less costly ambulatory care system so that there was a continuing demand for more and more factors in shaping our present health care dilemma. It is doubtful if history will look on them with unmixed favor.

Hill-Harris plans during the next 10 years to spend $9.75 billion for modernization of existing facilities. There will unquestionably be still more funds available for new facilities, and hopefully some of this influence will be channeled into ambulatory care facilities since Medicare encourages this type of service. Hill-Burton money was available for diagnostic and outpatient facilities in the past, but the restrictions were impossible. One of the stipulations was that, if an outpatient department were built, free care had to be extended. Who could operate an institution on that basis?

Regional health centers

The DeBakey Report, which was published in December 1964, resulted in a law passed in June 1965 known as the Regional Medical Program. Three diseases—heart disease, cancer, and stroke—are the subject of this famous report and the subsequent plans to implement it. It is a far-reaching plan, attempting to bring into active communication and support medical schools and universities, hospitals, practicing physicians, and all public health agencies and consumers. Regional health complexes, usually in connection with a university and a medical school, are organized strategically around the country.* Here specialists in the treatment of these three diseases are concentrated. Smaller and less specialized stations in the surrounding area then use these central complexes either for their more advanced techniques, as consultants for their more difficult cases, or as a referral station. Patients can be moved into the complex for special treatment and then returned again for follow-up by the original physician. The objective is better diagnosis and care in the treatment of these three diseases and, hopefully, others in the future.

Such a network is intended to stimulate a cooperation and a flow of information between the many health agencies and professionals that make up the medical world. The planning involved in the execution of such a program makes it necessary to survey the resources presently available and to stimulate the development of any that do not exist. The provisions for accomplishing such development are all contained in the program. Vast sums are being spent to develop training and education programs for all professional and skilled manpower. Training is being provided for everyone from research directors to nurses' aides and covers every phase of the health professions, including pharmacy, medical records, library research, and even the propagation of experimental animals. Federal money for scholarships and improvement loans is available for almost all categories of health workers.

The manpower shortage will be acute for

*The original bill called for these regional centers to be built around a university–medical school nucleus. This has since been changed to place less emphasis on the medical school as a nucleus.

some time. There is a need for many teachers and for a continuing education program for practitioners as well as academicians. This is one of the more valuable aspects of the program if it becomes workable; practitioners will no longer be sent out to operate in a world of their own, completely removed from the academic environment. There will be communication and interchange between the academic institutions and those physically removed from them, and this will result in better and more up-to-date care for everyone. Medical schools have been urged through the Coggeshall Report to enlarge their influence beyond the mere education of practitioners and to become actively involved with the university, the community, and most of all with the continuing education of its former students.

The Regional Medical Program was conceived to make use of all existing agencies, both public and private, with federal grants used to stimulate their maximum development and utilization. In practice the program has fostered regionalization by defining specialty service criteria for comprehensive health planning agencies. It has also been the stimulator in some areas for continuing education of private practitioners and has created interest in areawide continuing education centers, which extend the excellence of teaching hospitals and health centers to remote areas. Unfortunately, the plan has had difficulty taking hold, and the planned communication between the central complex and outlying centers has been slow developing. Much of the blame for this must rest with individual practitioners who are motivated by economic considerations and do not willingly send their paying patients to other specialists. Medical schools have trained them, and the A.M.A. has solidified their tendencies to become individual entrepreneurs or small shopkeepers rather than professionals.

Now the time has come for medical schools to change this emphasis. Too much attention has been paid to buildings and to individual reward. It is time to have a look at the system. We are now looking to the future and to large neighborhood health centers when we cannot run our own outpatient departments. They are still operating on an 8-to-5 system 5 days a week when there is a desperate need for them to be run 24 hours a day 7 days a week, especially in densely populated areas. One of the greatest boons to health care would be pediatric night clinics, especially in areas where there are large numbers of working mothers.

But we are thinking now of the "perfect system," one in which health care is available when it is needed and at a price one can afford to pay or prepay. This is what the buying public is looking for. It is also what the federal government has in mind when it attempts to stimulate such a vast interchange of information and technique and invest so much money to relieve the manpower shortage within the health care field.

It is very likely, however, that if these measures, which are intended to prod the existing health care structure into better performance, are unsuccessful more coercive measures such as Medicare will be instituted. The problem is not simple, and it is not likely than an antiquated health system will be allowed to continue unchallenged. The problem must be encountered head on, if not from within the system, then from without. At this point in time it would appear that the only effective pressures that can possibly be exerted must come from the consumer public.

Coggeshall Report

The famed Flexner Report of 1910 recommended changes that would bring medical education into better focus with the then recent developments in medical science. Since that report appeared, many noteworthy changes have taken place in medical education; standards and accreditation have been instituted and enforced.

Fifty-five years later in 1965 the Coggeshall Report, *Planning for Medical Progress through Education,* made its appearance. The study was undertaken under the auspices of the Association of American Medical Colleges with Dr. Lowell T. Coggeshall, vice president of the University of Chicago, as its director. Once again medical education was the target, but as might be judged by the staggering quantity of knowledge and techniques that has accumulated since 1910, this report was much more comprehensive in its recommendations.

Conditions have changed very much since 1910. Not only are we in the midst of a scientific explosion but a population explosion as well. There is an increasing urbanization and a growing number of elderly people. The population today is becoming evermore sophisticated about what it expects to receive from the health care system and what it considers a fair price to pay. Government involvement increases with each passing year, and the cost of care continues to rise alarmingly. Medical schools have traditionally avoided entanglements of any sort, limiting their function entirely to teaching and research. With these facts and trends in mind, the committee, headed by Dr. Coggeshall, in an effort to change the course of medical education, made some very specific recommendations.

1. There must be more attention paid to the medical needs of all society, with a consequent shift toward professionalism and away from entrepreneurial ends. The reputation of the profession has already suffered from severe criticism for clinging to its nineteenth-century concepts when the twentieth century is demanding a much more extensive involvement. To ignore this will not only damage the reputation of the profession but also bring further participation from government.

2. There will be an increasing need for more physicians and for better prepared physicians. New medical schools will be opened, but a study must be made to determine whether the enrollment of existing medical schools can be increased without affecting the quality of the teaching. Failure to attack will result in the establishment of substandard or marginal medical schools. It is strongly urged that medical schools be in conjunction with the main university and not isolated in hospital-centered institutions.

3. There is, of course, a manpower shortage in all of the related health professions. This training can be done in institutions other than medical schools, but it is imperative that something be done to relieve this manpower shortage. The Regional Health Program is making money available for education for all kinds of allied health professions.

4. Medical schools in their university settings are in close relationship with a number of other disciplines such as economics, business administration, sociology, psychology, and many others. They are in a position to coordinate these disciplines toward the objective of improved delivery of health services. Hospital-affiliated group clinic practice and family health requirements need to be perfected in a comprehensive health care setting.

5. Since no one physician can possibly be expert in all fields or even be acquainted with them, it becomes the responsibility of the medical school to foster a professionalism in its graduates to make an interchange of technologic and human resources possible. Only then can the vast fund of knowledge and resources be put to use.

6. The disciplines of research and instruction must somehow be made compatible. It is important for the physician to understand the complexities of research if he is to make use of new knowledge as it becomes available.

7. Medical schools must give up their positions of isolation and make use of the other university disciplines in the education of future physicians. The entire academic setting must be viewed as a continuum,

with the study of human biology being considered as only one aspect. The education of future physicians should be the responsibility of many schools and disciplines. This cannot be accomplished if medical schools are detached from the main university campus. The alienation that results from this arrangement is as real on the part of the university as it is from the standpoint of the medical school.

8. Instead of sending its graduates to seek internships and residencies where they happen to be available, each medical school should be responsible for its own graduates. Internship and residency must be considered a part of the physician's basic education.

9. The continuing education of its graduates must become the responsibility of the medical schools. No longer can physicians be sent out to practice without thought of refresher courses or updating courses. There must be a continuing communication between the school and its graduates if the public is to reap the benefits of new discoveries in technique and knowledge.

The Coggeshall Report is impressive in its vision and clarity. It remains for medical schools to implement its major recommendations. The unfortunate placement of certain medical schools away from the main campus, sometimes in distant cities, creates obstacles that are surely difficult if not insurmountable. It is not anticipated that any even standard of excellence among the schools could ever be accomplished. The incentive that makes the attainment of these objectives a driving force is that unless the voluntary system can chart its own course in a satisfactory direction, government will step in. This is a real danger, one of which those in the voluntary health field are well aware.

Millis Report[2]

The report of the American Medical Association's Citizens' Commission on Graduate Medical Education, under the direction of Dr. John S. Millis, president of West-

ern Reserve University, made its appearance after the Coggeshall Report and was a further study of graduate medical education. The Coggeshall Report and the Millis Report are in agreement that it is no longer possible for a physician to practice medicine isolated from the talents and contributions of other members of the profession or related fields of study. The knowledge and techniques available cannot be mastered by any one person, and there must emerge a team effort. Each specialty makes its contribution, but no one specialty is more important than any other.

The objective is to view the patient as a whole, a concept that will be the result of a comprehensive care program. At one time general practitioners functioned in this role, but the number of general practitioners dwindles each year for a number of obvious reasons. General practice has lost prestige as specialties have evolved. Educational opportunities for students who are interested in general practice are hard to find, and the conditions under which a general practitioner works are frequently less attractive than those that a specialist enjoys. It is a general feeling that the general practitioner has served a very useful function and that his disappearance leaves a vacancy in the health care field, but no one knows exactly what to do about it.

The Citizens' Commission studied this problem and came up with some specific recommendations.

1. Comprehensive and continuing health care is a very necessary part of the health care field, but there is no specialty qualified to function in this capacity. What is needed are individuals trained in psychiatry, internal medicine, pediatrics, preventive medicine, and medical gynecology who have access to all the specialties and supportive departments when the need for them is apparent.

2. This group of specialists will be known as primary physicians. At present the general population must do its own diagnosing and then decide what kind of

specialist to see. The primary physician would perform this function, but he would have continuing interest in the patient, and the complete health care of the patient would be his responsibility after the services of a specialist are no longer needed.

3. At present there are no medical school curriculums nor residencies to prepare students for this particular vocation. Therefore a new curriculum needs to be developed and a new residency pattern must be established.

4. It is urged that a new board specialty be created so that primary physicians could also become board-certified and enjoy a status comparable to that enjoyed by other specialties.

5. The Citizens' Commission strongly urges a study of the current methods by which physicians are educated. At present the medical school education, the internship, and the residency are three separate entities in three different directions. There is much wasted effort, overlapping, and many times serious omissions in the training. They strongly recommend that internships as they presently exist be discontinued. Instead, students should go directly from medical school into their residencies, but the first year of residency would be a specially planned educational year that would make the transition from undergraduate school into specialty training.

6. It is recommended that a commission on graduate medical education be established to plan, coordinate, and periodically review standards for graduate medical education and to approve the institution in which that education is offered.

These recommendations, although of undeniable merit, call for drastic revisions not only in medical school philosophy but also in the way that medicine is practiced in nonuniversity institutions and clinics. It is highly unlikely that such a revolution will occur quickly or easily. It is obviously the thinking of the members of this commission that these are not only desirable changes but workable entirely within the framework they have outlined. However, the practical implementation of these reports is doubtful. Some of the immediate and obvious problems are as follows:

The wide variance in remuneration between the academician and his brother physician, the practitioner, has almost taken on the aspects of a battle, sometimes identified as "town and gown," and academic and financial snobbery has resulted.

Another reason for this not being practical is that in the university, the theoretical hub for all this leadership, there is a continual power struggle for dominance of the various parts of this leadership. For example, control of the hospital is continually up for grabs by either the practitioner or the academician, and, in the matter of research grants, space determination sometimes takes priority over patient needs.

The charismatic nature of medicine has been translated into institutional life and into excellence's being associated with tangible evidence of materialism. To wit, the rug-on-the-floor, name-on-the-door complex is no longer reserved as a status symbol for the executive; it carries over into the pecking order of medicine.

Community medicine and family practice

Some medical schools and care centers are experimenting with curriculum and treatment changes focused on community medicine and family practice that seem to hold hope for correcting many of these problems. In one such situation research, development, and training programs are established by the school's division of community medicine. This division's aim is to unite the clinical disciplines in studying illness in defined communities, developing and analyzing health care delivery systems, and educating physicians and the health professionals in the provision of primary, comprehensive, family- and community-centered care. The division is crucially interested in assisting communities in developing health care programs, studying the relation of health and health care to education, housing, and employment, and focusing on ways in which health care can assist in social change.

The medical school is affiliated with four community health centers representing a variety of urban and rural settings and a range of ethnic and economic distributions. Each center serves a defined population and representatives of each community serve on a health center board. The school offers a clinical clerkship in community medicine at each center.

The clerk works in the community under the supervision of a staff physician. He cares for patients in a family- and community-centered setting. Beyond this he is expected to develop some knowledge of community organization and preventative, rehabilitative, and environmental programs. He learns to collaborate with other health-related programs through lectures and seminars on common problems in primary care, community mental health and community resources, cultural variations in manifestations of disease, and health care economics.

Students may also work as assistants to a staff member who is a community organizer, social worker, health educator, or administrator in a health center. Through the staff member, students learn the organization and dynamics of the community, the structure and authority relationships in the center, and the health-related problems of the center's clients. Students may undertake analysis of significant community problems and propose ways of coping with them and may, under supervision, provide psychologic support and problem-solving advice for individuals seeking care at the center.

Medicare

Perhaps the most implacable opponent of Medicare has been the A.M.A., but it has not always been so violently opposed.

In 1912 the issue was first discussed as a campaign platform plank by Theodore Roosevelt's Progressive Party. In 1917 and 1919 there were voices within the A.M.A. urging that group to give its most careful study to the problem and to make its studied recommendations toward the enactment of social insurance. It was apparent then that sooner or later such legislation would be passed and that it would be better to help lay the groundwork.

By 1920 these liberal voices had been silenced, and the A.M.A. took its unreasoning stand in opposition to any discussion of the subject. That year the A.M.A. House of Delegates passed the following resolution:

The American Medical Association declares its opposition to the institution of any plan embodying the system of compulsory contributory insurance against illness, or any other plan of compulsory insurance which provides for medical insurance to be rendered contributors or their dependents, provided, controlled or regulated by any state or Federal Government.*

The opposition held until the very passage of Medicare in 1965. When the Social Security Act was passed in 1935, it was recognized as only the beginning and that some form of compulsory health insurance should and would be eventually adopted. But social legislation is a gradual thing. It was another 30 years before the country was ready for it. Meanwhile every step of the way, whenever health insurance was urged, whether it was in California in 1945 when Governor Earl Warren proposed a compulsory health insurance program for the state of California or in 1949 when the President of the United States called for it in the State of the Union Message, the A.M.A. and the state medical associations fought it with ardor and money. When it finally became law it was a health insurance for the aged, but there was an awareness on everyone's part that other needy segments of the population would

*J.A.M.A. 74:1319, May 1920.

gradually be added to the list of beneficiaries and that government participation
would continue to grow.

The passage of this social legislation is
an example of the thoroughness with which
major legislation is debated in this democracy and it makes clear the reasons
why much of it is slow in passing.

Between 1961 and 1965 variations of the
King-Anderson bills were under constant
debate. Dozens of other bills were introduced and rejected. Among them were
the Kerr-Mills bill and the Byrnes bill.
When it became evident that some form of
legislation was imminent, even the A.M.A.
came up with a version called Eldercare.
What was finally passed was a combination of several of these bills, notably the
King-Anderson bill and the Byrnes bill,
resulting in a dual structure that is in
reality two separate insurance systems.

The first, Part A, which applies automatically to almost all people 65 and over,
is financed by special Social Security contributions by employees and their employers and by self-employed persons during
their working years. The second, Part B,
is a voluntary medical insurance plan that
is financed by a $4 monthly premium paid
by each participant, and this is matched by
an additional premium from the general
revenues of the federal government.

Nineteen million people were brought
into the program in July 1966 when it offi-
cially swung into operation. Before that
date each individual had to be contacted to
find out whether he wished to participate
in the voluntary Part B program. Informational booklets had to be prepared for all
of the providers of Medicare. An elaborate
machinery was made ready so that for each
participant the payment of deductibles and
the extent of the utilization under both
Part A and Part B could be known quickly.
This information had to be ready if participating institutions requested it.

The paper work, the quantities of mail
that had to be sent out to subscribers, the

information that had to be collected and
stored so that it could be retrieved almost
instantly—these were mammoth problems
for the Social Security Administration. But
Medicare is now in operation, and it is in-
conceivable that the direction will ever
be reversed. There is, however, an assurance that the benefits will gradually be extended to other groups.

It was the initial intent of Medicaid to
allow for payment for all comprehensive
health service to the low-income group.
But most states enacted what is called the
categorical parts of the medicaid bill, that
is, medical assistance program, aid to
families of dependent children, and aid
to the totally and permanently disabled.
Unless one met the narrow criteria and
the niggardly requirements, one was unable to get assistance from the program.

A specific section of the Medicaid Act,
Section 1315, allowed for demonstration
programs in state medicaid agencies to
waive the narrow requirements of the
categorical programs. Such a program is
being planned in the city of Newark.

This program calls for inclusion of 90,
000 additional low-income indigents into
a prepaid health care delivery system. The
plan would be administered by a local
authority on contract with various health
care providers. Catchment areas are being identified and various providers in
proximity to these catchment areas assigned. Capitation rates are fixed and payment to the providers is made on an annual
capitated basis.

In most states Medicaid has not been
able to satisfactorily develop a financeable
comprehensive care network, and state
legislatures have found it necessary to eat
away at funds available to the program.
These groups have continually picked
away at the range of benefits and the
financial levels of eligibility.

New legislation, referred to as HR 1,
which became Public Law 92-603, has
very wide ranging implication on Medi-

care, Medicaid, and maternal and child health. Among its most sweeping changes were its incentives to states to establish effective utilization review procedures for the programs. It allows for payments to health maintenance organizations. It eliminates the requirement that states move toward comprehensive health care programs. It speaks very strongly about the role of teaching physicians and how they should be paid.

One outgrowth is the development of professional standards review organizations (PSROs) under which practicing physicians assume certain responsibilities for evaluating the quality of the services provided under the Medicare, Medicaid, and maternal and child health programs. According to the Social Security Administration, the PSROs will be set up generally in geographic areas comprising 300 or more practicing physicians. Each PSRO is responsible for seeing to it that the payments are for services that were medically necessary and carried out under high professional standards. They will be limited to reviewing only institutional care, however, and will not be responsible for determining the charges.

It was not the purpose of the government to encourage or support substandard hospital or other institutional care. Quality is an elusive thing to define and measure in health care, but fortunately much progress has been made in this area before the advent of Medicare. The Joint Commission on Accreditation of Hospitals had gone far in upgrading the standards of hospitals, and the government relied heavily on their requirements for accredited institutions. Among the other groups that were consulted were the American Hospital Association, The American Nurses Association, The Health Insurance Benefits Advisory Council, and the American Osteopathic Association.

Hospitals that are accredited by the Joint Commission on the Accreditation of Hos-

pitals have only to comply with the additional requirement for utilization review. Those institutions that are not accredited can qualify as participating institutions if they essentially comply with the recommendations of the JCAH and establish a utilization review committee. This is a special utilization committee that reviews the admissions, the length of stay, and the professional services rendered for all those eligible for Medicare.

The utilization committee is the responsibility of the medical profession and either the medical staff within the institution or members of the medical society. This committee functions according to a well-defined plan that specifies the organization and composition of the committee, the frequency of the meeting, the type of records to be kept, the methods of selecting the cases to be reviewed, what constitutes extended duration, and the responsibilities of administration. Each case of extended duration must be reviewed, especially taking into account the availability and alternative use of out-of-hospital facilities and services.

There are two basic forms of Medicare protection against the costs of health care.* Part A, which applies automatically to almost all people 65 and over, covers the costs of inpatient hospital services, outpatient hospital diagnostic services and post-hospital care in the patient's home or in an extended care facility. Part B, which is voluntary and which was originally elected by over 90% of those eligible, covers physicians' services wherever they are furnished, home health services, and a num-

---

*The descriptions and amounts of coverage on the following pages relate to the original program and have been retained for historic purposes. These will continually change over the years. Anyone interested in current information should consult current government publications on Medicare, Social Security, and Welfare reform, available from the U. S. Government Printing Office, Washington, D. C.

ber of other medical and health services.

As previously stated, Part A is financed through special Social Security contributions of employers and by self-employed persons during their working years. Those who have elected to take advantage of Medicare, although they are not entitled to Social Security or railroad retirement benefits, will be covered by funds from the general tax revenue.

Part B is paid for by a monthly premium that each participant individually elects to pay. This is matched from the general revenues of the federal government. This money is paid into a separate trust fund that pays for all benefits and administrative expenses for this portion of Medicare. The premium is subject to increase as the cost of medical care rises.

Originally Part A covered the following four categories of care when the patient was in a participating hospital:

1. Inpatient hospital services up to 90 days per *spell of illness*

    A spell of illness began with the first day a patient received covered inpatient hospital or extended care service and ended when the patient had not been in any hospital or extended care facility for 60 consecutive days. Within each spell of illness the patient could use up to the full 90 days of hospital benefits and the full 100 days of extended care benefits.

    The patient paid the first $40 of charges for the first 60 days and $10 per day for the next 30 days. For the ninety-first through the one hundred and twentieth day the patient paid $20 per day. Included were room and board in a semiprivate accommodation, nursing care, drugs, supplies, most customary services, and whole blood beyond the first three pints. Not included were physicians' services, private duty nursing, or a private room unless it was medi-

cally necessary. The patient could elect to pay the difference between a private and semiprivate room.

2. Posthospital extended care facilities

    After the patient had been hospitalized for 3 days and before 14 days had elapsed since his discharge from the hospital, he was eligible for up to 100 days per spell of illness in an extended care facility. An extended care facility was one that was approved for participation in Medicare, one that had an arrangement with a hospital for the transfer of patients, and one that provided skilled nursing care or rehabilitation services. It paid all costs for the first 20 days and all but $5 per day for the next 80 days.

3. Posthospital home health benefits

    Up to 100 home health visits during the 1-year period after the patient's latest discharge from the hospital or extended care facility were provided. However, the patient must have been hospitalized for at least 3 days, the agency must have been arranged for within 14 days after the patient was discharged from the hospital or extended care facility. Services that were covered included visiting nurses, physical, occupational, or speech therapists, and medical social services and other health workers. Physicians' services were excluded.

4. Outpatient hospital diagnostic benefits

    These were paid on the basis of a period called a *diagnostic study*. All tests that a patient might receive from the same hospital for 20 consecutive days were included in a diagnostic study. If tests extended beyond 20 days, a new diagnostic study began. For each diagnostic study Medicare paid 80% of costs for covered services except for the first $20.

The contribution rates that covered

Part A were based on the first $6,600 of earnings in a calendar year and were equally applicable to employees, employers, and self-employed persons.

Part B covered the following services:

1. Medical and surgical services by a physician, whether given in a home, an office, or an institution

   This included incidental services and supplies that would ordinarily be included in the bill, such as consultations, diagnostic tests, medical supplies, and drugs that cannot be self-administered. Dental surgery was covered only if it related to the jaw or any structure contiguous to the jaw or to the reduction of any fracture of the jaw or facial bone.

2. Diagnostic tests such as x-ray examinations or laboratory tests
3. Prosthetic devices other than dental
4. X-ray and other radiation therapy
5. Necessary ambulance services
6. Surgical dressings, splints, casts, and other similar devices and the rental of durable medical equipment such as wheelchairs, hospitals beds, oxygen tents, iron lungs, braces, and artificial limbs and eyes for use in the patient's home
7. Home health services established by a physician

   After $50 deductible had been paid by the participant, Medicare paid 80% of the reasonable costs of covered services up to 100 visits in each year. This included part-time or intermittent nursing care, physical, occupational, or speech therapy, services of home health aids, and medical social services.

With the passage of Public Law 92-603, the influence of the Health Insurance Benefits Advisory Council (HIBAC) was modified. It still advises the Secretary of Health, Education, and Welfare on general policy matters for the Medicare and Medicaid programs, but this is the extent of its influence.

Certain state agencies are appointed to determine whether institutions and agencies providing health services and wishing to participate in the Medicare program qualify for approval. In most states this is the state health department.

In many states, certificate-of-need legislation has been enacted. This function frequently resides in the same agency as the state comprehensive planning agency. Certificate-of-need legislation was enacted in order to keep health care facility development in line with demand for services. The implementing of certificate-of-need in the various states has a direct effect upon the cost of health care services and particularly upon Medicare and Medicaid costs.

Efforts toward regionalization of health services will also help in reducing duplication of health care facilities and therefore have some effect on cost. This would mean that high-cost new services could not be permitted without approval by the local comprehensive health planning agency responsible for certificate-of-need and regionalization.

The Social Security Administration has chosen a number of public and private organizations to serve as fiscal intermediaries in paying the participating institutions for services rendered. Many hospitals have elected to deal directly with the government. The Blue Cross Association is the intermediary in many states and operates through its individual plans. Private insurance companies also do some of this work since Congress felt that a pluralistic and competitive system would have some advantages over a monopoly. Some of the companies involved are Travelers Insurance, Aetna Life Insurance Company, Mutual of Omaha, Kaiser Plan, Hawaii Medical Service, Prudential Insurance Company, National Mutual Insurance Company, and Coop de Salud in Puerto Rico.

The principal function of these private carriers is to reimburse hospitals and other institutional providers on the basis of reasonable cost for amounts due for services under both the hospital insurance and medical insurance programs. They determine the amount of reimbursement that is paid to the providers under national reimbursement principles. They also provide consultation and assistance to providers in maintaining and establishing fiscal records necessary to properly determine the costs of care.

Under Medicare the amount to be paid to the providers of care for services furnished to beneficiaries is the *reasonable cost* of such services. This was agreeable to everyone until it was time to actually establish the formula by which such payments would be made. It then became apparent that reasonable cost meant something different to each party involved. It took many months to hammer out a workable formula. These costs have been under review with fixed maximums and minimums imposed by state health and insurance regulatory bodies. Recently the health industry has been under federal control by the Cost of Living Council's Health Industry Body. In fact, the Cost of Living Council has an advisory council referred to as Health Industry Advisory Council (HIAC), which sets the controls on the health industry costs.

There was a time not too long ago when hospitals could give charity care and part-pay care because they could make up the deficit by charging their paying patients more. In effect they were the banker rather than the broker of services. Third-party payers usually paid on a contractual basis so that, although this was an assured source of income, it was not a source of funds for carrying on the "Robin Hood" practice, as this was known. As costs rose, the number of those covered by third-party payers rose and the number of those who could pay nothing or only part of their hospital charges increased while the number of patients who paid directly for their hospitalization became fewer and fewer. This source of income is now rapidly disappearing, and the day has arrived when hospitals will be unable to give free care. If price controls and price freezes continue in effect, it appears that only National Health Insurance will be able to save the health industry, particularly hospitals. The outlook at the present time is very bleak for salvation from this quarter.

There is an effort to develop health maintenance organizations (HMOs) as a substitute for present hospital and ambulatory care practices. The HMO has a positive connotation on the prevention of disease and the maintenance of health. Senator Edward Kennedy of Massachusetts has been a proponent of this type of organization and has pushed legislation supporting it. To date, few substantive results are evident. Briefly, an HMO is to cover a defined population on a prepaid basis, preferably a capitation basis.

The history of contracts that pay on the basis of cost (and sometimes on less than cost) goes back to pre–World War II days when the Children's Bureau conducted programs for the hospitalization of crippled children. During the war this system was further established through the Emergency Maternity and Infant Care Programs for dependents of servicemen. After the war, when Blue Cross rose to prominence, the same cost basis was used in varying formulas. Those plans that pay on the basis of charges do so by using certain controls that see to it that charges are reasonably related to cost. But Medicare changed this. It is now absolutely essential that hospitals know their costs and be able to calculate them accurately if they are to receive reimbursements through Medicare. This has been one of the better influences of Medicare because it has forced hospitals to abandon some of their obsolete business practices and to use modern business techniques.

After much debate the Social Security Administration published the booklet *Principles of Reimbursement for Provider Costs and for Services by Hospital-Based Physicians.* This is still under revision and changes are announced from time to time as experimentation goes on. It may be several years before a really satisfactory system evolves, and it is inevitable that hospitals will be forced to change not only their antiquated accounting procedures but their historic eleemosynary urges as well.

One of the hotly debated issues was the matter of depreciation based on the original or historic cost. Hospitals, however, wanted to use replacement costs that would reflect price increases and technologic advances in a rapidly changing field. Third-party payers have traditionally used the original cost in their contracts.

There were originally three principles by which depreciation can be added to cost. They are as follows:

An appropriate allowance for depreciation on buildings and equipment was an allowable cost. The depreciation must be (1) identifiable and recorded in the provider's accounting records, (2) based on the historic cost of the asset or fair market value at the time of donation in the case of donated assets, and (3) prorated over the estimated useful life of the asset, using the straight line method or accelerated depreciation under the declining balance or sum-of-the-years'-digits method.

Straight line depreciation is the method whereby the original cost of the building or equipment is noted. Some estimate is made of the price that it is expected to sell for when it has been used up, and an estimate is made of the number of years this will take. Schedules are available for this determination. For example, a piece of equipment costs $75,600. At the end of 25 years it is estimated that there will be a value of $600 left. By dividing $75,000 by 25 years, one arrives at the amount of depreciation for each year, or $3,000.

The sum-of-the-years'-digits method could be used as an accelerated method. Suppose that a piece of equipment worth $25,000 is to be depreciated in 5 years' time. First, add the sum of the years: $1 + 2 + 3 + 4 + 5 = 15$. The first year 5/15 of $25,000 is used, the second year 4/15, etc.

In the third, declining balance method, a piece of equipment worth $100,000 that is to be depreciated over 25 years would be depreciated at 8% a year. The first year $8,000 would be deducted; the next year the depreciation would be 8% of $92,000, etc.

The provider could choose its own method. It could use one method for one asset or group of assets and another method for others. It could change from one method to another with advance approval from the intermediary, but only one such change could be made on a particular asset.

On all assets acquired prior to 1966 the provider could choose an allowance for depreciation based on a percentage of operating costs, that percent being 5% for 1966-1967 and decreasing by 0.5% each succeeding year. This allowance was in addition to regular depreciation on assets acquired after 1965; however, when the optional allowance is selected, the combined amount may not exceed 6% of the provider's allowable cost for the current year. Depreciation on assets being used by a provider at the time it entered into Title XVIII was allowed and depreciation was allowed on assets financed with Hill-Burton or other federal or public funds.

The other cost principles were as follows:

1. Necessary and proper interest on both current and capital indebtedness was an allowable cost with certain restrictions: (1) that the loan be incurred for a purpose reasonably related to patient care, (2) that it was not an excess rate of interest, and (3) that it was paid to a lender not related through control or ownership or personal relationship to the borrowing organization.

2. Bad debts, charity, and courtesy allowances were deductions from revenue and were not included in allowable cost; only bad debts attributable to the deductions and coinsurance amounts were reimbursable under the program.

3. An appropriate part of the net cost of approved educational activities was an allowable cost. This included training programs for nurses, medical students, interns, and residents and various allied health specialties.

4. Costs incurred for research purposes over and above usual patient care were not includable as allowable cost.

5. Unrestricted grants, gifts, and income from endowments could not be deducted from operating costs. Those that were designated by a donor for paying specific operating costs could be deducted from that particular group of costs.

6. Discounts and allowance received on purchases of goods are reductions of the costs to which they related.

7. A reasonable allowance of compensation for services of owners was an allowable cost, provided that the services were actually performed in a necessary function. This applies to proprietary institutions, particularly extended care facilities, where the owners might act as managers, bookkeepers, and in other capacities.

8. In lieu of specific recognition of other costs in providing and improving services, an allowance amounting to 2% of allowable costs (with the exception of interest expense and the allowance under this principle) was includable as an element of reasonable cost of services. However, for proprietary providers the allowance was 1.5% of allowable costs.

This is the famous *plus* factor. It was bitterly debated as a bonus factor above actual cost, as an incentive to let costs rise, as favoring nonprofit over profit institutions, and thwarting proper planning of hospital facilities while providing no assurance of any net improvements in facilities.

Nevertheless, because of imprecise measurements of some costs, inadequate methods of measuring others, and a lack of adequate data, it was approved.

9. Total allowable costs of a provider was to be apportioned between program beneficiaries and other patients so that the share borne by the program was based upon actual services received by program beneficiaries. The provider had the option of using either of two methods: (1) the ratio of beneficiary charges to total patient charges for the services of each department was applied to the cost of the department or (2) the cost of routine services for program beneficiaries was determined on the basis of average cost per diem of these services for all patients. To this was added the cost of ancillary services used by beneficiaries, determined by apportioning the total cost of ancillary services on the basis of the ratio of beneficiary charges for ancillary services to total patient charges for such services.

All cost plans and revenue schemes used so far have developed nettlesome shortcomings. The hope for the future, however, could well be prospective budgets with accompanying prospective rates. This means that the provider, or hospital, predicts its budget for a specific period of time and sets rates in amounts to cover these expenditures. Then contracts are arranged between the various payers that specific services will be given at specific rates for a guaranteed period of time. This type of system, in order to have meaning, requires highly skilled and sophisticated managers. With the advent of more and more collective bargaining units, government controls and technologic advancements, managers are no longer able to guess about future costs but must be scientifically prepared to make accurate predictions, set targets, and manage resources to accomplish those ends.

Payment for physicians' services to hospitals and to individual patients is a particularly complicated area, especially insofar as hospital-based physicians are concerned. The law requires that medical and surgical services rendered to a covered individual by a hospital-based physician be reimbursed only under the supplementary medical insurance program, i.e., Part B of Title XVIII. Services that the physician renders to the hospital other than as direct services to the patients are referred to in other portions of the reimbursement procedure manual. This includes such activities as teaching, research, performance of autopsies, committee work, quality control activities, and administration. Determining the cost of such activities can be an arduous task.

Now that Medicare has been in operation over several years, it is possible to understand some of its strengths and weaknesses. The bed shortage that everyone feared did not materialize. It has now become apparent that Medicare did not affect the admission rate, but it did increase the length of stay of covered individuals. The Utilization Review Committee is not as potent a force as was originally hoped, primarily because the proprietary interests of the committee members are in conflict with their professional interests.

There is a cry for efficient health service, primarily concentrating on cost. As long as there are cost contracts and the method of reimbursement is based on costs, this efficiency cannot be demonstrated. When costs are increased, income is increased; and there is a strong incentive to increase costs. There are other subtle ways in which Medicare pushes costs up.

Since patients are able to pick their own physicians, who are then eligible for payment under Part B, and since patients must pay for a portion of the charges in an ambulatory care facility, the tendency is for them to seek a physician not affiliated with an outpatient department. This enables the patients to avoid long waits in these areas. It is driving costs up, since even the cost

of running the facility remains the same such that as the number of visits goes down the cost per unit up. Thus Medicare is driving cost up.

One of the most pressing problems that will have to be solved as government participation continues is the tremendous variance in cost for units of service in similar hospitals in the same area. How can one explain and justify the same or higher rates in a smaller hospital that has a limited range of services as compared to a large teaching hospital that offers a wide spectrum of services?

The true effects of Medicare on hospital costs will never be known completely because when Medicare became operational the basic wage law became effective for hospital workers. At the same time laboratory workers and nurses were becoming more aggressive in their demands for better salaries. Since personal care constitutes such a large portion of the cost in health care, when salaries go up, costs go up correspondingly. There was also an increased Social Security tax at the time.

A big cost of Medicare is in keeping records and reviewing regulations relating to them. These regulations will be under constant revision for some time to come until the system is effectively worked out. Most confusing, perhaps, for the hospital-based physician are the billing mechanisms centering around Part A (the hospital portion) and Part B (the physician portion). This troublesome portion of costing involves anesthesiologists, radiologists, pathologists, and EKG, EEG, and radioisotope specialists. In the past each hospital worked out its own arrangement with these groups. In some hospitals the specialists were salaried or worked on a percent basis. In other hospitals a lease or concession arrangement prevailed, with the specialist leasing facilities from the hospital but running the department on its own terms. Pathologists have traditionally been salaried or worked on a percentage basis because they have almost no patient contact. Before Medicare, the hospital usually made a single charge to the patient and did the billing for these groups. As soon as Medicare was enacted, the A.M.A. passed a resolution stating that hospital specialists should set fees and collect payments directly from patients.

The guiding principles as outlined by the Social Security Administration made no such recommendation. The arrangements between the hospital and the specialist groups were their own concern and could be worked out in whatever way that proved suitable to all concerned. However, "the law requires that medical and surgical services of a hospital-based physician be reimbursed only under Part B. Costs to a hospital for services furnished in the hospital by a physician that are not professional services to a patient will be included in the cost reimbursement under Part A."[3]

The law went on to define precisely what constitutes a professional service reimbursable under Part B. It is "an identifiable service requiring performance by a physician in person, which contributes to the diagnosis of the condition of the patient with respect to whom the charge under Part B is to be recognized, or contributes to the treatment of such patient."[3]

The pathologists were the most incensed since only a small portion of their work qualified for the *reasonable charge* reimbursement of Part B; most of it was reimbursable under the *reasonable cost* provision of Part A. The cost of training interns and residents is also reimbursable under Part A.

Some hospital-based physicians are in a position to make use of interns and residents as part of their training and to see many more patients than they would ever be able to see if they were working alone. This increases their income under the reasonable charge feature of Part B. The hospital enjoys no such bonanza with its reasonable cost provision under Part A.

By far the most difficult part of this whole complex operation is sorting out the costs. Which portions are applicable under Part B and which under Part A? These must be justified and are checked by extensive audits by the participating institutions and by the government auditors.

Medicare has removed the stigma of the wards, which is good. It pays only for semiprivate accommodations. Some of the older hospitals, however, find themselves with a large number of ward beds (because of demands from an earlier era) and a shortage of semiprivate beds. If patients under Medicare are not given semiprivate accommodations, a penalty is levied against the hospital. The penalty is the difference between semiprivate and ward charges. If the semiprivate rate is $79 a day and the ward rate is $70, then a $9 penalty is assessed against the reimbursable cost; this is $9 less than the actual cost of the care.

In one large city hospital this resulted in a loss from cost of $114,000 annually. In order to correct this situation and to meet the requirements an immediate cash outlay of $150,000 would have been necessary to convert the ward beds into semiprivate rooms. This would have resulted in a loss to the hospital of 60 beds. It is inevitable that such a squeeze will push prices up one way or another.

Other losers are bad debts of patients other than Medicare patients and also nursery and delivery room costs. The nursery and delivery rooms never have been able to pay their way. They are used predominantly by young families who do not have a lot of money, by women from lower income groups who tend to have larger families, and now by unmarried mothers who frequently cannot pay. These areas of the hospital have always relied heavily on other areas to make up their deficit. By removing the extra income involved in charges and by reducing all charges to cost, how can hospitals support these areas of heavy deficit? If a solution is not found, hospitals must inevitably go bankrupt.

Medicare requires that patients be placed in nursing homes when the need for acute care is past; this is based on the supposition that nursing home care costs less. However, in large metropolitan areas with a shortage of nursing home beds, nursing homes will pass up Medicare patients in favor of private pay patients whom they can charge more than cost.

Medicare has for the first time made hospitals truly accountable, both internally and to the public. Antiquated accounting systems have been forced to modernize, and this has been an influence for the good. Just keeping up with the revisions is a good-sized task, and these revisions will continue to come.

The Social Security Administration is looking constantly for more efficient and less costly ways of running this vast program. To that end, one of the 1967 amendments has been a program of incentive reimbursement experiments. Money is available to institutions to experiment with plans whereby new methods of providing the care and reimbursing for that care can be tried. The plans must function under a set of guidelines outlined by Social Security Administration, and they must be able to be evaluated on some well-developed statistical design.

The goals are admirable in that any creative talent that lies hidden is being sought out. The chances for success seem limited, however. All participation in the programs is to be voluntary, including physicians, institutions, organizations, and beneficiaries. This calls for a wide consensus. At the same time there does not appear to be anything in it for anyone, not even a copyright for an ingenious plan.

States have been encouraged to develop their own comprehensive medical plans through Public Law 89-749. The money available is for planning on a wide range of health service, including mental health. This has received very little publicity, and whether there has been any participation is questionable.

To date, the government plans have been courageous. Programs concerning particular segments have done well, but there is no overall plan. What is needed is less emphasis on accounting methods and more emphasis on economic means. This calls for participation by both public and private sectors of the economy to recognize that there must be total involvement by individuals in financing their care rather than political, expedient methods to appease certain voting segments of the populace.

Medicare is ahead of its time. A total blueprint should have been established before it was implemented. Not every person over the age of 65 is poverty stricken or unable to pay some portion of his health bill. There should be some private responsibility involved.

Surely a large part of this problem is attributable to the fact that third-party payers like Blue Cross and organizations like the American Hospital Association that are not really concerned with the operation of hospitals have been the negotiators for hospitals. These intermediaries will speak most emphatically from their own interests. In the future, every hospital must speak for itself, each from its own set of circumstances and needs. Unless this happens, the quality of care given to all segments of the population will become questionable.

CASE HOSPITAL

In the early 1960s it had become evident that the American dream was changing. A country that had virtually attained visions of masterful technology and abundant material possession was finding that, in the balance, the quality of life and environment was declining. Moreover, as social pressures began to mount for directing technology and wealth toward human good, it saw that the same institutions that had propelled success thus far must facilitate the balance, for it was doubtful that new organizations directed to social and environmental achievements could start and mature in time to move technology in necessary future directions. Yet these giants, designed for other times and conditions, seemed grossly unprepared to undergo the immense change required. Indeed, those in education and health were reluctant to engage at all at the threshold of an epoch demanding two changes at once, a change in mode of service to improve immediate contribution and a change in perspective from reacting to immediate circumstances to acting to meet future requirements over periods of 10, 20, or 30 years or longer.

This is the environment in which America is emphasizing health care. It is insisting that the health care industry marshall its resources toward a high-caliber product. Increasing demands for continuity of care, reasonably priced, in convenient packages, require that the industry create entire new approaches to providing service. Every resource and program must be utilized to its maximum. Every agency, institution, and leader must collaborate to overcome waste and duplication.

Historically, American health services developed in organizational structures fashioned after industrial models in the early stages of bureaucratization, using charismatic or traditional modes of operation. One or two men carried the responsibility or most of the decision making. These health services have been autonomous organizations with vested interests. The result has been inefficient use of money, manpower, facilities, and equipment. Health technology and specialization have reached a degree of development that cannot tolerate this type of situation.

Today's health care potential requires that decisions be made by groups of people who possess or have access to specialized knowledge and who can ferret out the information needed, weigh it, and draw conclusions. These people must be arranged into an organization that coordinates them toward common health care goals. Health

science, technology, and, more recently, financing have advanced to the point where their full potential for society cannot be realized unless new ways of organizing, coordinating, and utilizing them toward common objectives can be found. This can be effected through a partnership between free enterprise and government.

The industry has been challenged to improve its existing ways of providing service and at the same time to experiment with new ways of packaging and delivery. It has in essence been told to do two things that it is not prepared to do—first, to substantiate what efficient/effective health care is, and to provide it that way; second, to innovate.

Efficient care, effective care, and *quality of care* are terms that have been wrestled with for many years. The question has been raised, "Who should accept responsibility for establishing standards?" Answers have included private citizens, individual hospitals, hospital associations, and governmental agencies. No one has pursued the responsibility with sufficient vigor.

This is the environment in which Case University and Case Hospital found themselves faced with change, and credit must be given to the president of Case University for sensing the need and redirecting the university's interests. Urban Case University was founded to educate the working and immigrant population in a large American city. As technology paved the way to upward mobility in the late 1940s and early 1950s, however, the university followed the aspirations of its administration, faculty, and clientele, away from original purposes. The trend continued until John Kennedy's administration, with legislation driven forward by convictions such as "the rights of man come not from the generosity of the state but from the hand of God" provided new emphasis on social thinking. In the words of men who shared the university president's conviction: "He began to see Case's role in quite different terms, terms more consonant with its beginnings and with the times. He embraced the idea of action-oriented education and a policy of assistance to the school's black neighbors."

It was a period of diverse views when conservatives and activists struggled with choices between existing paths or practicing responsible citizenship in the immediate community. It was, too, a period that left little doubt that people and government shared with physicians and administrators a growing concern over the existing state of human health and the "system" of delivering services to promote its wellbeing. In this particular arena, attention was focused on university medical centers that were struggling to improve current programs at the same time they sought innovative strategies for providing a newly declared essential right of the American people.

University medical centers drew attention because they commanded health resources and political, academic, and research platforms. Undertaking improvement and experimentation, however, required new arrangements between hospitals, the schools for which they provided clinical settings, and management. Usual organizational structures required new forms of better integrated resources and programs. Prospects of new curriculum and facilities, expanding clinical services, better understanding of organization and management, and changing social, political, and economic environments introduced new ways of constructing fresh missions and alternatives for meeting them.

At Case University the president placed new emphasis on health by appointing a new vice president for a health sciences center. Under the auspices of this office, the university's loosely confederated Schools of Medicine, Dentistry, and Pharmacy and the University Hospital were brought together as a center. To round out and diversify programs, two OEO neighbor-

hood health centers were created and strong affiliations were entered into with many of the city's hospitals to eliminate duplication of skills and facilities. In the mid-1960s the College of Allied Health Professions was begun, and in 1967 the regional health affiliates incorporated to initiate, stimulate, aid, study, evaluate, and provide for coordinated programs in education, research, and community action in the field of health. Major health institutions were attracted because they shared a philosophy of team programs and recognized that it could be implemented through integrated services in a health complex.

Broad health center missions were defined as (1) the creation and formulation of new knowledge (research), (2) transmission of knowledge to students (education), and (3) social application of knowledge to the public (service). Of these, the third related most directly to the hospital and embodied a philosophy that direct participation in provision of health services is an essential aspect of the broader educational and research objectives. In fact, the process of professional education and the milieu of health-related research necessitate selective and judicious involvement in health care.

In carrying out the university's role in direct health care, the role of the hospital and clinics was expressed as threefold:

1. As stated in the state Hill-Burton plan, hospitals that are operated as training facilities of a school provide a clinical service or facility necessary for health profession education and will enable the school to provide additional or improved clinical education. Only as a singular commitment to the highest standards of education, both basic science and clinical, as integrated into all levels of professional education, will professional practice serve its ultimate goals.

2. Recognizing that the basic responsibility for direct service is not im-

mediately met through universities, the hospital and clinics of the health sciences center accept the responsibility for demonstrating ideal and practicable forms of organizing and applying newer knowledge to clinical science.

3. Again, as recorded in the state Hill-Burton plan, university hospitals and clinics must be peculiarly equipped to offer specialized services that attract patients statewide and from other states. In addition, they can provide specialized educational programs in graduate and continuing education.

Goal and policy statements in support of fulfilling this role included the following provisions:

Goal—*Emphasize excellence of service to patients while maintaining a balanced commitment to research and education as part of the university's role in the community, state, and nation.*

Policy—Excellence of service will be maintained by providing that amount of service necessary to maintain high standards of inpatient care programs, clinical research programs, basic research programs, and outpatient programs as related to a faculty sized and composed to serve the needs of the medical school, significant research areas, and model programs that illustrate an optimal method of delivering health care services. This balanced concept is in distinct contrast to commitment to service for its own sake.

Goal—*Recruit a full-time staff balanced between different fields of concentration and between patient care, education, clinical research, and basic research.*

Policy—This is a corollary of the preceding goal. It is also a necessary consequence of a health care goal of supplying a single level of care to all patients. Instead of faculty and hospital staff serving part-time with hours divided between

private and hospital patients, the full-time staff member would be a salaried professional operating within the context of the center.

Goal—*Maximize the potential for creating new health knowledge, its teaching, and its application by integrating disciplines traditionally outside the health sciences.*

Policy—New programs, particularly those including social and environmental scientists, will be developed to broaden the concerns of health care to include as many factors as possible to provide comprehensive care programs.

Goal—*Cooperate with the school board in the establishment of special educational and health programs in neighborhood schools.*

Goal—*Centralize administration to set unified policies for education, research, and service.*

Policy—Augment the staff at the office of the vice-president for health sciences in order to assure its capability of developing the functional unity and conceptual integrity of the health sciences center. The activities of research, administration, program and community planning, continuing education, and development and public relations will each be represented by an associate vice-president.

Goal—*Limit the total expansion of the health sciences center.*
Policy

1. Limit the number of beds at the health sciences center to no more than 1,500 but no less than 600 in accordance with national experience relating to efficient operating size.

2. Review the size of medical programs to assure that none is too small to operate efficiently or too large for its medical significance to the health sciences center.

3. Limit the size of health sciences center programs to that commensurate

with its commitments to research, education, and health care.

Goal—*The health sciences center will concentrate its efforts on those activities directly related to the support of its primary goals of research, education, and delivery of health care.*

Policy—All supportive services that can be supplied more efficiently and less expensively from outside sources will be utilized. Thus it will:

1. Promote the establishment of a central laundry to serve the hospitals of the area.
2. Purchase preprocessed foods from outside suppliers, thereby reducing the food service functions to an assembly and delivery of food only, consequently reducing the size of the dietary staff and the amount of space required for food purposes.
3. Contract for any maintenance services that may be purchased economically.
4. Provide student housing only for minors and women students for whom the university has a parental responsibility in order to maximize the allocation of land and money toward education, research, and service.

Goal—*Increase student enrollment at undergraduate, graduate, and postgraduate levels in response to national needs and to Case University's status as a state-related institution.*

Policy

1. Enlarge the student body without a concomitant increase in bed ratio by affiliation with other medical institutions.
2. Expand the medical school enrollment.
3. Expand the pharmacy school enrollment.
4. Expand the dental school enrollment.
5. Expand the allied health professions' school enrollment.
6. Introduce new paramedical training

programs at all levels to alleviate the manpower shortage in the health professions.

Goal—*Relate clinical teaching programs to all schools of the health sciences center.*

Policy—The clinical teaching experience of all the health professions will assume an importance equal to that now given in the training of physicians.

Goal—*Develop care concepts and programs to fulfill the promise of modern medical science and emerging national health policy.*

Policy

1. Establish a community health program that will serve the primary medical care needs of 50,000 residents in the area. This program will offer high-quality family care. This will be done in a group setting. Appointments will be on an individual basis.
2. Participate in regional health care programs such as heart, stroke, and cancer projects in order to marshal the collective resources of the region's medical institutions in attacking national health problems.

Goal—*Give special attention and priority to the interests, convenience, and amenity of the public and of patients, while maintaining the highest level of professionalism in the delivery of health care.*

Policy

1. This goal reinforces other goals. It implies that the distinction between classes of patients (i.e., private and other) will be done away with. It also is consistent with other qualitative goals regarding the level of patient care. Concern for the patient's dignity and comfort is to be considered as important as his health problems.
2. Establish the single room as the basic inpatient room. Multibed will be used only as medical needs of the patient indicate.

3. Institute a preprocessed food **system** capable of serving the patient at the patient's convenience and of providing him with a wide choice of foods.

Goal—*Establish cross-disciplinary patient-care programs consolidating various specialties having related concerns in order to maximize contacts in education, research, and patient care.*

Policy—A neurosensory program (neurosurgery, neurology, otorhinology, and ophthalmology), a human growth and development program (obstetrics, pediatrics, and gynecology), a musculoskeletal program (orthopedics, rheumatology, and physical medicine and rehabilitation), a cardiopulmonary program (thoracic and cardiovascular surgery, cardiology, chest disease and inhalation therapy, and bronchoesophagology), a general surgery program, and an internal medicine program shall be established in which each program will find on a single floor, to the extent possible, offices, clinical research, outpatients, inpatients, diagnostic facilities, treatment facilities, related service laboratories and operating rooms, and x-ray facilities when necessary and practical.

Goal—*Establish throughout the hospital a single level of high-quality care based on best professional judgment and patient need and not on socioeconomic factors.*
Policy
1. Visits to all outpatient facilities shall be on an individual basis.
2. Provide equal physical facilities for all patients regardless of the source of payment for medical services.
3. Provide the amount and nature of medical care to the patient based solely upon medical need.

Goal—*Shift the emphasis of care for the patient from continuity with a particular physician to continuity within a system involving teams of health care personnel.*
Policy—This goal is another of the mutually reinforcing systems of goals for the center. It implies some of the same policies described earlier.
1. The eradication of the distinction between social classes of patients.
2. The health sciences center will embrace the responsibility for treatment of the whole patient. This will mitigate the trending for specialists to pay inadequate attention to health problems not related to their specialty.
3. It implies that the present erosion of the traditional "doctor-patient" relationship will be eased by teams of mutually reinforcing health care personnel responsible for the patient's general health needs as well as for specific complaints.

Goal—*Maximize the convenience of access to health care facilities for patients.*
Policy
1. Provide adequate and properly located parking for outpatients and for arrival of inpatients and emergency cases.
2. Schedule outpatient visiting 8 hours daily and include some time on evenings and weekends.

Goal—*Employ every possible means to make the most rational use of scarce, qualified personnel.*
Policy
1. Organize the location of hospital activities so that most personnel will find most of their needs on a single floor most of the time.
2. Provide the professional staff with new supporting personnel to relieve them of administrative and logistic chores. A unit-manager system should be adopted and a special logistic force developed.
3. Include labor-saving equipment to reduce or eliminate time spent in hand-moving items within the hospital.

Goal—*Cooperate with the school board and the department of health in establishing and staffing community health centers modeled after the community health program.*

Over the years the hospital had grown in a situation common to most university teaching hospitals, i.e., under the direct responsibility of the dean of the school of medicine. During the past several years the university, cognizant of changing social needs, reevaluated its teaching, research, and service programs in light of projected future trends and commitments. In so doing, an executive director who is a co-equal of the several deans in the health

sciences center was appointed for the hospital. All report directly to the same vice president for health sciences.

The hospital's formal organization exhibited the pyramidal characteristics common among health care organizations. The bulk of authority for decision making rested on the top (Fig. 3-1). The influence pattern prescribed to coordinate such an organization may be compared to a wagon wheel (Fig. 3-2, *A*). Administration is the hub; departments are at the outer extremities of the spokes; the rim and spokes represent established interaction and communications. The existing pattern of coordination is represented in Fig. 3-2, *B*. The bulk of authority for decision making rested at

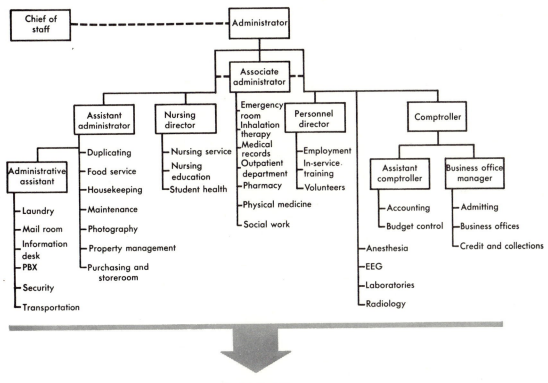

Services to users

Fig. 3-1. Existing hospital organization. Practically all of the shops of this class are organized upon what may be called the military plan. The orders from the general are transmitted through the colonels, majors, captains, lieutenants, and noncommissioned officers to the men. (From Taylor, F. W.: Scientific management, New York, 1947, Harper & Brothers, pp. 92 and 93.)

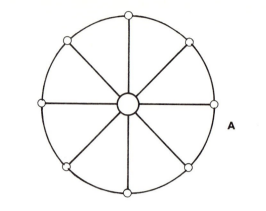

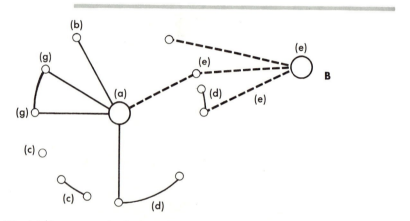

Fig. 3-2. A, Wagon wheel of coordination. **B**, Scattered wagon-wheel effect (see text).

the hub *(a)*; a heavy dependency on the hub had developed among some departments *(g)*; others had withdrawn in isolation *(d)*; and still others had sought or been infiltrated by authority from outside the hospital's administrative structure *(e)*. The hub lost contact with some departments and became too involved in the operations of others. As the hub, administration, became overburdened with day-to-day operational detail, it limited the interrelation of the departments involved. It minimized the initiative of department chiefs. It blocked personal development of personnel. Departments were isolated. Problem solving was a shoot-from-the-hip matter of expedience with little forethought

of future consequences. Leadership, supervision, and communications were lacking. Since this type of organization limited department chiefs in their authority to fulfill their responsibilities, department decision making was concentrated in administration, where an attempt to do too many things had developed. Policy development, long-range planning, and procedural improvement suffered from inattention. Horizontal communication at lower levels was practically nonexistent.

Administrative coordination was not good. As a result, when administrative solutions to routine departmental problems were sought, the action taken reflected the inappropriateness of the level of decision.

They did not consider the consequences to other areas. Uncoordinated activities between departments developed. Cooperation lagged.

A good example of this lack of coordination involves the activities of the department of nursing. This department had taken on overall administration and some medical administration and set out to build its own hierarchy. The emphasis was not on the profession of nursing but on striving for power. A strong central nursing hierarchy evolved. Individual head nurses would not act unless word was received from the nursing office. Training and career development were replaced by a staunch militaristic hierarchy. Nurses were always trying to win their point, not on the basis of ability, but on the basis of right to decide; whether or not the facts supported their action was not important. Control and power by threat and dictate became the objective. Once in trouble, they ran to the weak administrative structure for support, and when this was not forthcoming because of the ridiculousness of the decision, a pouting type of behavior resulted along with cries of an inconsistent policy and weak administration.

Staff size had not been determined for many departments. It was not known how many man-hours were available to work or how many should be required. Standards of performance, quality, and cost were nonexistent. There was little flexibility for the sharing of employees among departments. Supervisory trainers and managers acted as "lead" workers with no time for management. Department heads and personnel were uncertain as to what their jobs were. They felt unappreciated.

An organizational philosophy with commensurate goals and objectives was lacking. Consequently there was a lack of understanding and identification with the hospital as an organization. There was frequent reference to "I—they," which upon examination mean "I" work here and

"they" are a gray area of administration who tell me what to do. This disassociation was a combination of unwillingness to change, lack of coordination, and failure to have or to understand a relationship with the hospital as an entity. A state of normlessness and a lack of organizational values existed that was thwarting and frustrating.

Planning or predicting change and need was done on a daily basis. Crisis administration was practiced, and direction by default was encouraged. Ignore a problem or talk it to death was the pattern of decision making.° Fire fighting was the byword. In the absence of planning, similar problems presented themselves over and over again; the same solutions were sought over and over again.

This situation, which was internal to the hospital, was somewhat indicative of needs of the entire health sciences center. For many years the schools and the hospital operated in an autonomous manner, and there was very little interrelated coordination. The recent reorganization formed some sense of direction, but its newness also caused confusion. The hospital became overextended and provided administrative and resource services well beyond what could be considered legitimate hospital responsibility. For instance, the bulk of dietary, personnel, maintenance, purchasing, laundry, mail, telephone, and security services were provided and administered by

°This form of administration could be tolerated if this type of behavior could be communicated to those expecting a precise definition or decision in all cases. However, sporadic "lowering of the boom" as the result of certain actions leads only to confusion. Consistency is not necessary in decision making, but a consistent philosophic application in problem solving is necessary. This is imperative to allow all concerned to play the same game, with the same interpretation of the rules of the game. The administrator's role then becomes one of interpreting the ball park and assuring that the same game with the same rules applicable to all are followed and enforced.

the hospital for the entire center. There was no common accounting mechanism to distribute the cost appropriately, and the effectiveness of these services for the patient was diluted. In addition an overall coordination of the use of these services at the campus level was needed. Hospital administration carried responsibility for provision, but it had little influence on utilization. In effect it was a banker when its role should have been that of a broker.

Even patient care services sometimes developed in limbo without adequate coordination toward the goals of the overall campus setting. A community mental health center had been made operational with sparse and very informal agreement as to who was administratively responsible for its operation. Although most of the money for staffing, renovation, and equipping came from federal, state, and university funds, the hospital was responsible for providing support for operational costs. In its efforts to establish accounting and financial arrangements to assist in meeting this responsibility, it became evident that the authority to guide the operation was not being adequately accepted by any administrative center; not by the hospital, the department of psychiatry, the school of medicine, the center administration, or the mental health center itself.

In this state, day-to-day operations were extremely difficult. Progress and change were stymied. It was in this setting that the hospital found itself challenged to substantiate what efficient/effective health care is and to provide it. In this setting, it was challenged to innovate. It did not find itself well prepared to do either. Immediate, dramatic reorganization was imperative.

A word about dramatic reorganization and change must be added. As attested to by the many and varied "change agents" circulating organizations today who rely upon their own personality qualities to promote change, change is not a well-understood phenomenon. To be highly benefi-

cial to the organization change must not only have cause and hope but also direction; it must have this from its onset. And it should also have a potential of benefit for the organization. Change for the sake of action that has not been thought out in relationship to the organization in which it occurs may not have only neutral effects; it may well be detrimental.

Case Hospital experimented with a change agent. Results were less than satisfactory. The change agent used group dynamics and other counseling techniques and appeared to only pacify and strengthen the status quo. The reason for this lack of success, it is believed, is due to the noninvolvement or nothing-at-stake role of the change agent. In Case Hospital it was found that supervisors were not communicating or getting involved with their people. It would appear that the only way change can be effected is total commitment and involvement in all levels of management and face-to-face relationships with the people affected by the change. Approaching the bare facts with some identifiable objective in mind before change is initiated is imperative. It must involve those people searching for alternative courses of action and must allow a ruling-out process rather than issue a dictate. Facing the reality of the situation, not sugar-coating the pill, is "tough on the stomach" in the short run but makes a more permanent result in the long run. The face-to-face relationship must be visible to all involved in the change, and the willingness to listen to the other person's side is imperative.

The use of information in the form of facts with measurable outcomes is a mechanism. It is definitely uncomfortable for all concerned. Telling half-truths and glossing over the nitty-gritty details with vague assumptions is disastrous in the overall plan. Therefore to effect and implement change, the plan must be made available with its objectives, and the details of the implementation must be spelled out in understandable terms to those implementing the change and to those effecting the change.

Alternative courses of action must be explored by that same group and then the chips must be allowed to fall where they will. The key word here is *involvement* and having something at stake for each contender. Managers who delegate this nasty task rather than involving themselves will soon find that what looked like the perfect answer is in reality the beginning of a series of minor problems resulting in major collapse of the idea or the plan.

Some organizations and some sections of our society (often geographically identified) are so in the habit of doing things the traditional way that even a disaster fails to produce enduring change, or change with enduring effects. This state of affairs is referred to as being in a rut. Sometimes those in a rut will feel that change should occur or will want to project an image of change. New blood in the form of experts or consultants is brought in. In cases where the people who "seek" change want only an image or are not willing to support it, the new blood will be so saturated with the old blood that it becomes ineffective or will leave in order to preserve its virility. In many such institutions,° even a major catastrophy such as the threat of bankruptcy fails to generate change. In these situations the organization is well on its way to decay.

°Conversion of means to ends becomes so institutionalized that, unless the organization has symbolic value, its ability to be productive is lost and it no longer is able to make a contribution to the larger society in which it was created for specified purposes.

This could be called the bad people–good people theory. If a status quo is maintained in the environment, the bad people will drive out the good people. To avoid this, the administrator's role becomes one of changing the environment in order to create an organizational structure that can accommodate all types of individuals. His real and only objective will be to create an environment able to accommodate people with all types of ability and motivation. Once created, the organization becomes able to place people in their respective ability and motivational niches. The organization moves, then, toward a self-directing and self-regulating organism. At this point it reflects individual and group philosophies and human behavior. It is in effect a living organization, or better, a human organization. It is life itself, not a cold materialistic thing. Service organizations committed to individual betterment for both consumers and providers must strive for this type of organization and administration. Once this is attained, the need for catchy phrases and high-sounding slogans will diminish, and the organizational acts, expression of human abilities and emotions, will speak for themselves.

The end results or the acts of the organization will be identifiable. No interpretation of intent or results will be required.

REFERENCES

1. Durbin, R. L.: Do new hospitals attract new doctors? Mod. Hosp. **100**:98, June 1963.
2. American Medical Association: The graduate education of physicians, Chicago, 1966, The Association.
3. Principles of payment for services of hospital-based physicians, Washington, D. C., 1966, U. S. Department of Health, Education, and Welfare, Social Security Administration.
4. Durbin, R. L., and Springall, W. H.: Systems organization for a hospital, Hosp. Manage. **104**:36, Sept. 1967; **104**:57, Oct. 1967; **104**:38, Nov. 1967.

chapter four

REORGANIZATION OF A HOSPITAL

In undertaking reorganization of Case Hospital, it was believed that an orientation must be established toward the larger spectrum of health care. It was apparent that the formal organization was rooted in the classical approach. Existing practices were neither adaptable to change nor compatible with current organizational commitments.

The organizational pattern needed was one that could provide a framework for routine, technical, innovative, and professional activities, allow flexibility in correcting existing operating problems, and stimulate experimentation. A new environment was needed, one that stressed the value of innovation among all personnel. This environment must accommodate a diversity of personnel while stimulating creativity and encouraging participation at all levels. Broad organizational values and information must be provided for interpretation to be used as guideposts for challenging people to experiment with causes of success.

In the existing organization, authority and leadership were dependent primarily on charismatic or traditional influences. Seldom did it stem from ability. It did not have the basic characteristics that promote efficient/effective routine; it did not have the characteristics that stimulate and coordinate professional judgment; it did not encourage experimentation.

The new horizontal reorganization was structured with a view toward accommodating the complex pattern of human relationships and communications necessary for the efficient delivery of health services. It represents a synergistic organization of resources into **systems** that provide component parts for coordinated **programs** of service. It is a formalization of philosophy, theory, and practice that sets forth certain propositions about systems and programs.

SYSTEMS AND PROGRAMS

If, according to the definition of a hospital established earlier, the primary characteristic of a hospital is care, then a question must be directed to the legitimacy of the various departments that are found there. Is it necessary for the hospital to operate these activities; and, if it is, is it necessary to arrange the activities within traditional departmental boundaries?

Hospitals are notorious for departments. Among those commonly found in a large hospital are nursing service, nursing education, personnel, in-service training, pharmacy, central sterile supply, dietary, baby formula room, laundry, radiology, housekeeping, maintenance and grounds, laboratories, hospital administration, public relations and fund raising, purchasing, storeroom, physical and occupational therapy, admitting, social service, business office, emergency room, surgery, anesthesiology, and postanesthesia recovery. Most of these departments exist solely for the purpose of obtaining and allocating resources and materials to programs of care. Often organizations outside the hospital can provide the same services efficiently, although effective application remains the responsibility of the hospital. Hospitals have been extremely reluctant to turn to these outside sources, preferring instead to produce their own.

Considering all of the activities that the hospital chooses to operate, is the usual departmentalization the best way to arrange them? Departmentalization finds its prescriptive roots in the work of such men as Luther Gulick, L. Urwick, Henri Fayol, and J. D. Mooney. Others such as Alvin Gouldner, Philip Selznick, and Robert Merton have discussed its effects on the organization.

Departmentalization is often oriented to the tasks performed by workers on the division-of-labor basis. The total group of tasks assigned to a department is accepted as determined in advance by the organization and is characterized by purpose, process, persons, or place. This type of departmentalization is heavily dependent on a pyramidal organizational structure* and the assignment of workers as the property of a given department. Such an orientation does not recognize or allow flexibility to deal with the psychologic effects of minute reduction of work into tasks. It often overlooks the possibility of combining sets of tasks into new jobs to be performed for several departments by one group of employees. Since tasks and the procedures for carrying them out are handed down from above, the operation of a department often becomes mechanical, and the initiative of the department head and personnel withers.

Mechanical means of operation becomes

the primary goal of the department, and it eventually loses sight of overall organizational goals. Moreover, higher organizational echelons lose their ability to relate to departments. The accumulation of employees and resources within a department becomes a prevailing interest, and empire building is encouraged. Functional contribution to the larger organization is lost sight of. Emphasis on the pyramidal structure does not leave flexibility for innovation and judgment and is thus limiting to innovators and professionals. It also hinders relationships with other departments, clients, the public, and other organizations to which it must relate.

Departments vary, of course, in the intensity of their autonomy or interdependence with other departments and the organization as a whole. They also vary in the degree to which they strive to maintain their autonomy and the reasons for which autonomy is sought. Professionals create privileged information, confidential communications, and a professional vocabulary in order to insulate themselves. Skilled workers organize in order to limit the number and types of tasks assigned to their jobs.

It is possible that a degree of departmentalization may be necessary. If so, the hospital will be faced with competing departmental demands. This will be disrupting to some extent, but, when understood and accounted for, may serve to move the organization toward its goals. This means that administration must recognize and effectively deal with these factors within an organizational framework that is nonmonolithic and nonpyramidal.

To deal effectively with these problems a broader and more feasible arrangement of activities must be designed for health care organizations. Traditional departments may be rearranged in a manner that relates them to a common, functional characteristic or specialty. These several common classifications are as follows:

---

*Departmentalization is also created by professionals and other groups as a means of insulation from the pyramidal structure.

Patient care
Professional service departments
Logistics
Business and finance
Quality control
Security and medicolegal affairs
Environmental services
Personnel and education
Medical staff
Programs of care

The grouping of departments in relation to these classifications creates systems (see Fig. 5-1, p. 80) and programs, the function of systems being the channeling of resources into programs (see Fig. 6-1, p. 98). These are definable units of input available to programs on an accountable basis. The introduction into each group of a capable manager/coordinator who has special ability in relation to the common denominator will facilitate the identification of units of departmental service to the common end product.

At the upper administrative levels, however, there is one characteristic among the systems' administrators and program directors: to work effectively among their groups and themselves to attain organizational goals. The administrator and his associates should be coordinators among the assistant administrators for systems and program directors.

The relationships of each of the sections in this chapter, as placed into context therein, form a synergostructure. A synergostructure provides a framework for action among discrete entities so that the total effect is greater than the individual effects taken independently. In the field of health care it is particularly dependent on establishing the relationship between theory, practice, and environment as described throughout this book.

As applied to health care, a synergostructure provides the perspective and flexibility for constantly pursuing organizational goals at the same time that it deals effectively with the changing nature of the environment in which health care packaging and delivery occur and with the changing need for new organizational forms and processes.

STRUCTURE AND SPECTRUM OF ABILITY, BEHAVIOR, AND VALUES*
Spectrum of ability

The organization should provide a framework that is flexible enough to match the abilities of the people with the objectives of the organization. The formal structure may range from a straight vertical line to a straight horizontal line. Between these two extremes lie many gradations, and a complex organization may utilize many of these within a broad framework.

The reasons for using such a variety of structural patterns lie in the attempt to maximize the potential contributions of many different individuals and groups in many different situations. These individuals and groups include unskilled and semiskilled workers, technical specialists, innovative specialists, and professionals. The activities of the former two may be classified as being largely routine and those of the latter two as being mostly nonroutine. This characterization will vary, however, particularly in relation to the division between technical specialists and innovative specialists. Additionally, people throughout the organization will tend to fill a variety of routine and nonroutine roles during their employment regardless of the nature of the activities related to their primary job assignment.

The routine task worker and the nonroutine task worker tend to differ in six major ways; special ability, background, work environment, motivation, control, and loyalty responses. A comparison of each of

---

*This section incorporates parts of Professions Within an Organization: Conflict and Adaptation, an unpublished master's thesis by John C. Aird, University of California, June 1967. (Recipient of the Stull Award.)

these indices gives greater insight into their relationship and effect on organizations. Analysis of the difference in the tasks performed suggests the difference in ability between the participants. The routine task is characterized by standardness of form that lends itself to repetitiveness of performance. This will occur when and if unpredictable conditions can be minimized and the situation can be made constant. Often, removal or minimization of the human element in the situation will achieve this result. Once done, the task can be easily routinized and ultimately, perhaps, even automated. Performance of this type of task requires the ability to act time and again in a standard, uniform way. This demands the abilities of concentration, consistency, conscientiousness, and perseverance on the participant's part. Little creativity, imagination, or intellectual depth is required. The challenge lies in the successful completion of the task on the basis of a sound, prescribed approach.

Conversely, those variables in a situation that cannot be made constant define an operating milieu in which the application of expert individual analysis, interpretation, and judgment is the best method of maxi-

mizing the potential for completion of the task. Thus the nonroutine task is vastly different from the routine task. The variability of the nonroutine task demands exercise of expertise and application of appropriate nonstandard activities to ensure completion. The power of assessment and the ability to act wisely upon it requires a great depth of knowledge founded on a sound educational background. This being the case, we find that certain activities demand certain approaches to ensure completion. The specific abilities, backgrounds, and personality inclinations tend to fall within particular task areas, which in turn require different organizational structures, environments, and motivational approaches.

A physician, for example, is seen as a certain type of individual with a certain background, performing tasks within the nonroutine task area.* Conversely, a dietary tray line worker is seen as a different type of individual whose background and abilities lend themselves to performing

---

*In other than diagnostic areas the tasks appear to be tending toward routinization (e.g., operative procedures). The effects of computer application on routinizing diagnostic evaluation are as yet unclear.

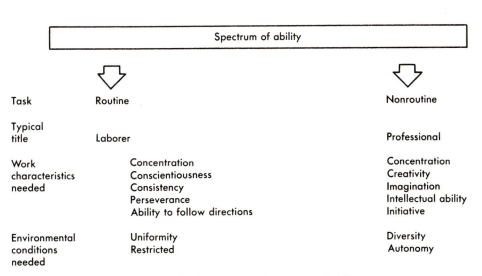

	Spectrum of ability	
Task	Routine	Nonroutine
Typical title	Laborer	Professional
Work characteristics needed	Concentration Conscientiousness Consistency Perseverance Ability to follow directions	Concentration Creativity Imagination Intellectual ability Initiative
Environmental conditions needed	Uniformity Restricted	Diversity Autonomy

Fig. 4-1. Structure and spectrum of ability.

tasks within the routine task area. Organizational approaches to these two "groups" of people should differ. Routine tasks should be assigned to people whose abilities link them with this task area, and their performance should be closely guided by standardized procedures and adequate supervision. Analytic people with judgmental capabilities should participate in the nonroutine task area, an area characterized by freedom of movement and activity. These extremes of the structure and spectrum of ability are portrayed in Fig. 4-1.

This distinction on the spectrum lays the groundwork for a deeper analysis of the organizational implications involved in the areas of control and loyalty placement. Such an analysis gives insight to the need for a broad and flexible organization.

Implications of professionalization

As an occupation moves from the routine toward the nonroutine extremes of the spectrum and tends to become more and more professional, it will break more and more of its organizational ties in favor of those of its professional association. Often the result of this development is a conflicting relationship between the profession and the organization. This conflict can develop in many ways, but perhaps one of its central origins is the fact that as a group becomes more professional the organization has less and less control over the group. By defining how their members may be used in organizations, restraints are imposed on management by the profession. In this way the profession becomes the master of its own ship, and the self-esteem of its members is raised. Tasks once performed but now considered to be of a nonprofessional nature are dropped. The profession thus limits itself to an area of functional specificity within which it considers itself to be the ultimate authority.

Thus the organization must be willing to limit its control over the group in return for the group's contribution of its professional expertise to the organization. Theoretically a state of equilibrium is reached. The organization gives up that amount of control necessary to obtain the valuable expertise that a profession is uniquely capable of delivering. However, equilibrium seldom occurs, for the relationship is not static but is one filled with undercurrents of strain periodically soothed by accommodative mechanisms. Ironically, once their expertise has been organizationally recognized, professions seem to exhibit still less commitment to any organization. For, granted such expertise, professionals generally achieve increased job mobility and can fill jobs in many different organizations. As a result, their control by and loyalty to any one particular organization becomes limited at best.

Other implications arise from the need for freedom to apply judgment required by the professional. If we consider the application of judgment as an art, then, in contrast to science, it may not be reduced to routine. Efforts to overlay scientific routine on professionals may have a restrictive effect.

Art relies heavily on judgment, the results of which are not always predictable. Science, on the other hand, involves the application of proved methods, the results of which are usually predictable. The physician, for instance, relies heavily on professional judgment while applying proved, scientific tools. The accuracy of the results of each scientific tool such as laboratory tests and x-ray films is predictable, but the interpretation of the meaning of the results relies upon judgment and is less subject to scientific accuracy. The consequent course of treatment and its outcome are also heavily involved with many subjective and sometimes unpredictable variables.

Efforts to overlay the routine pyramidal organization on the medical staff of the hospital usually bring about a dichotomy between the hospital organization and the medical staff.* One of the principle reasons for this may be that the effects of the routine performance may be judged against demonstrable, objective standards based upon predictable results—the ends. If the results are bad, the routine was not performed in an acceptable way. Since the results of professional judgment are often not predictable in the same sense, the judgment itself cannot be evaluated in the same fashion. Instead, an analysis of professional judgment can only be done by those familiar with similar decision situations—peers. Thus collaborative peer assessment is the most effective means of determining the acceptability of a physician's use of professional judgment. Pyramidal organizations that use scientific standards are not conducive to peer judgment. Thus the effects of a collaborative medical staff organization in a pyramidal hospital organization is conflict, often emotional and unobjective.

Consider now the application of one administrative tool, industrial engineering, in an organization where both unskilled em-

*This dichotomy is also seen in universities in the faculty-administration split and in industry in the research scientist–administration split.

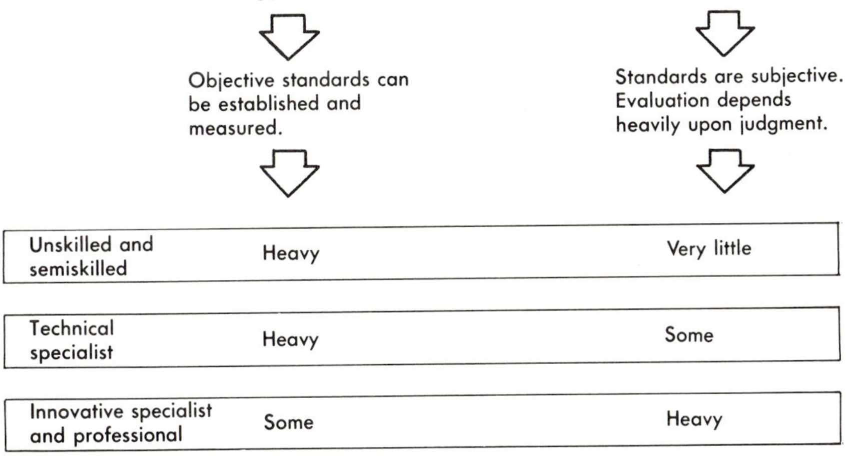

ployees and physicians work. Industrial engineering techniques drawn from scientific management and specifically adapted to hospitals can be used very effectively in some parts of the organization but not in others. Looking at this application to the spectrum of science and art, industrial engineering is most applicable in those categories that rely heavily on science (Fig. 4-2).

Pursuing the effects of having professional groups in an organization further, it has been noted that these groups will increasingly place their own professional or even departmental interests ahead of those of the total organization. They tend to lose sight of the goals of the organization and to identify and push their own goals and work as being the most important. With many departments in an organization, competition inevitably occurs, for such groups will seek to protect their own status and autonomy.

In some of these instances the attempt at professional growth may *exclusively* reflect a concerted effort by the group to gain the advancement of its own status and position in relationship to other departments within the organization. Thus the department interfers with the overall

Fig. 4-2. Spectrum of science and art.

coordination of the organization. The whole organization becomes a mass of competing groups pursuing their own interests regardless of their effect on the organization. Often isolation or insulation results.

These control and loyalty considerations lead us to two subsidiary continuums reflecting degree of control and loyalty relative to occupational position on the spectrum (Fig. 4-3). Both these continuums support the statement that the extremes are distinct in both organizational position and treatment and occupational response, making delineations in approach comparatively easy. It is for this reason that most organizations have been able to achieve at least crude organizational distinctions between the two. But what about the area between the two extremes? This is where the ambiguities of treatment and competing loyalties occur. Only through a more rigorous examination of the contributions

these groups make to the organization and the type of situation that is required in order to maximize those contributions can we more effectively deal with this problem area.

Moving to the right from the routine task area, one can postulate further categoric breakdowns that affect both control and loyalty. These are the semiskilled worker, the tradesman, the specialist, and finally the professional. A closer look shows the relative differences among these groups (Fig. 4-4).

Loyalty-wise, center groups will constantly feel the pressure of competition between organizational commitments and trade association ties. Additionally, personal needs for status and pay often cause them to forsake the area of their expertise for areas where these needs are more readily met. A good example of this is the bedside nurse who could become a true

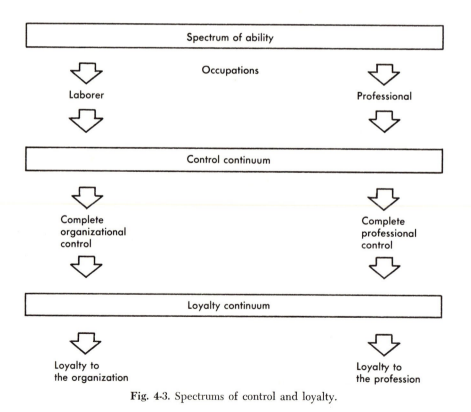

Fig. 4-3. Spectrums of control and loyalty.

nurse specialist, but who, for pay purposes, status, and prestige, must join the competition in the superordinate-subordinate structure in order to survive. Again, ability is not recognized, and the old-fashioned master-servant relationship does not give way. This situation produces strain and tension, which affect total productivity and effectiveness.

What does this analysis tell us? First, it indicates the significance of spectrum position and movement in terms of organizational consequences. Second, it demonstrates the need for further analysis of the center occupational groups if the ambivalence of their position is to be clearly understood. In organizational terms, their position must be made more tolerable and secure if concerted and sometimes spurious attempts at occupational movement along the spectrum are to be adequately dealt with. Third, it is clear that in the tradi-

tional organizational model there is a built-in, natural conflict between the professional person and the organization. Since a range of organizational models is being proposed here, let us pursue this conflict, see what causes it, where it occurs, and how it might better be accommodated in a new model.

Conflict

The professional-organizational conflict is an outgrowth of the difference between the two institutions: bureaucracy and professionalism. More precisely, it is between the primary functions of these two.

For the profession this consists of the protection of the opportunity for the autonomous exercise of individual judgment that is essential to the proper carrying out of the work of the profession. For the organization this consists of a rationalistic approach to management that will ensure

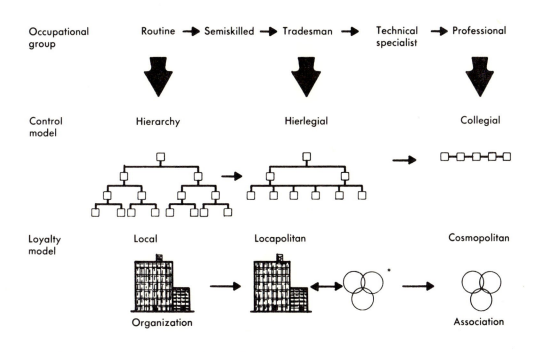

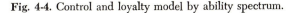

*Loyalty to organization or occupational association, guild, or union is a factor of the balanced effect of the other upon it.

Fig. 4-4. Control and loyalty model by ability spectrum.

the efficient coordination of diverse activities. Both look upon the trend toward opposites, i.e., the bureaucratization of professions and the professionalization of bureaucracy, with almost fanatic apprehension. One might then wonder why both the professional and the organization tolerate any collaborative relationship, particularly when it seems to involve inevitable conflict.

The professional has discovered that without organizational help he simply cannot afford many of the sophisticated technical devices, with accompanying facilities, that his expertise requires. A further advantage is the availability of specialist consultation and other professional assistance when needed. In addition, the professional has found that within an organizational structure he has not lost but gained flexibility and freedom of activity. For, whereas strict conformity to local customs and amenities was necessary in private practice, such is not the case within an organization, where the structure itself serves to buffer close scrutiny. The main control is that exerted by the organization itself; typically, this takes the form of limited peer supervision.

The plight of the organization has been equally effected by developments in modern technology, for specialized services are now demanded and must be made available. Years ago Saint-Simon predicted as much when he stated that, as modern society developed, an organization would be able to rely less and less on coercion, force, or violence to accomplish its ends and therefore must rely more on obtaining and keeping those experts whose specialized skills are needed.

[To do this, the organization grants a] large measure of autonomy to some occupations . . . because experience has shown that in order to get important kinds of jobs done effectively, they must be done by the experts who in turn are the competent judges of the needed expertness. If the laity were to judge what is legal procedure and what is not, society would be even more of a scramble than it is. If the laity were to judge what

is appropriate medical therapy instead of the medical expert, then our national health record would be even worse than it is. And so, through the list of all professions.*

Today it is evident that hospital organizations can no longer entirely rely on a monistic approach to management and goal determination. It is equally evident that no new approach has been made operational and that what has been accepted as "inherent" tension is considered undesirable but continues to be tolerated because of mutual need. The picture of conflict usually presented is one of an organizational monster unilaterally draining out the lifeblood of professionalism. In reality the relationship is reciprocal.

In terms of the organization, the problem is getting the needed experts and professionals into the organization without giving up so much organizational control that the professionals actually determine the goals and direction of the entire organization. The professional and innovative specialists, on the other hand, would like to enter the organization and yet not compromise their own autonomy to such an extent that they are entirely organizationally controlled.

[As a result of these reservations] the system tends to acquire a pluralist character. This means that there are multiple centers of power. The organization does not wholly absorb the professionals, nor do the professionals wholly absorb the organization. To the extent that a system of relations is pluralist, it tends toward a balance of freedom and power or, in functional terms, between the conditions conducive to creativity and those conducive to control.†

The existing tension is thus not necessarily dysfunctional and should not be considered unilaterally so. To the extent that it is an alternative approach to complete absorption of one by another or isolation

*Merton, R.: The search for professional status, Amer. J. Nurs. **60:**663, May 1960.
†Kornhauser, W.: Scientists in industry, Berkeley, 1962, University of California Press, p. 197.

by one from the other, it suggests the need for a pluralistic, synergistic structure.

To keep the conflict within acceptable nondestructive limits it is mandatory that a deeper appreciation of its origins and likely areas of occurrence be gained by organizational administrators and managers, for only through such increased awareness will come the needed organizational alternatives in which each—the organization and the profession—can be accommodated to a productive if sometimes uneasy partnership.

Origins of conflict

Within the last 15 to 20 years in the United States tremendous advances have been made in technology that have stimulated the professionalization of various occupational groups. Because this has been a relatively recent development, it is only in the last few years that many organizations and institutions are realistically beginning to confront the problems stemming from this fact. This emphasis, however belated, has not been misplaced, particularly in the case of the hospital, for there has been a vast proliferation of professional groups, with its inevitable consequences not only on the organization but sometimes more tragically on the patient. Professionals have developed to bring specialized skills in the form of more sophisticated and better techniques of care. It is unfortunate and somewhat ironic that this development often leads to fragmented, less personal, and poorer care because of the lack of organizational integration. Obviously then, this subject is of critical importance to hospital organization. The range of conflict that is described here obviously does not occur in every case involving a professional in an organization. However, it is possible to hypothesize that as an occupational group moves further and further along the spectrum, it will simultaneously tend to experience more and more of these types of conflict situations in its dealings with current forms of organizations.

Goals. The objectives of professionals and organizations vary in many instances. This is in large part attributable to the differences in the mental attitudes of the professional and the organizational man. The professional's training, intellectual inclination, and emotional composition tend to make him seek finite solutions to all problems and finite answers to all questions. He categorically rejects compromise in this area as being unprofessional and therefore unsatisfactory. The organizational man, on the other hand, is constantly forced to utilize the techniques of compromise in giving substance and solution to the intangibles and variables present in every problem. As a result, most organizational solutions have the unfortunate and ironic characteristic of being classified as illegitimate by at least one of the contributors. The aura of illegitimacy is compounded by the often incomplete or temporary nature of the solution. Everyone is thus left dissatisfied. The "compromiser" is looked upon by the professional as being a spineless creature whose only saving grace comes in the bitter acknowledgment that, after all, he is an "organization man" from whom little better could be expected. In turn the organizational man reacts by labeling his continuously uncompromising assailants as unrealistic prima donnas whose idealism is only exceeded by the narrowness of their vision. With regular and, in the sense described, mutually unproductive contacts, labels become fixed, and what began at latent attitudinal polarization becomes manifest.

As mental attitudes differ, so do goals. The professional constantly seeks to know *why* and not just *how*. His energies are expended toward technical excellence and not just quantity of output. Productivity coefficient may serve the utilitarian aims of operational efficiency, but it is anathema to creativity. These differences in goals define an operational environment in which the component parts are constantly either overtly or covertly at conflict with each other. The professional tends to approach work's problems and decisions in terms of their professional implications whereas formal organizational leadership looks at the same problems and decisions in terms of their organizational consequences. In this fashion their goals are split. The professional considers his work an end in itself; the organization sees it only as the means to larger organizational ends.

With each professional group simultaneously pursuing its own goals in this way, one can readily see how the situation becomes a great deal more complex. Gouldner[1] has addressed himself to this problem, suggesting that Parsons and Comte may have been mistaken in presenting groups in an organization as being of sufficient interdependence as to have a common goal or goals. It would seem that Gouldner's position is a slight overstatement, for an organization does have certain prescribed goals. The important thing to remember is that these do not have to and may not necessarily be in agreement with any or all of the specific goals of the groups of which the organization is made.

Autonomy. A basic source of friction in an organization may concern the organizational need for control and the professional need for autonomy. As the professional has only limited loyalty to the organization, the latter is even more reluctant to grant such freedom than it might ordinarily be. The professional, to show his motives are pure, traditionally claimed total responsibility for any and all actions taken in his work. A substitution of peer control has been the final strategic step.* In this way the professional has essentially unburdened the

organization of the responsibility for anything he personally might do. Despite the strategic importance of this maneuver in the obtainment of the desired autonomy concessions from the organization, the professional has nevertheless often resented the fact that he alone then must bear the total risk. So at present the doctor "does the cutting" and not the organization. However, the now famous Darling case in Illinois and other recent legal decisions seem to indicate an alteration in this relationship.*

One can be sure that if the hospital is going to be held liable for decisions made by doctors in the latter's areas of expertise the hospital as an organization will demand more control over the practices in those areas. It is predicted that this will take the form of the imposition of its own rules on the professional, the upgrading of

---

*This is in great contrast to Weber's theory. He felt that administrative superiors would be more technically proficient and thus better able to judge in this area specifically than the expert himself. Gouldner and Parsons disagree with him on this point.

---

*Darling vs. Charleston Hospital, 33 Ill 2d 336. Damages sought by Plaintiff for allegedly negligent medical and hospital treatment. The court ruled that it is the duty of hospital staff to see that all medical procedures are followed and that nurses have responsibility to report developments in medical care to the attention of the administrator, who in turn must notify medical staff for action. The ruling states that "The conception that the hospital does not undertake to act through its doctors and nurses, but undertakes instead simply to procure them to act upon their responsibility, no longer reflects the fact. Present-day hospitals, as their manner of operation plainly demonstrates, do far more than furnish facilities for treatment. They regularly employ on a salaried basis a large staff of physicians, nurses and internes, as well as administrative and manual workers, and they charge patients for medical care and treatment, collecting for such services if necessary by legal action. Certainly, the person who avails himself of 'hospital-facilities' expects that the hospital will attempt to cure him, not that its nurses or other employees will act on their responsibility." Also, "The standards for Hospital Accreditation, the state licensing regulations and the defendant's by-laws demonstrate that the medical profession and other responsible authorities regard it as both desirable and feasible that a hospital assume certain responsibilities for the care of that patient."

the requirements for the granting of staff privileges, and a generally reduced area of discretion in which the professional remains autonomously able to exercise his own judgment. Thus, if subsequent legal rulings should continue in this new trend, this particular area of conflict will warrant close observation for serious friction.

Incentive systems. Many social scientists and organizational theorists have recognized the inherent problems in the imposition of organizational incentives on professional persons. The question of whether economic and hierarchic "raises" constitute motivational forces in the mind of the professional is certainly one worth consideration. It is suggested that the professional is committed to his professional work; thus incentives that are caused in organizational terms are at best ignored and at worse prove dysfunctional to professional loyalty. The professional's frustration is compounded by the fact that there is little organizational recognition of professional excellence in professional terms. Sooner or later, if a professional wishes to advance within an organization, he must give up his professional allegiance and climb aboard the hierarchic ladder.° At present this is the only way up!

Administrative procedures and detail. Although this is somewhat related to the means-ends conflict mentioned earlier in the area of goals, it is an area that is significant enough in its own right to warrant separate comment. In many organizations the most common complaint heard from professionals is that administrative procedures interfere and even obstruct their professional work. Interestingly enough, a common complaint from organizational

---

°For example, a registered nurse who is skilled and enjoys giving bedside care can only be recognized in the hierarchic ladder if she goes into management, usually as a head nurse. The result is the loss of a good bedside nurse and the addition of a supervisor who is not administratively trained.

management is that lack of professional cooperation in administrative matters results in reduced efficiency and increased cost, effort, and time.

Nature of authority. The professional appears to recognize authority only proportionate to demonstrated ability within a certain area of specialty. In his mind, deference is shown to the comptroller not because of his position within the organization but because of his superior knowledge and competence in financial affairs. In contrast, the organization considers authority as an integral part of a hierarchic position in the bureaucratic structure. Thus a boss's decision is followed not because of its intrinsic value or appropriateness to the situation in question but rather because he is the boss and should be obeyed by a subordinate without question. Extending such reasoning, one arrives at this axiomatic circular syllogism:

The boss is boss because he makes wise decisions.
The decision is wise because it was made by the boss.
Therefore, do what the boss tells you to do.

As a result, the conflict lodges between the professional, who is checking every organizational order for its academic validity, and the bureaucrat, who is checking its origin. The differences can be even more clearly seen in those instances when an order is believed to be poor or inappropriate. The professional objects on principle and refuses to obey, whereas the bureaucrat makes what minor alterations he can before acquiescing.

Individual self-actualization. Sociologist Chris Argyris contends that normal individual development within our culture involves growth from infant passivity to adult activity. Organizations have long pursued the course of control of individual behavior in the interest of achieving coordinated, efficient, and united action. By encouraging passive behavior, the organization gives the self-actualization principle little chance to flourish. As a result, the individual may feel frustrated in his desire to express his own unique personality. The organization, however, realizes this and offers sufficient material rewards for behavioral acquiescence to offset the dissatisfaction felt. As long as these rewards exceed the personal injury sustained, the individual complies with the system. Yet the organization pays a high price for such a system, for individual creativity, motivation, and self-development are largely stifled.

Specialization and professionalization. As our technology becomes more and more sophisticated, professions grow, specialization occurs, and new professions are born.* As a result, much intraorganizational conflict and strain is engendered. As an occupational group grows professionally, there tends to be a great deal of infighting that goes on as other professions defend the interest boundaries of their particular functions. As a result, an established professional group may actually block the advancement of a new profession because of fear of job infringement.

Historically, this can be clearly seen in the case of the doctor and the nurse. The doctor has blocked the nurse's professional advancement for years in fear that some of his cherished tasks would be usurped, undermining his total role. He has looked upon her as a handmaiden or personal servant. Although this is not a professional-organizational conflict per se, it is one that greatly adds to general organizational tension and strain and is worthy of note.

Having diagnosed a range of professional-organizational conflict areas, one might define and create a corollary range of *conflict accommodators* through the implementation of certain policy changes and/or structural changes in the management of professional persons. In this way

*The use of the term *professions* here simply indicates an occupational group that is moving along the spectrum of ability.

both the organization and the professional can best achieve their respective goals. These suggestions should not be looked upon as infallible panaceas. Rather one hopes that they will serve to stimulate serious and constructive thinking as to potential mechanisms available in dealing with professional conflict situations.

Suggestions to facilitate professional-organizational adaptation

There appear to be three basic approaches that organizations can take in their dealings with professionals. First, they can resist any and all professional activity within the organization proper, excluding the medical practitioners, who are not actually part of the organization. For example, in those areas in which a certain amount of expertise is needed, the functions can be divided into technical subunits so that no one group can obtain a monopoly over any one function. In this way the issue of having professionals within the working part of the organization can be totally avoided. A criticism of this approach is that it might prove unsatisfactory because of lack of continuity and comprehensiveness of expertise. Second, one might suggest the total envelopment of the organization by one or more professional groups. Conflict between organization and profession is avoided because the professional so dominates the situation that organizational identity no longer exists as a separate entity. Unfortunately it is likely that with specialization intraprofessional cleavages will develop that will contribute toward conflict in the organization once again. The third approach is a compromise between these two. Where professional existence is needed and deemed appropriate, it is strongly supported. Where it is not, it is strongly resisted. Because of the reservations cited in reference to the first and second approaches, it is assumed that the third offers relatively greater potential in alleviating or accommodating the inherent conflict relationship between professionals and the organization.

It is in this frame of reference that the following suggestions to accomplish this end are made. One should note that in no way are these suggestions intended to eliminate all organizational friction, even if this were possible. Instead one hopes that they will provide the boundaries within which an acceptable range of conflict and tension can exist within an organization. The effect these suggested strategies have on the original conflict will determine the type of conflict the organization will subsequently experience. In considering these suggestions, remember that there is no perfect correlation between conflict area and accommodative suggestion, but rather that there is an overlapping, extension effect at work as well in these instances.

Organizational recognition of the conflict problem. Honest confrontation of the existence of conflict by all within the organization is in itself a major step forward. Thompson has stated that organizations have historically ignored the fundamental conflict situation that was ever present in their midst.

[For] to legitimate conflict would be inconsistent with the monocratic nature of hierarchy. . . . Modern organizations, through the formal hierarchy of authority, seek an administrative consensus! Conflict resolution, therefore, must occur informally by surreptitious and somewhat illegal means. Or else it must be repressed, creating a phony atmosphere of good feeling and superficial harmony.°

Yet it is obvious that conflict *must* be legitimized through recognition before any sort of accommodation for it can be developed. This means that management must gain a greater understanding of its origins, its organizational implications, and its potential of positive rechanneling.

°Thompson, V. A.: Hierarchy, specialization and organizational conflict, Admin. Sci. Quart. **5**:521, Mar. 1961.

Organizational recognition of frustrations and motivations of the professional. If professionals are to be a positive part of an organization, there must be value satisfiers for them within the organization. Because organizations have typically skirted the major issues of professional-organizational relations until quite recently, there is a dearth of organizational knowledge as to what motivates the professional and what in turn he perceives as rewards for excellent work. It is clear that only through acquiring such knowledge can organizations hope to attract and hold competent professional personnel. One area of motivation potential is linked to the earlier suggestion that the professional has a need to know *why* and not just *what* and *how*. This reflects the fact that modern organizations are very dynamic and create feelings of insecurity among many of the groups within it, making it important that personal contact be instituted along with explanations of future plans and objectives. If such explanations were consistently made to the professional, there would most likely be at least three beneficial outcomes: (1) feelings of "not being considered," of suspicion, and of resentment would be allayed; (2) the ego needs of the professional would be satisfied; and (3) a potential valuable source of expression will have been solicited. This then might be one professional motivator. The ability of the administrator to perceive others and to limit those factors that are a source of frustration to the professional groups within the organization is critical to his success. False assumptions concerning their motivational needs and points of frustration can be sufficiently disruptive to the total organization as to endanger its very existence.

Encouragement of greater professional involvement and participation in the total organization. Dr. John H. Knowles, general director of Massachusetts General Hospital and author of *The Teaching Hospital*, has stated that the practicing physician is responsible for approximately 79% of all hospital costs. This is based on the fact that the doctor is the decision maker who initiates these expenditures. He decides that a patient should be admitted to the hospital; he decides what operative procedures, tests, or treatments should be performed and what equipment and supportive personnel are needed; and it is he who decides when and if the patient should be discharged from the hospital. Thus the physician alone is the primary factor in determining what services in what quantity, at what quality, and at what cost the patient will receive in coming to the hospital. In this sense he is not only the controller but the comptroller of care. Recognition of this fact has led the President's Commission to Improve the Effectiveness of Hospitals to state as one of its recommendations that the physician be brought more fully into the formal management process of his institution.

A number of organizational studies have also demonstrated the value of bringing the professional into the management field. Where participative professional leadership is allowed within the organization, significantly more positive professional-organizational relations were found.* This is understandable when one thinks of the ego structure of the professional. In this instance he is led into the "inside picture" of the operation of the organization in a meaningful way that satisfies him. In this way his opinions on issues are not only heard but are also seriously considered. It should be noted that with young scientists this method of organizational contact is found to be particularly helpful. Others have proposed similar involvement on the grounds that it will expose the professional

to the goals and some of the business facts of the organization as well as make him realize why certain policies and procedures must be followed. It is intended that communication and a feeling of mutual understanding will result from such a program.

Another strategy that has been propounded as a way to reduce organizational conflict, particularly among professional specialists, is to construct interoccupational project teams whenever feasible. Although this may be an excellent mechanism for developing cross-organizational loyalty ties, its value is qualified by what several studies have pointed out—that low-status groups prefer little contact with professional persons.[2] Therefore, when done with the right groups, the separation of groups may prove as productive in alleviating conflict as does the joining of others. This suggests that any intraorganizational teams that are formulated must come from the ranks of those groups that tend toward professionalization. Since these are most often the most influential groups in the organization anyway, this limitation may not be dysfunctional for organizational purposes.

Dual-control system. Administrators should critically analyze the necessary jobs to be done in their organizations, especially as to who can best perform these jobs. These will be split between those of a nonroutine nature requiring a high degree of judgment to ensure proper fulfillment and those of a more repetitive nature requiring a maximum of efficiency in completion with a minimum need for reflection and judgment. For the nonroutine task the organization desires a quality approach and a correct diagnosis, irrespective of efficiency in terms of supervision or control. To achieve this, expertise and judgment are needed so that autonomy of work situation is allowed. This is the price the organization pays for the right answer. But in those areas where such judgment is not needed because the procedural techniques

---

*See Baumgartel, H. W.: Leadership as a variable in research administration, Admin. Sci. Quart. **2:** 344, Dec. 1957; and Marcson, S.: The scientist in American industry, New York, 1960, Harper & Brothers, pp. 151 and 184.

and appropriate steps are both routine and known, the organization is concerned with efficiency in terms both of time and control. As little expertise or individual judgment is required in this type of job, standard techniques of operation and efficiency controls are instituted through organizational supervision.* With this in mind, the administrator should analyze his specific organization and guarantee professional independence in those working areas where such expertise is required. In contrast, he should consciously and conspicuously refrain from similar support where the tasks constitute no more than repetitive functions. In all of this it is essential that the administrator be cognizant of the basic implications of professionalism on organizational control and loyalty, for only with such knowledge does he differentiate on a sound basis.

The importance of separating *treatment* in organizations has been the subject of much writing. It has been suggested that professional satisfaction is a direct product of the relative control the professional has over his own work. It might be noted here that this same principle applies to the nonprofessional as well; except in this case, studies have shown the circumstances to be reversed to such an extent that restricted autonomy is more conducive to producing feelings of satisfaction than the more autonomous approach.† Under these conditions it seems that a dual or multi-control system best fits the needs of the different groups within a complex organization. One reservation to this suggestion is

the threat of splintering organizational objectives. However, the chances of this happening can be greatly reduced if management retains the sole right, though perhaps in conjunction with professional consultation and guidance, to actually determine what the organizational objectives will be, whereas the professional is granted complete autonomy to pick the means whereby those objectives can best be reached.

Dual-authority system. To the extent that a dual-control system exists, it is natural that a dual-authority system will exist as well. One line of control remains in the traditional superior-subordinate mold, whereas the other develops into a collegial relationship based on education and influence rather than the threat of punishment. In this fashion the hierarchy of authority is counterbalanced by the hierarchy of influence. In the latter, decisions are reached only after proper representation, consultation, discussion, and integration of ideas among the respective colleagues. It is hoped in this way to place the occupational groups in the system that best suits their needs.

Several additional comments have been raised in regard to this system. Litwak[3] has emphasized that, although the existence of these two authority lines may be functional for the organization as a whole, they must continuously be kept separate and distinct (occupationwise) to remain so. Strauss,[4] in contrast, has turned toward F. Taylor's model, maintaining that lines of control can be implemented simultaneously within the same occupational group or even in the case of a single individual. This appears to be based on the theory that man is not a single disciplined type but one capable of having many different kinds of authoritative relationships at the same time. Thompson[5] has pushed both these ideas even further in saying that any formulated authority lines may be broken down and restructured as the occasion demands. Thus when problem solving or

---

*Sometimes limited and harmless autonomy is allowed. For example, a man mopping a floor may have limited autonomy of movement or procedure but may be allowed extensive autonomy of speech and expression at the same time.

†See Abrahamson, M.: The integration of industrial scientists, Admin. Sci. Quart. **9:**211, Sept. 1964; and Litwak, E.: Models of bureaucracy which permit conflict, Amer. J. Nurs. **67:**178, Sept. 1967.

planning is needed, a loose collegial structure is formed; when the time for the implementation of a program comes, the hierarchal structure is turned to. One stimulates creativity; the other, conformity and efficiency. Whichever line is deemed most suitable, it is anticipated that their simultaneous existence will reduce conflict in the organization because the environment will be one equally balanced by the conformity demands of the organization and the autonomy demands of the professions.

Dual-incentive system. To the extent that there are in an organization different occupational groups with different backgrounds, different areas of expertise, and different contribution potentials, it is logical to assume that different incentive systems will exist to stimulate and motivate the totality of the organizational range of human variation. Unfortunately this has not been the case. At the present time organizations have few meaningful incentives for the professional worker. This contributes in large measure to the insecurity that the professional feels within the organization. His position is not only tenuous, but his nonadvancement possibilities in the area of his expertise is organizationally assured. A therapeutic step might be the construction of multiple career lines for professional people. Where previously there was only one ladder of advancement within the organization, the administrative one, which not unsurprisingly was rejected by a majority of the professionals, now there might be several ladders so that greater flexibility and choice could be ensured.

This in itself might help lessen much organizational conflict; a dual system of rewards might be created to lessen it even more. The rewards of the regular organizational employee would remain essentially the same, but a whole new list must be devised for the professional. There has been considerable experimentation in this area

already, particularly by industrial research organizations. One of the rewards might be as follows: instead of granting greater authority in the form of a higher administrative position, greater freedom to engage in his professional specialty could be ensured.

Other professional rewards might include recognition for professional work; the opportunity to do research, to consult, and to teach while being organizationally paid; the allowance of organizationally financed opportunities for further professional development; the provision of more professional help, more work space, and better facilities; the opportunity to see individual ideas carried out; more discretion in the selection of programs in which to work; and assistance in handling the administrative details required by the organization—all of which should add variety, challenge, and a chance for creativity to his work in the organization. In a sense these rewards are centered on those areas in which the professional places the greatest value: autonomy and professional development.

A warning should be made, however, concerning the application of too many rewards, for, as the number of rewards increases, the relative value of each proportionately decreases. Thus a reward system that is overused will soon become functionally impotent. An additional principle is that, as the number of obstacles or barriers overcome in the obtainment of a reward increases, the commitment to that reward increases as well. Though rudimentary in terms of applied psychology, these two principles form the cornerstone of any reward system. And, even in this modern day and age, with a plethora of personnel management guides and manuals, it is significant how many organizations lose the vitality and potential benefit of their reward systems by ignoring just these two principles.

Looking beyond the methodology of reward applications, the institution of a system of specific professional rewards at all augers well for the organization, for it is the first substantial step toward guaranteeing the professional a meaningful role in the organization without threat of being overwhelmed by the total institution. This will provoke multidimensional loyalties on the part of the professional, one of which will be toward creating an atmosphere of respect and understanding between the two, and in fact may be *the* deterministic force in organizational behavior.

Alleviation of administrative procedure load. There seem to be three basic approaches to the reduction in the administrative load for professionals. One might develop the position of scientist-administrator. Such an individual, with a background in both these areas, should be capable of effectively bridging the gap between the professional and the organization, thus taking much of the administrative load off the individual professional under him. There are several complications and disadvantages to this proposal, not the least of which is that such dual-trained individuals are difficult to come by. Another approach might be that each professional or group of professionals have an administrative assistant who does nothing but take care of administrative details. Although this is an appealing idea in many respects, it is likely that such an individual will only be capable of operating as an administrative clerk and nothing more since the remuneration for such a job is not likely to be sufficient to retain a top administrative individual. A third approach is one where the administration's job is fragmented downward as much as possible. This means that most operational decisions are reached at a lower level. Policy decisions, on the other hand, might be submitted to an interoccupational committee that is responsible for all decisions of an organizationwide basis. The problem here is that it can probably be accurately predicted that managers will not tend to com-

mit occupational hara-kiri in such a fashion. A further reservation is that if this delegation of administrative procedures downward is not done very carefully the organization can experience traumatic results. Despite these reservations, it appears that some beneficial results can be obtained by reducing the professional's administrative load, whatever the means.

Careful recruitment. It is possible to attempt to bar entry of those professional individuals who the organization feels would act in a disruptive way within the organization. To the extent that this is done, the organization can establish perimeters to potential organizational conflict. There are, however, certain legal restrictions placed on the organization in this regard. For instance, since Hill-Burton funds and Medicare apply to most private hospitals, the courts are beginning to look upon the private hospital as semipublic. Thus the board may not keep a doctor from treating a patient in the hospital, although actual staff privileges may be denied; and even when they are denied, they must not be done so in a capricious or discriminatory way. Yet certainly within the limits prescribed by law this is a worthwhile mechanism for reducing conflict, particularly of the most consistent and troublesome kind.

In-service education. It is suggested that through a good in-service education program of some sort the professional can be made more aware of the goals and complexities of the organization. Such education will hopefully elicit a more sympathetic and understanding attitude toward the organization. In addition, a good orientation program is helpful in placing the organization and the professional on common ground. A program should not be undertaken on admittance to practice, however, as the professional is primarily interested in getting his own work started. But, after a suitable adjustment period is past, such a program may prove beneficial to both the organization and the professional.

Achievement of self-actualization. One would anticipate that, when dual-control, dual-authority, and dual-incentive systems exist, the opportunity to self-actualize will be greatly enhanced. If self-actualization does occur either individually or in a small work unit, feelings of satisfaction will result, and the tendency to conflict with the organization that provided such an opportunity will be greatly reduced.

• • •

We believe that such approaches, if strategically employed, will tend to create an environment where conflict is approached with objectivity.* We hope that, through selective recruitment, proper in-service education and organization orientation, involvement in all phases of the organization, and the creation of interoccupational teams for specific projects, a professional-organizational relationship can evolve that will cut conflict between the hierarchal structure and the professional. A joint dual-systems approach in the areas of control, authority, and incentives apparently has great potential for encouraging more efficient and effective intraorganizational relationships and for maintaining continuity of effort, both of which are absolute necessities if attainment of organizational goals is to be achieved. To the extent that this occurs, the administrator's function within the organization has been fulfilled, for the administrator's primary job is the establishment of goals and the creation and coordination of appropriate programs to ensure their attainment. Should these

_____
*We recognize that the foregoing suggestions are totally organizationally oriented. Since this is the area with which most of the readers are concerned, this direction has purposely been taken. Note, however, that for even further alleviation or accommodation of conflict the professional must have a corresponding series of suggestions as well.

suggestions contribute toward this end in any way, they will have served a valuable function.

In addition, three approaches to introducing innovative specialists and professionals into the hospital may be considered:

1. Obtain them for the organization by hiring them from consulting firms. In this way the organization obtains the needed expertise without getting them intimately involved in the administrative process.
2. Bring them into the organization as line **executives.**
3. Structure the organization in a manner that is conducive to their judgment and innovation; at the same time this coordinates their activities toward common end objectives.

In either of the first two situations, in the absence of the third, erosion of respect for administration occurs, and the specialists leave the organization as they lose respect for line authority.

The need of the individual to judge and innovate appears to be the basic cause of this problem. The individual in today's professional and innovative training and educational programs is encouraged to be creative. He leaves his studies with a much different ability than did his predecessors, who received how-to-do-it instruction. Having thus been encouraged to innovate in their formative years and having been forced to form a philosophy based on a theoretical framework, they become frustrated on the job in a rigid pyramidal organizational environment where their needs to exercise judgment and innovation are resisted. The practice of shadowing and counting the mistakes of others is not satisfying to their need for exploration and experimentation, and they begin to look to professional associates for support and help in changing their environment. As a result, the professional organization takes this opportunity to promote its own objectives and to give purpose to its reason for existence.

It takes up the case, and the organization becomes split between the professionals' objectives and its own. Such conflict in objectives results in either anarchy or compromise, and the division between the ivory tower and the workshop broadens.

There are two approaches to a solution: (1) to bridge the gap between the ivory tower and the workshop and (2) to rework the organizational structure to allow for the inclusion of professionals and innovators. The first approach is not an attempt to remove the theoretical from education but to allow the practical to participate in the theoretical phase of the student's preparation and, in addition, to allow the theoretician or academician to participate in the practical development of the student. In effect this is a cross-fertilization between university faculty and organizational managers. The second approach, that of organizational structure, involves replacing the hierarchy with an organization that places emphasis on the ability to act rather than the right to decide. The steep chain-of-command type of organization is replaced by a flat type of organization where professionals and innovators are reorganized and respected on the basis of individual ability. This in essence means decentralization and identification of specialty and subspecialty sectors rather than the arbitrary building of an organization on a strict hierarchy.

In summary, the importance of this discussion is related to the posture of the traditional organizational model rather than structuring a model that allows flexibility in dealing with the abilities of people and their environmental needs.

The latter aproach hinges on recognition of individual ability, background, and inclination. If the suggested approach of spectrum of organizational differentiation based on ability is followed, the abilities, needs, and inclinations of the individual members will have been adequately encompassed.

Spectrum of behavior and values

In recognizing the differences in individual ability and in organizing to accommodate these differences, the following propositions have been taken as generally true:

1. Work is a natural human function; under the right conditions most people like to work. People are creative; under their own direction and control they will work toward given objectives.
2. Work and behaviour in the organization are the result of a person's interaction with the environment that he finds there.
3. Interaction with the environment is the result of human motivating factors. Among these motivating factors are needs for involvement and respect. The environment in which organizational members work must be realistic, responsible, and right, both in contribution toward organizational needs and their own personal needs.
4. A person will interact with his environment in the way which he believes will come closest to satisfying his needs.
5. An environment should be established in which people will interact in the manner that they believe will meet their needs and that will contribute efficiently to meeting organizational goals at the same time.

Realistic behavior is that which, in its long-run effect, contributes both to organizational and personal good. People who behave realistically will endure short-run hardships and some failures as long as the long-run perspective is good.

Responsible behavior is that which fulfills personal and organizational needs without preventing others from fulfilling their needs. Responsibility begins at the top of the organization and extends downward so that the organization acts responsibly toward its members, and they in turn act responsibly toward each other and the organization. As responsibility grows, the integrity of the people and groups will grow, and the development of self-discipline results.

Right behavior is contingent upon a basic establishment and demonstration of values and standards in the organization that are acceptable both to the individual members and the organization as a whole. Through evaluating behavior as right or wrong against these values and standards, individuals and organization strive to improve. Without articulated values and standards and recognized efforts to improve ethical neutrality, a sense of normlessness develops that tends to destroy feelings of personal worth and erode organizational structure and function.

In working toward positive development and exercise of realistic, responsible, and right behavior, the organization and its members need to coordinate their singular interest with those that best promote the welfare of all; only in this case will both obtain the best possible fulfillment. The organization cannot compromise, however, to the point where it is no longer legitimately meeting the needs of the society of which it is a part. It is not a complete democracy with complete freedom of dissent, where the major purpose is finding those goals that are popular among the majority of people working there. The goals of the hospital are determined by its purpose in society. Its major purpose is to find an effective way, not necessarily the popular way, of achieving those goals. Democratic means are valuable in determining internal objectives, but the purpose of effectiveness must not be sacrificed for complete democratic popularity.

ADMINISTRATIVE RESPONSIBILITY AND INTERRELATIONSHIPS

It is the responsibility of the administrator and his associates to (1) develop a broad, overall philosophic framework that is a system of values and principles; (2) establish overall, organizational goals that are points of ultimate achievement within the philosophic framework; and (3) delineate organizational objectives that are accepted points of achievement and operation in the never-ending effort to meet goals.

It is the responsibility of the administrator and his associates to work as a team with the assistant administrators and program directors who have special ability in specific areas to interpret organizational philosophy, goals, and objectives in terms of policy.

The application of the spectrum requires an administrative team that has a philosophy and that understands human organization. This team must be willing to innovate and to risk its own organization's future. Survival is a key issue, both individually and organizationally. Administration is the means to that end.

Striving for equilibrium is the objective of administration. This is best pursued by creating an air of freedom where innovation by the individual and the organization can occur and wherein the ability and individualism of the members can be recognized and used to their fullest. There are many differences because of educational, physical, emotional, psychologic, economic, and motivational backgrounds, but the organizational structure and the administrative approach must accommodate them. No one pattern will suffice; the entire spectrum must be considered.

This requires an administrator (or administrative team) who is a leader in every sense of the word. In moving the organization toward its goals, he must deal fairly with many internal and external needs and influences. He must consider the consumer, the unskilled and semiskilled workers, the technical specialists, the innovative specialists, the professionals, the volunteer organizations, the board of trustees, the governmental agencies, and the public media. He must be a man who thinks for himself, who has organization, management, and administration at his fingertips, who accepts the responsibility to function ethically and fairly with every group in turn, and who understands the human need for a leader and the human desire for individuality and can incorporate all within the organization.

There are very few administrators in the sense that they can cope with people and ideas at the same time that they are coping with economics. It is much easier for an administrator to be a specialist in one particular area where the need for his counsel will contribute to his own sense of security. This is the day of specialists, it's true, but not in the manager's chair. The manager must be a specialist only in making things happen through people. What is needed is a philosopher. He must employ expediency toward an objective, but not toward solutions.

Instead of dehumanizing every situation and reserving all authority, authority and responsibility are pushed down to a level where problems originate, are understood, and can be handled. This does not eliminate the need for top management by any means. But the administrator of such a system becomes a coordinator and a catalyst, and not a dictator. He will make the organization tick by using every available bit of talent on every level where it happens to exist.

In the new organization the assistant administrators and directors are specialists in the functional area of operations represented by their respective systems and programs. It is their responsibility to work with department chiefs within their areas of special ability to interpret policy in terms of operational systems and procedures and to ensure that the systems and procedures developed are compatible with those of other areas of specialization. The administrator and his associates should be available to participate in this process when appropriate, but to act as catalysts,

not to become engrossed in the details.

It is the responsibility of department chiefs to work with department members so that particular services can be produced efficiently and effectively. At the grass roots of the organization are the people who work with the problems. They must have a say in innovation, problem solving, and implementation if they are to take an interest in their work and find satisfaction in it. Department chiefs must ensure, however, that their operations and methods of producing services are compatible with other areas that are affected by their operation. The administrator and his associates and the assistants and directors should be available to assist in this process as coordinators when appropriate.

Finding people who are capable and willing to handle prescribed areas of responsibility is one of the administrator's most important and difficult tasks. Once they are placed, it takes still more resolution to give them the freedom to manage their areas and the support they need to see them through their failures, but it is amazing what new life emanates from such a virile organization. Planning becomes a united effort. It is not an organizational booklet published every year or two; it is a natural outgrowth of the aspirations and the needs of many areas with one controlling factor; it must fit within the framework of the philosophy.

Although the philosophy must come from many sources in a complex organization, it must be evolved, articulated, and interpreted through the central administrative core. This takes endless communication and interpretation. Eventually every employee knows where he fits in the scheme of things; he knows how much creativity he can exercise in solving his problems. Those who do not stay within the framework of the philosophy will feel the pressure from the other employees and either get back in line or eliminate themselves. This negates the use of much firing and hiring, a technique that has never accomplished anything very positive, although granted, no organization can survive without at least an occasional use of it.

It is the individual who emerges as the really important component, i.e., the individual and his means and goals. The environment must constantly encourage the betterment of each individual by allowing him to interpret his place within the general framework of the philosophy. Individual satisfaction and personal relationships are paramount. Efficiency is not getting people to mechanically reach a predetermined standard, but rather getting them to use their full potential.

This means interpreting philosophy at all levels. It is futile to tell the yardman that if he does a good job he will improve patient care, for he is too far removed from the patient. Tell him that if he does a good job he will be promoted or given a raise, or that his service will be much appreciated by the visitors, nurses, and doctors. These are things he understands. It also means involving every group in the planning and the objectives, sometimes through the use of committees.

Much controversy has arisen as to the role of committees. There have been those who want committees for purposes of decision making and, at the other extreme, those who want committees for nondecision making. Here again the spectrum comes into play, based on the abilities involved. In a hierarchal situation committees will have a strong appointed chairman who may "sandbag" or use coercion and threats to accomplish the committee's activity. The membership is made of a cross section of the organization and their abilities are not necessarily needed or used.

In highly sophisticated organizations where there is an abundance of special ability, there is less need for a formally developed committee. Experts seek one another out informally and continually seek to find the best solutions to the situations

at hand. The membership is comprised only of those persons whose abilities are required for the occasion. The need determines the composition of the group. The individual members are interdependent, and a leader arises as his ability is indicated and desired.

In effect the committee structure itself adheres to the spectrum. Small issues concerned with simple tasks require a committee membership that differs from that needed to deal with large issues concerned with more specialized talents. The greater the issue or decision to be made, the more the need for nondirected leadership. This leader will arise when the need requires certain ability, and the possession of that specific ability will determine the required leader.

DECISIONS

Following the philosophy of delegating authority and responsibility according to ability and accountability, decisions should be made at the point closest to activity where the following criteria are met:

1. The personnel who are most expert in the matter at hand participate in making the decision
2. The personnel making the decision ascertain that it is compatible with other operations
3. The personnel making the decision ascertain that it is within their scope
4. The personnel making the decision will stand accountable for it

Herbert A. Simon discusses this type of decision making in his book *Administrative Behavior.**

Decisions made in this manner are contingent upon the establishment by the or-

---

*See Simon, H. A.: Administrative behavior, New York, 1961, The Macmillan Co., pp. 79-109. Of interest also are pp. 123-129. Note, however, that the values influencing decisions in Simon's theory seem to arise largely from within the organization; attention should also be given to values reflecting the external organizational and social structure.

ganization of stable and understandable expectations and upon the provision of information about values, assumptions, goals, and attitudes that should enter into and influence the decision. Decision makers must ascertain and be guided by what is a realistic, responsible, and right decision in reference to themselves and the organization. The following discussion establishes the outline within which decisions are made.

This outline is based upon the belief that the process of rendering service should arise from decisions made by the personnel rendering that service whenever possible. Using this philosophy, the outline encompasses the determination of philosophy, goals, and objectives and their implementation and evaluation at the organizational level, systems and programs levels, and personnel level.

The organizational level includes the board of trustees and administration. Although the board of trustees is the ultimate legal authority, the two must work together to form the philosophy, goals, and objectives as a whole and to spell these out in terms of policy. Many health care organizations operate with no clear philosophy, goals, or objectives and with few policies. If they, at their initiating, organizational level, are going to set the framework within which both their formal and informal structure may function compatibly with their legitimate purpose in the community, they must clarify this purpose.

Organizational implementation is the process of mobilizing the policies and procedures, putting them into action, and moving the organization toward its goal. Implementation is facilitated by a strong communications system and by authority as the means by which implementation is molded and directed to ensure that policy, allocation, and coordination decision are consistent with organizational goals. Information about philosophy, goals, and objectives is fed into the communications sys-

tem that relays it through the organization in such a way that systems, programs, and individuals identify with them. By using the communications system in this manner to constantly relay information, knowledge, support, and evaluation throughout the organization, they may determine more detailed goals and objectives. These objectives should be compatible with those of the entire organization while allowing decisions to be made at the appropriate level.

Organizational evaluation is a means of appraising philosophy, goals, and objectives and their implementation and determining how well the purpose of the organization is being effected. Evaluation includes crystallization of evaluative information for consideration of improvement and change; this should occur throughout and should be passed on to the proper recipients.

Systems and programs correspond to areas of activity identified by ranges of authority and accountability, groups of policies and procedures, and methods of implementation and evaluation through which they might conduct one or several specialized functions. They further define organizational philosophy, goals, and objectives along with broad instructions for implementation, applying expertise in establishing system and program goals and objectives. Every effort must be made to impress upon them that they are not independent of the overall operation but rather are fulfilling an internal function within the totality.

Implementation at this level follows much the same process used at the organizational level, with the exception that primary implementation is largely within a system or program, even though their authority may be limited by their own bounds and may be superseded by organizational authority.

Evaluation is most important here. The system and program alone are in the critical position of being able to assess their particular area of operation and interpret that assessment in light of their expertise. Since they cannot relate this evaluation to the overall organization as well as those at the operational level, it is important that they undertake it with an ever present awareness of their position in the organization.

One set of policies and procedures established at this level will relate to the rendering of service by personnel. The survival of the philosophy of decision making previously stated requires that these be sufficiently broad and have enough latitude to allow those who are most expert in the specialized function of service to derive more specific goals and objectives of their own at the personnel level.

REFERENCES

1. Gouldner, A. W.: Organizational analysis. In Merton, R. K., Broom, L., and Cottrell, L. S., editors: Sociology today, New York, 1959, Basic Books, Inc., p. 420.
2. Pelz, D.: Interaction and attitudes between scientists and the auxiliary staff: I—viewpoint of staff, Admin. Sci. Quart. 1:4, Dec. 1959.
3. Litwak, E.: Models of bureaucracy which permit conflict, Amer. J. Nurs. 67:178, Sept. 1967.
4. Strauss, G.: Professionalism and occupational associations, Indust. Relat. 2:26, May 1963.
5. Thompson, V. A.: Bureaucracy and innovation, Admin. Sci. Quart. 10:1, June 1965.

PART THREE
RESOURCES AND APPLICATION

Reorganization involves the creation of systems and programs. Systems form a commonality among diverse parts—they channel resources into programs. Programs are means at the point of service of coordinating resources from systems into care, teaching, and research packages to meet projected ends.

chapter five
SYSTEMS

A horizontal type of organization was established, creating an environment that takes into account the variation of abilities of people working there. In such an organization, decision making takes place at the appropriate decentralized point. Assistant administrators for systems, program directors, and employees make many operational decisions that were previously made by top administration alone. These decisions are based on overall organizational objectives translated into systems, programs, and personnel objectives.

In terms of organization structure one prominent characteristic of the old organization was departmental isolation, a deterent to any synergistic framework. Departments had been identified and operational tasks had been assigned, but there was no commonality among them. This resulted in great departmental discrepancies both in the economy of personnel utilization and efficient/effective performance of tasks. Relationships between units and departments had not been considered; means-ends similarities had not been sought out.

As presented in Figs. 5-1 and 6-1, reorganization involves the arrangement of departments into systems and programs, each of which relates to a common characteristic. The grouping of departments in this manner encourages collective evaluation of resource utilization as input to coordinated programs. This holds the potential of eliminating organizational barriers and evaluating functional possibilities of systems and programs in a synergistic framework. It views the aggregate of health resources and programs as just that—**resources** and **programs.** Like-function centers are created and allocated upon demand by systems, and their resources are coordinated and utilized by programs.

An examination of each of the systems reveals its specific potential for contribution.

PATIENT CARE SYSTEM*

The patient care system is the most human oriented. It is the one system in which the characteristic of delivering services by human beings to human beings will not be obviated by automation in the near future. However, it is expected that significant changes will occur here. In fact, these changes will perhaps have a more far-reaching effect on hospital services than anything going on in any of the other systems. Two of the most important areas of change are the future of nursing as a profession and the utilization of nursing service personnel.

In Chapter 3 the existing patterns of

---

*The patient care system contains the social service and nursing departments.

79

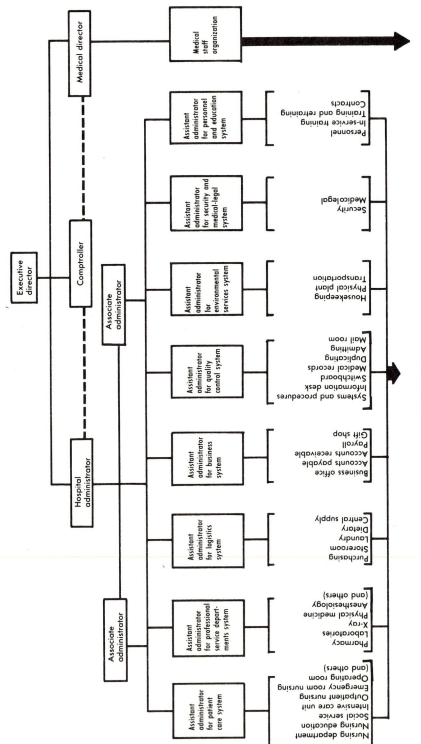

Fig. 5-1. Systems.

coordination at Case Hospital were identified by singling out (1) departments with a heavy dependency on administration, (2) departments that had withdrawn in isolation, (3) departments that depended on other departments for contact with the administration, and (4) departments that had strong contacts with authority from outside the hospital structure. The department of nursing was identified as having isolated itself from the formal administrative pattern.

For many years the department of nursing had provided informal leadership in the solution of many day-to-day operating problems. It was this department that often made decisions that would have been more appropriately made by administration or the departments in which the problem existed. Having grown up in this manner, it was often looked to as the leader in lieu of the administrator.

Faced now with a new organization pattern that had been formulated by the higher levels of administration and presented to assistant administrators and department heads as a new scheme of operation to which they must adjust, nursing reacted by isolating itself from change. As the systems organization gained strength and began to take on meaning in terms of operating policy and procedures, it became more and more apparent that the patient care system, into which the department of nursing had been placed, was a crucial and pivotal point of translating the benefits of the departments in other systems into meaningful service to patients and clients. If this system would not participate in the change, if it would not work as part of the team, if it would not innovate in order to improve its own operations, then it would act as a block to the effectiveness of other systems no matter how well their operations were carried out.

After considerable pressure had been placed upon the department to identify its operating problems and deal with them objectively, a 2-year *plan of change* was offered. This plan of change was outlined along the lines of a human relations approach and was based upon problems such as the following. Personal interrelationships and the relationships between the nursing office personnel and the personnel on the nursing units were so bad that they had to be worked with and changed before any organizational or administrative changes could be undertaken. Indeed it was believed that the nursing office and the nursing units were so much at odds with each other that a planned change in organization, such as assessing responsibilities and creating new programs, would increase feelings of insecurity, isolation, inadequacy, overwork, frustration, and lack of reward to a height that would absolutely prevent success. Personnel were directing much of their time and energy toward "fighting" administration, service departments, physicians, and the organizational structure. Areas of responsibility and authority were poorly understood and needed to be redefined; there was inadequate support for nursing from other departments, physicians, and administrative superiors. The nursing staff was inadequate in both number and quality; personnel orientation and training programs were inadequate; nursing personnel felt that they were not rewarded for their efforts; and the department had operated for many years in a position of isolation from the rest of the hospital. There had developed many intricate systems and interrelationships to "get the job done." The fact that they could get the job done despite the problems previously stated was their main source of security. Therefore any proposal to change the way in which they were presently operating was a threat to their security and survival.

Once these problems had been identified, a 2-year plan of change was proposed that would establish an overall philosophy for the nursing department's activities, i.e., examine the literature; involve hospital administration, public relations, and the personnel department in creating and initiating new programs for recruitment; check to discover how the unit supervisors and head nurses view their positions in the nursing organization and elicit their problems, irritations, and frustrations; discover the same things about each nurse member of the nursing service office; and create a program that will revitalize the total nursing department at each and every level.

Considering the situation out of which this proposal grew, it was an admirable attempt to establish a program of self-renewal, but, as one can see through examination of the outline, its primary cause, hope, and direction were self-centered and did not relate the department and its activities as an integral part of the overall organization. Additionally, the period of time proposed for getting the department to a point where it could begin to experiment with any real changes in programs, administration, or staffing was 2 years. This was far too long in view of the speed with which reorganization was moving in other systems and the pressure that was being placed upon the patient care system for more adequate delivery of service.

Approval by administration of the principles of change proposed by the nursing department and strong encouragement accompanied by pressure from other systems failed to produce evidence that anything more than a facade of change was being generated from the scurry of activity that was taking place. This type of activity could be equated to Parkinson's Law, which states that work will be expanded to fill the time available for its accomplishment.

After the appointment of a new assistant administrator for patient care and some other personnel changes, administration moved to generate definitive changes in nursing programs, staffing patterns, and personnel utilization. These changes were to be made despite previous years of

causing frustration and discontent among nursing personnel. After considered deliberation, administration and the assistant administrator for patient care concluded that many of the problems outlined were caused by a feeling of isolation from the rest of the hospital organization and to a realization that, although present operations were inadequate, nothing was being done about it. That these were the valid problems rather than a fear of changing the old way was later fully borne out.

Changes undertaken so far find their genesis in the following statement by the new assitant administrator for patient care:

Since my arrival at Case Hospital, I have been greatly concerned over the state and progressive direction of nursing. I have observed, as you have as well, that the existing pattern of delivering nursing care services no longer adequately meets the needs of our patients. If this observation be apt, I feel an analysis of our activity, development, and future direction is imperative. To be meaningful in terms of stimulating "progress" in nursing, such an analysis must be accompanied by a readiness to adopt new ways and means of doing things where so indicated.

As an additional step, I would suggest that a written philosophy be formulated for the department. A portion of this should be devoted to a definition and priority categorization of departmental objectives. A further step would involve determining set standards of care with suggested methods of implementation. Such standards would include an outline of safe and therapeutically effective techniques of nursing care.

In developing both of these (the analysis of nursing and the departmental philosophy), the role of the director of nursing service is obviously crucial, for it is this one person who more than any other must accept this challenge if any movement forward is to take place.

With this introduction, I would like to take the opportunity at this time to state my evaluation of the department and its needs. These fall into three basic areas: the definition of nursing office responsibilities, the clarification of various programs overlapping or cutting across the department, and the analysis of specific functional procedures presently followed by the department.

DEFINITION OF NURSING OFFICE RESPONSIBILITIES

Director of nursing service. Major responsibilities include planning, organizing, directing, coordinating, and evaluating the activities of the nursing department. Strong emphasis should be given to developing an environment within the department that encourages creativity, stimulates the development of new knowledge, techniques, and systems of nursing care, demands full utilization of personnel skills and motivates those individual abilities on which quality service depends.

Assistant directors of nursing service. The focus of these jobs surrounds the functions of coordinating and supervising all nursing activities. More specifically, this would include in-service educational participation and counseling of the respective head nurse, the initiating of such shifts in staff as are necessary because of inhouse patient composition, and the formulation and initiation of specific nursing projects. One possible area for significant contribution would be the establishment of one or more graduate nurse seminars in which various subjects could be presented or discussed under their leadership. It is anticipated that competent pursuit of these functions entails a reduction in those tasks presently carried on that are clerical in nature.

Assistant director of nursing service for non-professional employees. This job carries the total responsibility for the recruitment (through personnel), training, staffing, and even discharging of all nonprofessional employees. The position must have full authority to handle all affairs in this area. An opportunity to meet with the aides and orderlies at regular intervals for both information and discussion of procedures and problems must be developed if this position is to become an active force in nursing administration.

Assistant director of nursing service for the student-exchange program. Although it is the intent of this program to be service focused, it should be emphasized that the service experience presented to each student should be such that she will gain new knowledge and develop new or improved nursing skills as a result. At no point should the student be used to plug holes in straight service because of an inability within the nursing department to provide graduate nurse service coverage. The assistant director will be totally responsible for administration of this group, including student scheduling and assignments.

CLARIFICATION OF VARIOUS PROGRAMS

School of nursing program. Up to the present time we have assigned nursing students according to *our* service needs rather than to *their* educational benefit. Naturally this practice has frequently resulted in educational deficiencies. Correction of this problem will occur only if the faculty assigns and schedules service experience

to the students. Nursing service personnel must be made to realize that the student is *not* to be exploited for service benefit but is on the floor purely for educational purposes and is expected to get the widest possible exposure to patient care. In this sense, what was previously the apprentice's workshop becomes the student's laboratory.

With the anticipated change in the nursing educational program from a 3-year diploma to 2-year and 4-year degree programs, additional complications will arise. Only if nursing service and nursing education leaders plan jointly for this transition will there be a smooth exchange of responsibilities for the students in the classes involved.

Nursing recruitment program. The recent study of staffing patterns by each department clearly showed the extent of a nursing personnel shortage at this hospital.

This shortage unquestionably restricts flexibility, maneuverability, and quality of nursing service at this time. Therefore all efforts must be spent in attempting to attract and recruit more professional and licensed practical nurses. We must ask ourselves why Case Hospital has been unable to attract more graduate nurses and licensed practical nurses thus far. Salary is a factor, but is not always a determining one. Job satisfaction is usually a more important need with these people. It is my belief that nurses seek employment where there is latitude for independent thinking, where there is an atmosphere both challenging and receptive to innovation, and where there is creative leadership in administration. In this sense, I feel we must redouble our present efforts to create such an environment.

Program for better utilization of personnel. One of the contributing factors to our present nursing shortage in our poor utilization of available personnel. Why can't some of the less demanding, less skilled tasks now performed by graduate nurses be assigned to less skilled personnel? A utilization study would help to clarify the present use of our personnel and might even give us a rough index of the quality of our service. With this knowledge we would be in a better position to decide between alternative steps toward upgrading the level and performance of our nursing service.

In similar fashion, I feel it is mandatory that the head nurse be released from nonnursing functions so that she can devote her time and energy to supervising her staff and unit. This release will occur when someone else can demonstrate that he can adequately take over these functions. One of the real gaps is a lack of substantial preparation for or experience in supervision on the part of the head nurses. This is a skill that, with exposure and practice, one can learn. Recognizing this need, a plan is being developed for a 3-day workshop in supervision for all head nurses.

To release the head nurses from their nonnursing responsibilities, it is eventually intended that a unit-manager system be introduced in all patient units. It will be this individual's responsibility to supervise all "hospital care duties," i.e., those nonnursing supportive services that are connected to the overall maintenance of the unit.

Orientation program for new employees. A well-planned orientation program for all new employees is an essential part of any nursing service. A new employee has a right to expect a thorough orientation to the department and its philosophy, its personnel, its procedures, and its standards. Case Hospital has never had such a program. It is the responsibility of nursing service to help structure such a program and see that what is not part of a centralized presentation be covered decentrally by each nursing unit to which a new employee is assigned.

Job description program. Job descriptions are almost totally completed. They still need to be reviewed and discussed with each category of nursing personnel so that all are aware of their job responsibilities. Once completed, these descriptions should be used for reference on the nursing floors.

Team nursing program. I am eager for us to begin developing a plan for instituting the team nursing concept into nursing service. Team nursing is a means of providing more comprehensive nursing care to all patients. It will provide the head nurse with a method of delegating responsibility to nursing personnel within her unit. Initial responsibility for planning this should be assumed by someone in the nursing office.

Committee participation program. Nursing representation on almost all committees is provided by nursing office personnel. It is my feeling that, while some of this is necessary and valuable, some of it could easily be covered by head nurses. Although it is important to have someone that is knowledgeable of the total nursing situation on a few of the committees, most of the committees do not demand such breadth of knowledge and would gain valuable assistance by hearing from a person who is functioning on the operational level. It is also clear that head nurses would then be more of an integral part of the planning and operation of the hospital. In addition, such exposure would help them to develop their leadership potential as well as allow them to have greater exposure to other disciplines and people

in the hospital, thus expanding their views and orientation. It is my hope that this involvement, the appointment of some head nurses to serve on some of the various committees, be instituted as soon as possible by the director of nurses. A mechanism for reporting back to nursing as to the developments in these committees is provided for in the head nurses' meeting.

ANALYSIS OF SPECIFIC FUNCTIONAL PROCEDURES

Transcribing orders. First, the existing method of transcribing orders from patient records must be carefully reviewed by service and educational personnel with the expressed intent of developing a better, more efficient procedural method that includes individual nursing care plans and excludes all unnecessary repetitive transcriptional steps.

Second, the specific purpose for having unit clerks is to relieve nurses of clerical duties. Unless all clerical activities are assigned to the unit clerk, including the transcribing of orders, the head nurse will continue to spend time on desk work rather than on supervising her personnel.

A training program for teaching unit clerks how to transcribe patient orders must be implemented and delegated to one person who will assume responsibility for their training.

Change will have to occur also in that area of social work associated with the poor. With more and more of the low-income groups' being covered by cost contracts, the job of social work will change from one of taking long histories of patients, placing poor people in charitable facilities, and providing them with funds to buy drugs, glasses, and other needed medical supplies to one of being the link between the health care team and the community.

The role of the social worker in the past has often been that of a shipping clerk trying to remove from the paying hospital the burden of the economically unstable poor to some other segment of society. The social worker will more and more work under the direction of the captain or the quarterback of the health care team and take her instruction as part of a master plan determined by the total team.

PROFESSIONAL SERVICE DEPARTMENTS SYSTEM*

The trichotomy of professional, semiprofessional, and administrative activities that occur in departments such as radiology and laboratories makes this system one of the most challenging to coordinate. The primary objective is to coordinate the administrative and supportive responsibilities of the other systems with the professional practice in these locations to the end of creating organizational unity and comprehensive service.

In many situations, particularly university teaching settings, well-coordinated administrative relationships and communications in these areas have been extremely difficult to establish, the end result being fragmentation, isolation, and waste. It is the responsibility of the assistant administrator to coordinate these activities and relate them effectively (budgetarily and administratively, within a framework of quality) to the entire organization. As a member of the administrative team, the assistant becomes the pivot point around which these areas may interact effectively with other areas of service and operation.

LOGISTICS SYSTEM

The objective of the logistics system is to weave the departments of purchasing, transportation, storeroom, laundry, dietary, and central supply into a common logistical base within the complex in which supplies and equipment are procured, stored, processed, transported, and delivered. Considerable sharing and dovetailing of resources and manpower may be accomplished among these departments when they are coordinated toward the end of a unified logistical system.

---

*The professional service departments system includes pharmacy, radiology, physical medicine and rehabilitation, inhalation therapy and pulmonary function, anesthesiology, electroencephalography, electrocardiology, cardiology, all laboratories, and various other specialized work areas.

Central to the logistical process is a common, mechanized delivery system that can be controlled and programmed to make automatic pickups and deliveries. Such a system can be supported by centralized bulk storage and predetermined points of use or substorage. Thus transportation and delivery becomes a service shared by all departments to provide physical delivery of their items of service when and where necessary. This type of logistical system lends itself to many computer applications.*

There is appearing on the hospital scene from various manufacturing sources a piece of equipment that forms a mechanized network for the transportation of supplies, pieces of equipment, and possibly even human beings throughout a health care

---

*Take, for instance, the supply of 8 × 14–inch sterile, gauze bandages to a 30-bed medical-surgical nursing unit. Twenty-four hours in advance the number of patient discharges and admissions and the ratio of surgical to nonsurgical cases on the unit can be predicted with reasonable accuracy. This information is fed into a computer that has a programmed correlation between the ratio and percentage of occupancy and can indicate the supply of bandages that must be added to the existing stock on the unit in order to fulfill the next day's needs. Having determined the resupply required, the computer adjusts its record of supplies on hand in the nursing unit, directs the storeroom to deliver the needed quantity of bandages to the unit, charges the supply to the appropriate expense account, depletes the perpetual storeroom inventory file, and creates a purchase record for storeroom resupply. At the next predetermined delivery time, the bandages are sent to the nursing unit for storage and use. When the actual ratio and percent of occupancy for the unit is known, the computer is informed and adjusts its record of supply on hand in the unit accordingly. At this point it is ready to repeat the cycle. Since the computer program is based on average use, it should adjust to reflect significant changes in use-ratio-occupancy correlations. It may be programmed to make such changes automatically from time to time, or it may be changed manually. The resupply might be calculated and delivered biweekly or weekly, and the degree of statistical and automated sophistication may vary according to need and hardware availability.

complex. Successful installations have been made at Loyola Hospital, Maywood, Illinois, and McMaster University Teaching Hospital in Ontario.

This system is primarily made up of an overhead rail type of conveyor or is programmed to run on casters that are directed by a magnetic tapelike substance on the floor. It can handle the movement of a variety of items, from the smallest needle to bulk food to ultrasonic ovens, with which food can be prepared at the patient's bedside. The logistics system can use this equipment and schedule delivery of various items of supply and equipment to requesting floors, both vertically and horizontally, from a central warehouse area.

The positive factors, of course, are in its labor-saving potential and its availability both day and night, 7 days a week, for service. The drawbacks are basically threefold: noise, cost, and space requirements. As far as noise is concerned, the equipment would have to be programmed to operate during waking hours of patients and in times of low personnel and patient traffic. Concerning the cost involved, it is estimated from one source that its installation is about 6% of building costs. Space requirements on the overhead system are quite large where corners are involved. The space required for the storage of the containers for transporting the supplies also constitutes a problem.

Basically the system is comprised of three elements: (1) a network for picking up, transporting, and delivering equipment and supplies; (2) a container for transporting the supplies; and (3) either a track (overhead or ground-level) or a magnetic tape fastened to the surface of the floors for horizontal movement and within elevators for vertical movement.

This system provides a means of combining requests and demands of various areas and of sending, in toto, their requirements on a scheduled demand basis. It is conceivable that a network encompassing many buildings within an organizational complex could be devised. Once installed, maintenance for continued operation becomes mandatory since existing pools of employees needed to transport carts with supplies and equipment hopefully would be eliminated. Major breakdown of a logistics system would create quite a crisis. However, this form of mechanization, although costly at the time of its original installation, can theoretically effect great savings in personnel costs.

One of the problems of hospitals is the turnover in personnel employed in logistical types of job classifications. From the standpoint of the individual, the retraining of these "pushers and pullers" would be a step toward betterment of the individual and a shift in emphasis from the strong-backed, weak-minded employee to an employee who has a respectable place in society with reliance on the human mind.

Mechanization in hospitals, along with its more sophisticated form of automation, can definitely be accomplished away from the patient's bedside. However, when we consider using this mechanism as a form of substituting the personal touch with the sophisticated machine, we had better seriously consider the effects of the decision on the humanization of the health care industry.

BUSINESS AND FINANCE SYSTEM*

The business and finance system includes the responsibility for creating financial management information and for managing the activities of all business operations. Beyond this, it reworks the accounting and budgetary mechanisms so that budget programs, performance budgets, cost accounting, and performance classifications become integrated. In the latter area it works

---

*This area includes departmental offices, inpatient and outpatient business offices, payroll department, accounts payable, and various other programs as assigned.

closely with the quality control system in developing statistical correlations between performance classifications, measures of productivity, and costs. This assistant is always available to systems, programs, and departments to give consultation on business and financially related matters.

The role of the accountant, or comptroller, in the past has been twofold: (1) to accumulate the facts relating to fiscal affairs and (2) to recommend the decisions based on these financial facts. With the broadening interests of health care and the financing of care based on costs, there arises a need for an economist decision maker instead of an accountant decision maker. The accountant's role will be confined to presenting facts to the economist, who will incorporate them with effects of social and economic values in the decision-making processes. Accountability for funds and proper bookkeeping is the accountant's area of expertise, but organizational decision making takes more training and experience in economic and social terms than the accountant has received.

Many accountants are still used both in a fact-finding role and as an interpreter of future fiscal planning. Many are fully aware of the effects of legislation directing payment for cost alone. As a result, income continues to be based on setting charges on a percentage of a population who could be overcharged, and the impact of cost controls is overlooked. The result is over-financing of programs. In this situation the comptroller, with his accounting background, believes that the only way to provide solvency is to cut costs and restrict expenditures. This not only affects the morale growth of individual employees but creates a lag in program development, making large capital outlays imperative at some time in the future. Another consequence of this practice is one of restricting income by cutting the wrong costs since a majority of patients are covered by contracts carrying cost reimbursement.

An economist who is provided with facts can choose alternative courses of action and make decisions that will give long-range economic stability. The economist must replace the accountant in decision making and become a social and economic planner who is cognizant of social needs and has an awareness of potential funds from varied sources. This means that the role of the accountant or comptroller will be restricted to identifying proper accounting techniques that will allow the financial facts to be presented in an understandable fashion, and his role will include internal and external auditing coupled with better internal controls. The economist will be the real fiscal policy maker, and because of his special background and training he can match expenses with proper sources of income in order that accountability at all levels will be assured.

QUALITY CONTROL SYSTEM*

The quality control system is a new approach intended to make available reliable information in usable format. It provides a setting in which proved and experimental methods of productivity and quality measurements, administrative research and information flow, and storage and retrieval can be combined with operations and made generally available to all who need them.

The system is concerned with three major functions:

1. Coordination of ongoing operations of the departments that are grouped in the system
2. Provision of information and communications in the hospital under the concept of the case information system

---

*Composing this system are the hospital departments of systems and procedures, information desk, mail room, switchboard, medical records, duplicating, and admitting. All are related to the common denominator of information flow and documentation.

3. Establishment of expectations and indicators of productivity and quality

The assistant provides consultation to the entire organization on establishing good information flow and documentation and on establishing expectations and measurements of productivity and quality. He should not attempt to dictate to any department what their expectations should be. The necessity for developing and measuring expectations of quality of service is part of the organization's philosophy and must be done by each department.

Establishing expectations and indicators of productivity and quality begins with administration itself. Broad goals must be spelled out along with the general mechanisms that are acceptable in attaining them. It follows that when goals have been specified all systems and programs should strive toward them. All personnel, departments, systems, and programs must be given sufficient knowledge, support, and evaluation by administration so that they can develop detailed goals at their operational level. Some of these goals will be individually oriented and others will be group oriented; all should be legitimate in their relationship to the major organizational goals.

The entire responsibility for the development of information flow does not lie with the assistant administrator for quality control alone. His primary consideration is within the realm of current ongoing operations and the connection of these to a larger information project, which is discussed in Chapter 7.

During this period of change the role of the record librarian is expanding in scope and importance. She is becoming not only the guardian of the medical records but a collector of information, for the records contain the vital information that reflects the quantity and quality of the care. Any change for the purpose of improving that care will be based on statistics, many of which are contained in the medical rec-

ord. This could be the number of patient visits, the number of "occasions of service," the space required, or the number of people involved.

There is an increasing number of outside agencies who are interested in this information. State and regional planning groups are interested in an increase in the volume of visits. Certain state and city agencies compile their own statistics in the form of mortality and morbidity tables. When any government agency is involved in the financing, statistics are vital. Every program in education is interested in a breakdown of the volume of patients. Medical schools must assign students where the volume makes it profitable to the student. Their applications for research grants require information that is statistical and accurate, especially when government grants are involved.

The Joint Commission on Accreditation of Hospitals attaches great importance to medical records. In 1967 it announced the standards for accreditation of extended care facilities, nursing care facilities, and resident care facilities. Once again, medical records are given prominent attention. Complete medical records are required for extended care and nursing care facilities. This includes nursing notes and a social service summary. Resident care facilities must have a rudimentary chart with an identification sheet, a medical summary, and a history. A yearly reevaluation is required; this includes laboratory reports, x-ray reports, and a social service summary. These records require at least part-time supervision by a qualified record librarian. It could raise cost, but, since it is also likely to raise quality, it is a step forward.

Perhaps the most important function, when all is said and done, is keeping track of the charts. This takes constant vigilance. Well-meaning physicians often take them to their offices to work on them and then forget to return them. A tactful clinic coordinator knows how to get the work on them finished and still know where they are. Laboratories can also mislay reports of tests, and unless the physician sees the results of the tests it is a waste of time to have them done.

Transporting of records is another problem. When 700 records are used in one day and there are records from the previous day in a state of semicompletion, this is a heavy, bulky stack of papers. Pneumatic tubes have been in use for some time, but they have certain shortcomings. Because these tubes are a maximum of 8 inches in diameter, an active chart may be too large to be transported by this system and thus will need to be carried by a messenger. It is a slow process also when many charts are needed.

The system of the future may not require the charts to be moved at all. An electronic system will automatically transport the chart to a television camera. Operated by remote control from the physician's office, the system will select the correct page and the camera will convey the picture to the television screen in the doctor's office. It will be possible to make entries by marking on a video matrix with an electronic pencil. Hard copies can be made automatically by pressing a button. A duplicator will process the hard record.

There are some legal implications that are holding back the development of this type of system. Records have always been treated as highly confidential matter. It will be so easy to view or obtain a copy of a record that its confidential nature may be negated. One systems consultant has overcome this by coding and keying the card, which is carried by the physician, that gives access to this information. It may also be more difficult to obtain signatures with this type of system. It is very likely that these objectives will be overcome. New buildings under construction are being wired for this purpose. The convenience will be the reason for its eventual acceptance. The problem of lost and mislaid records is a nagging one which consumes much valuable time. It sometimes takes a tremendous effort to locate them.

Records are kept current usually for 5 years before they are stored in an inactive file. State laws require that they be kept on an average of 7 years, either microfilmed or hard. Children's records are kept until a child reaches legal age. Microfilming reduces the amount of space that old records require, but they must be expertly stored so that retrieval is possible. There should also be microfilm viewing equipment in each clinic for the convenience of the physician.

The charts are important not only to the immediate medical facility but to outside agencies as well for health statistics, for litigation proceedings in criminal and civil suits, for justification of payment, and occasionally for use by the Internal Revenue Service for checking the volume of income reported by a physician. Because of the many demands made upon the medical records department, in the future the medical record librarian will need longer periods of education and training. At least a 4-year college degree with a good background in liberal arts and biologic sciences is usually required. The ambitious individual may acquire a 2-year master's degree in systems and communications, followed by a management training program.

This will not eliminate the need for medical record technicians. There will be several levels of responsibility within the department, and those persons with advanced degrees will assume a role in management. This need has been emphasized by the work done in quality control, communications network development, and systems analysis.

There are government funds available for training record librarians. At present, there are 33 schools offering programs in this area, and some schools grant a bachelor of science degree. The American Medical

Record Association offers a training course. If the results of a test are satisfactory after the course is completed, the student becomes a registered medical record technician. There are several degrees of training within the field in an effort to enlist much-needed manpower. Institutions interested in training and up-dating their record employees can obtain short-term traineeship grants.

The record librarian is the logical person for quality-control activities since she is the guardian of statistics. Indices must be defined if quality is to be defined and measured. An excellent example of this occurs in nursing, where medication errors can be very upsetting. When the number of medication errors that are allowable has been set for a nursing unit, the quality-control area sets up the device for recording the number of errors. If a correlation can be set up between the number of nursing hours and the number of medication errors, changes can be made in the procedure to see whether the variation of some ingredient might reduce the number of errors. For instance, one such study revealed that after a certain point more nursing hours usually produced more medication errors. There may be some point where the number of nursing hours in relation ot the number of patients is optimal, but this needs to be discovered, if indeed it does exist.

This procedure could be applied to other problems also. What is the optimal number of occasions of service for an outpatient visit? In one study concerned with the quality of care rendered by the physician, certain indices defined by the Joint Commission on Accreditation of Hospitals, e.g., autopsy percentage, quality of medical records, and the number of unjust tissues, were correlated with the consultation rate, the length of stay of the patient, and the death rate. Only a rough profile of quality was discerned in this study, but it opened the way for many other similar studies. Studies of this nature will ultimately influence the way in which outpatient care is delivered.

Management looks for alternative courses of action when it is necessary to make a decision, but it must have enough information to know in advance what will happen if one course or another is followed. This means that information must be classified and stored so that it can be retrieved and distributed as it is needed. As one of the focal points for gathering information, the medical records department becomes a crucial link in the comunications network. This information must be distributed as needed, it must go to the right people, and it must be accurate. This is an absolutely essential operation if resources are to be used to their maximum.

Medical record librarians figure heavily in the systems approach to hospital management since quality control is one very important system. Quality control covers medical records, admitting, information desk, switchboards, duplicating, systems, and procedures. It must eventually include the use of a computer in the light of a total information system. This system is responsible for developing indices of productivity and quality, storage and retrieval systems, and distribution. It is involved with video matrix, microfilm, and magnetic tape.

Indices and methods of collecting information will eventually be extended beyond the patient care aspect into teaching and research and then beyond the hospital into programs of service. It will involve recruitment, training, and continuing education of the professionals and extend into home care, community mental health, and neighborhood health centers.

Technical programs do not teach management. This requires study and experience, as does any other discipline. But there are still plenty of technical problems to be confronted, some of them old and familiar, such as getting charts to the outpatient areas on time. Medical record librarians now have a choice: they can limit their activities to those day-to-day technical problems, or they can obtain the education and training that leads them into management and deal with those problems that are changing the quality of packaging and delivery of tomorrow's health care.

SECURITY AND MEDICOLEGAL SYSTEM

The security and medicolegal system concerns itself with the security of the entire physical complex and the medicolegal problems of the institution. The prime purpose is the security and protection of patients, employees, and property. Security personnel must be carefully selected, trained, and oriented to the problems of a large complex. Their responsibilities are for safety, prevention, detection, and investigation. Integrity, tactfulness, and firmness are indispensable characteristics for these employees.

The security system is designed for central control of all situations requiring its services. A control station is strategically placed in the area of greatest need, manned for 24-hour coverage, and equipped with centrally supervised indicators of fire and burglary. The system is broad in coverage and has access to the personnel and plant of all systems. It must be involved in the screening of new employees.

In addition, all matters with medicolegal implications are handled in this system. The assistant administrator acts as the primary contact with legal advisors and insurance agents.

ENVIRONMENTAL SERVICES SYSTEM

The environmental services system includes the housekeeping and physical plant departments. Since the housekeeping department employs large numbers of unskilled and semiskilled individuals, it is fertile ground for training and educational programs. Mechanisms for upgrading and rewarding employees for a job well done will provide strong motivation. The goal of the housekeeping department is to create the cleanest, brightest, most aseptic environment possible.

The direction of a physical plant in a dynamic, changing facility is both maintenance and construction oriented. The care and operation of existing buildings is important, but it is perhaps not so critical a management problem as the construction phase because expenses related to maintenance are more readily within the means of the institution.

Demands of a constantly changing plant require leadership with construction expertise as well as maintenance. Critical money decisions involve design, planning, budgeting, contracting, subcontracting, and buying. To do this properly requires the use of business methods of the construction industry. Since people with this type of ability may not be attracted to full-time institutional work, a consulting service that specializes in such work may be retained to organize the physical plant, to establish policy, to advise, and to supply leadership as required. This consultant would organize the department, emphasizing the difference between maintenance and construction work. After this, expert direction of the operation is still required but may be carried out by capable staff members. However, the expert should continue to be available on a consulting basis.

It is anticipated that the information system will include programming of manpower needs, housekeeping schedules, and preventive maintenance.

PERSONNEL AND EDUCATION SYSTEM

Today personnel administration, education, and training are in the spotlight in the health care industry. This is borne out in the Health, Education, and Welfare report by Secretary Gardner to President Johnson in 1967, in which he confirmed that rising hospital charges can be attributed largely to rising wages and an increase in the cost of hospital supplies. One of the areas of hope for the moderation of these increasing costs is a greater supply and better utilization of health manpower. The personnel and education system can contribute immensely toward this area of hope by improving all aspects of employment.

This system should expand the total training effort to facilitate adjustment of employees to the organization and the job and to provide opportunity for development, growth, and promotion. Efforts must include new approaches to training, such as programmed instruction. Training classes may also be established in conjunction with the Bureau of Vocational Rehabilitation, Manpower Development and Training Act, and other federal, state, and local programs. Other programs such as supervisory training must be developed with assistance from this system. Its role is also to administer existing benefit programs, to research new benefits, and to constantly keep abreast of changing benefit practices among hospitals in the region and of changing needs of the work force so that appropriate changes in the current program can be realistically recommended.

Job breakdown is a must before human resources can be inventoried. This does not require definitive job descriptions since responsibilities vary with individual ability. Only those requirements needed to accomplish the general task need to be listed. The psychologic requirements as well as the physical and skill requirements should be identified. In addition, personnel interviewers must be aware of program requirements for manpower today and also of new program requirements and their personnel demands. The job being filled today will no doubt be obsolete in the future. With the increased knowledge and technologic advances, the backbreaking labor jobs in health institutions are decreasing and are being replaced by tasks that require people with higher educational levels and more sophisticated technical abilities. The housekeeping worker is being replaced with machines, and even the laboratory technician's work is becoming automated. Nurses will do less paperwork and will carry on more human relation activities.

Much of the system's effort is spent in counseling and coaching supervisors and others who have a particular problem that requires discussion. It is important to realize that the aim is to help find the solution through exploration of possibilities rather than to effect the solution or to insist upon a certain course of action. In this way supervisors can be developed and their growth promoted.

If personnel needs are to be met and individual talents are to be improved, a career development program must be developed. This program will inventory the skills and education of each employee and will also define the employee's potential. This potential will not be for the present employment alone but also for future job opportunities. A blueprint including this information will be maintained on each employee. Training and education will be afforded the employee in an orderly fashion in order that his full potential can be realized. When this information is cataloged, the personnel system can rapidly adapt training programs to the employee's need and select personnel for advancement. With technologic advances coming at the rate that they are, many present jobs will be changed and new requirements will demand different personnel skills.

The development of a career program will cause employees to have a sense of permanency and a feeling of ownership in the institution. With this personalized interest, each employee will feel that management is interested in his welfare. In addition, definite salary scales and job breakdown will allow for a planned program of the employee's educational and economic growth. True loyalty will be increased, and job turnover will be reduced. The addition of planned training and education will then become an investment in the individual's growth and worth to the organization and less of a punishment and reward type of system.

With this type of personnel and educational program, a profit-sharing incentive plan becomes both a necessity and a meaningful experience. In addition, job standards and productivity measures are used for true indices of productivity. By this measuring system of productivity, personnel and training directors can determine objectively the training requirements for the individual employees to determine what specific type of training and experience is needed to allow the employee to do his job better.

With this built-in, long-range planning, employers will be less resistant to spending resources on meaningful training and education. The employee will develop a sense of well-being in regard to his feeling that management cares and that his employer is really interested in the employee's worth to himself and in turn to the organization. The inventory system will allow for meeting current job classifications and will allow for identification of personnel able to be utilized for new job demands. The practice of bringing in outsiders with some charismatic ability will decrease since a built-in supply of experts will be available. Emphasis will be on developing individuals within the organization rather than seeking so-called "outside experts." The practice of employing consultants on a short contract basis will become more acceptable. Career planning will help to formalize training programs and to identify those employees who need further training and work experience. This type of indexing of employee talents will help assure that the best person, based on ability, is doing the right job. Promotion from within then becomes a reality. The work situation will become more meaningful to both the employee and the individual employer.

MEDICAL STAFF SYSTEM

To fully develop the concept of total resource allocation through systems, physician's services must be included. The medical staff system is the means of channeling physician's services into programs.

The medical staff system becomes the basis for organizing physicians' activities around research, teaching, and clinical service. The underlying motivation of each is to provide the best possible service to the consumer, with the patient as the ultimate beneficiary.

Within the framework of decentralized responsibility established for systems and programs, peer self-government is undertaken through formal bylaws, rules, and regulations that extend the overall organizational philosophy to the functions of the medical staff.

Traditional organization of the medical staff has resulted in a dual-power health organization structure: administrative power and medical staff power. Conflict has been inescapable and unobjective, as both parties have sought monistic control. A more viable approach is to view the organization in its entirety, with the system of physicians' resources feeding into programs. In the past, medical and administrative functions have been only loosely tied together by informal agreements and by standing formal offices and committees often created solely for the purpose of licensing requirements. In place of this, an arena of collaborative action must be created in which all resources are placed into perspective with organizational goals. This arena is the total organization that is conducive to collaboration, with concentration of effort in the joint conference committee, the executive committee, and the operational advisory committee.

The following statement by the American Hospital Association provides the basic orientation of the joint conference committee:

A. Composition: The joint conference committee shall be a standing committee composed of . . . members of the medical staff and the governing body. The chief executive officer shall be an *ex officio* member without voting privileges. The representatives from the medical staff shall include the president elect, president, and immediate past president. The chairmanship shall be alternated between the governing body and medical staff every two years.

B. Duties: The joint conference committee shall conduct itself as a forum for the discussion of matters of hospital policy and practice, especially those pertaining to efficient and effective patient care, and shall provide medicoadministrative liaison with the governing body and the chief executive officer. It shall have the following specific duties:

1. Accreditation: It shall be responsible for acquisition and maintenance of JCAH ac-

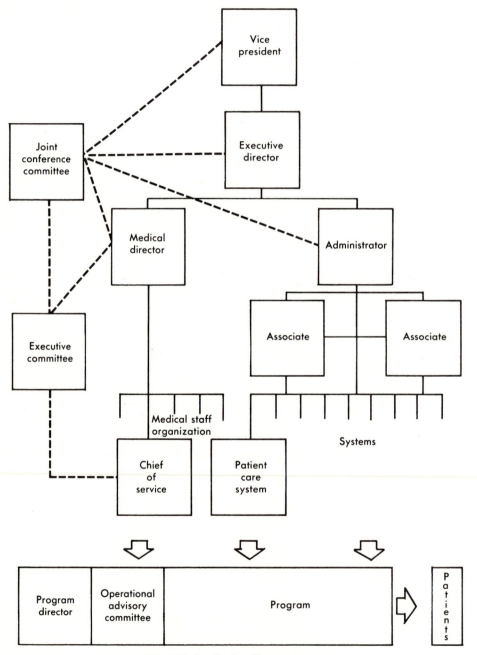

Fig. 5-2. Medical staff organization.

creditation for which purpose it shall form a subcommittee that includes key hospital personnel who are important in implementing the accreditation program. From time to time, it shall require that the Joint Commission's survey forms be used as a review method to estimate the accreditation status of the hospital and it should supervise a trial survey during the interim year between regular JCAH surveys for purposes of constructive self-criticism. It shall identify areas of suspected noncompliance with JCAH standards and shall make recommendations to the executive committees of the governing body of the medical staff for appropriate action.

2. Disaster planning: It shall be responsible for the development and maintenance of methods for the protection and care of hospital patients and others at the time of internal and external disaster. Specifically, it shall form subcommittees to:

adopt and periodically review a written plan to safeguard patients at the time of an internal disaster, particularly fire, and shall assure that all key personnel rehearse fire drills . . . (periodically); and

adopt and periodically review a written plan for the care, reception, and evacuation of mass casualties, and shall assure that such plan is coordinated with the inpatient and outpatient services of the hospital, that it adequately reflects developments in the hospital community and the anticipated role of the hospital in the event of disasters in nearby communities, and that the plan is rehearsed by key personnel at least twice yearly.

C. Meetings: The joint conference committee shall meet . . . (periodically) and shall transmit written reports of its activities to the executive committees of the governing body and the medical staff.*

Concentrating on organizing the medical staff for the provision of patient care, we find a major organizational division between the level of the executive director and the vice-president (see **Fig. 5-2**). Whereas the executive director is concerned

with the organization of physicians for patient care, the vice-president is involved, as well as the deans of the various schools, in the use of physicians in other activities such as teaching and research. At this level it is envisioned that the activities of the joint conference committee can be expanded beyond those recommended by JCAH to provide an arena for, first, interaction between the several entities and, second, and more to the point under consideration, interaction between the several administrative bodies involved with patient care.

As the chief administrative officer concerned with patient care activities, the executive director employs a medical director to serve in a pivotal position between administration and the medical staff. He is responsible for ensuring meaningful staff self-government and organization and must carry out the formal organizational responsibility for adequate medical care. To fulfill this responsibility, he must have jurisdiction over all physicians when they are engaged in service activities related to all patients. This authority accrues directly from the vice-president (acting in lieu of a hospital governing board) through the executive director. A close and effective relationship with the executive committee is essential.

The executive committee is the coordinating arena for the entire medical staff and its departments as they endeavor to render patient care. As such, it is the most authoritative representative of the medical staff in its relationships with all higher levels of organization, both professional and organizational. Its primary functions are outlined by the American Hospital Association as follows:

The executive committee shall coordinate the activities and general policies of the various departments, act for the staff as a whole under such limitations as may be imposed by the staff, and receive and act upon the reports of the medical records, tissue, and such other committees as the

*Joint Commission on Accreditation of Hospitals: Guidelines for the formulation of medical staff bylaws, rules and regulations, 1971, Chicago, 1971, The Commission, pp. 39-40.

medical staff may designate. The executive committee shall meet at least once a month and maintain a permanent record of its proceedings and actions.°

In the same reference, the Association goes on to say:

Doctor Thomas Ponton, in his book, *The Medical Staff in the Hospital*, says, "The executive committee is the most authoritative body of the medical staff, and one of its duties is to consider all business before it is brought to the attention of the full medical staff. In so doing, it will take action on all but the most important matters, hereby facilitating the transactions of business and saving much time at the meetings of the medical staff. It should report its actions to the full meeting of the active staff for confirmation, and when it presents matters for discussion it would usually recommend a course of action."°

In the program operational areas, where the physician renders service, further collaboration is provided for through an operational advisory committee composed of physicians, nurses, the unit manager, and other appropriate persons from the program. Working with the program director, it forms a sounding board for the peer group, a review mechanism, and a self-regulating body for ethics. In carrying out the director's policy, it sets quality standards and defines compensation. It sets the standards of research loads, the level of academic excellence, and the quality of care practiced in the service section. One of its

main missions is to examine and evaluate working relationships between physicians and other personnel to the end of promoting teamwork and professional standards.

In a medical center, health university, or regional setting, the medical staff system should be related to a corresponding system at the higher level. In this setting, a provost would head up the whole system, and it would come under a vice-president or overall regional manager. Another board could be superimposed upon the system in order to define professional qualifications expected, the amount of research time allocated to each man, his personal development record, and in-service training or continued education required. Any review of the effectiveness of the inputs into the various programs could be set up and administered at this level. All committee work should be able to be reviewed by the director for this particular system, and all program directors should have a voice in evaluating future needs for this system. The program directors would then form a body or a committee of the whole to collectively review, in their perspective, the activities of the professional system as related to the entire organizational scheme.

In all of this organization of physicians and medical staff through delegation of authority and responsibility, the source of delegation must actually possess the authority and responsibility that it acts to delegate. Delegation of responsibility without authority is pretense.

°American Hospital Association: Hospital accreditation references, Chicago, 1964, The Association, p. 58.

chapter six
PROGRAMS

Systems form a commonality among diverse parts—they channel resources identified by function into programs. **Programs** are means at the point of service of coordinating resources from systems into care, teaching, and research packages to meet projected ends. These resources are allocated in the form of personnel, equipment, finance, and expertise. Once injected into a program, they are molded by a program director to fit the program's needs (see Fig. 6-1).

The primary consumer designation of resources should be made according to the purposes for which the resources are used, i.e., teaching, research, and service, and according to the activity location where they are used, i.e., a nursing unit or program floor. Thus a record is kept and budgetary information is established relevant to research, teaching, and service expenditures. Furthermore, since these activities often occur side by side in an intermixed fashion at specific locations, information about their aggregate use is furnished to those responsible for the overall management of designated areas such as the program floors, which is discussed in the next section.

In this sense the systems and programs lend themselves to the concept of a linear flow of resources for research, teaching, and service purposes into program management units of interrelated activities. Although the goals and efforts may vary, the management unit exhibits essential underlying similarities for planning, coordinating, and controlling, with program and performance budgeting as a matrix. The ultimate goal is to structure and meet commitments that are within the limits of available resources when their use is *management*. This provides a means of visually demonstrating organizational structure and is an aid to decision making in allowing trade-offs and alternative courses of action.

Just as each system has an expert administrator in its own field, the program or management unit must have a director who is a coordinator of the inputs. The director concentrates on seeing that all inputs are working for the benefit of the total program. He is not identified with any single input, therefore he is not responsible for the internal functioning of an individual system input. He must, however, be responsible for seeing that the planning and daily operation of each system input is in accord with the program objectives and that the program is in accord with organizational objectives. Thus program directors are the authorities on design and coordination of programs. The systems are responsible for ensuring the availability of quality resources through recruitment and education; the program is responsible for

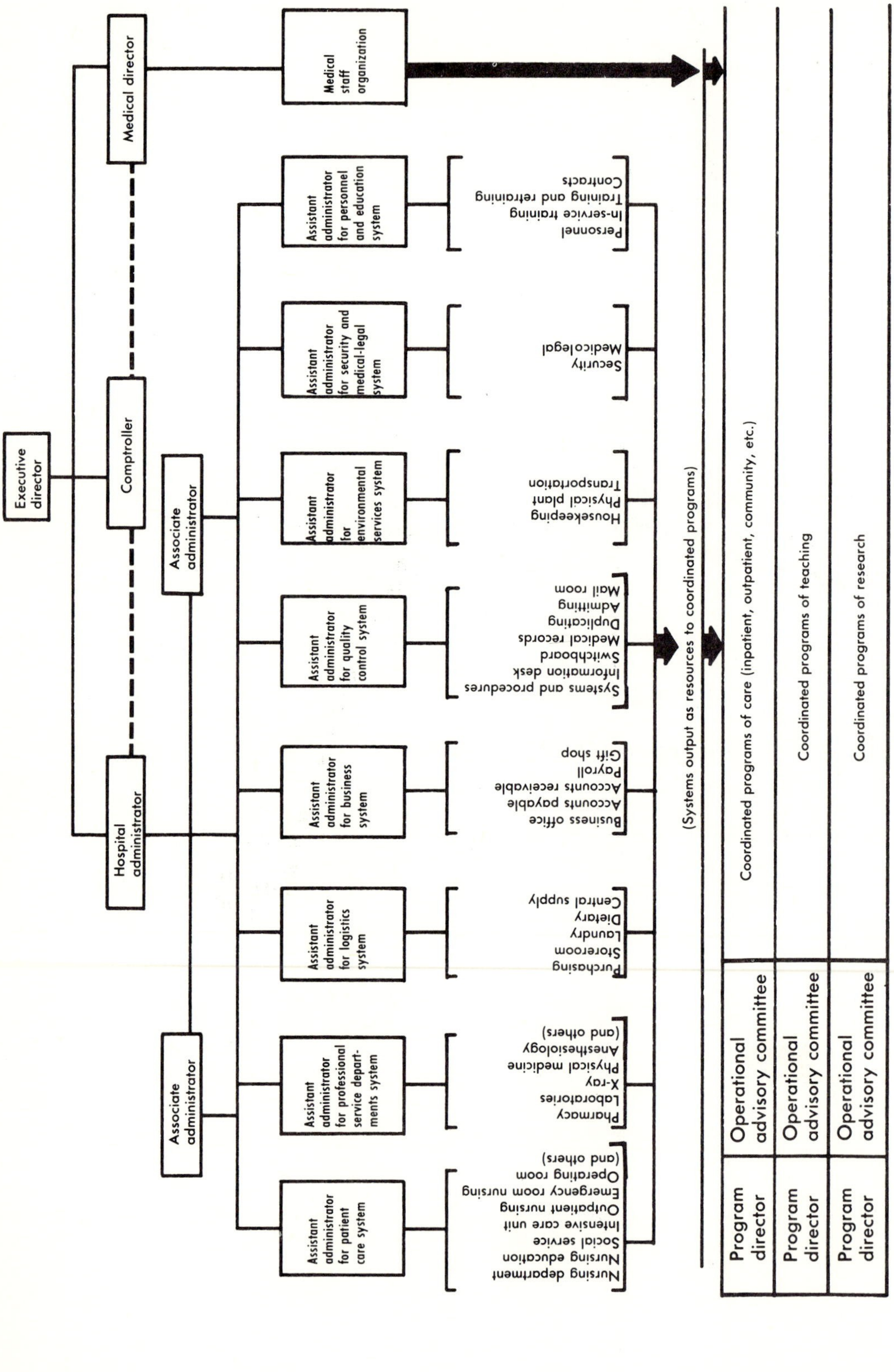

Fig. 6-1. Programs.

incorporation of resources input in effective ways to ensure program goal attainment.

For example, ambulatory care activities in a program serve as a framework for service to ambulatory patients. This service is composed of multiple system inputs coordinated to deliver care to the patient in an expeditious manner and, at the same time, to provide the necessary information and revenue to support this care. Although all of the systems provide input to ambulatory care, there are four principle inputs: (1) the business system, (2) the quality control system, (3) the patient care system, and (4) the professional system.

The business system is responsible for the collection of fees from patients or third parties either by cash or by billing. This function is supervised by a business manager who is aided by cashiers and by billing and insurance clerks. The quality control system is responsible for establishing medical records and for rating patients to determine fees to be paid. This system also works closely with the business and patient care systems in expediting proper communications flow. The patient care system supplies input of nursing personnel and needed social service assistance. The fourth significant operational input is the professional service provided by physicians. Although difficult to do, it is absolutely necessary that these services be organized and coordinated if the program is to operate as a unit and not as a series of sporadic independent clinics.

The remaining systems play supportive roles in the program. Of particular importance is the personnel, training, and continuing education system, which assists in the training and recruitment of personnel. It goes without question that logistics, environmental services, and maintenance are necessary elements, although none may have full-time representatives in the program area.

PROGRAM FLOORS

Unique in physical and functional arrangement will be the program floors of the clinical sciences teaching building. Each will house inpatient and outpatient services for the care, teaching, and research program associated with a particular "body system."* Taking the neurosensory program floor as an example, consider the interrelationships and interdependencies between neurologists, neurosurgeons, ophthalmologists, and otolaryngologists, all of whom work with the nervous system.

In the program floor approach they are brought together in the neurosensory program. Since the program needs specialized diagnostic and treatment equipment and associated experts and technicians, they are brought together at the program location. Much of the time and effort wasted in the movement of patients from patient floors for diagnosis and treatment and by professionals and nonprofessionals in moving from one area to another is eliminated. In effect, the framework for a specialty hospital is created. The clinical sciences teaching building will be a series of these specialty programs stacked one upon another. It provides a more suitable environment for a multidisciplinary approach for solving medical-surgical problems of a patient, for teaching various kinds of students, and for clinical investigation.

Supportive services must be organized. The patient is admitted and discharged on each floor. Demands for logistics and sup-

---

*For example, the human growth and development program will focus on areas of care of the neonate, i.e., obstetrics and gynecology and pediatrics; the muscoskeletal program on orthopedics, rheumatology, and physical medicine and rehabilitation; the cardiopulmonary program on thoracic surgery, vascular surgery, pulmonary function, cardiology, bronchoesophagology, etc.; the neurosensory program on neurology, ophthalmology, otolaryngology, audiology, and neurosurgery. Also included are the general surgery program and the general medicine program.

ply, nursing service, medications, food service, medical records, and administrative services must also be met on a decentralized basis. Such decentralization requires flexible organization with adequate information for planning, coordination, and control. This is accomplished through systems and program organization.

AMBULATORY CARE

One matter of significant difficulty in creating programs at Case Hospital was how to combine inpatient and ambulatory care responsibility under each program director. A review of some of the historic aspects of clinics and outpatient care will help in understanding this.

Specialization has been practiced for ages. Herodotus wrote that medicine was divided, with each physician treating a single disorder. Later another Greek historian noted that the patients were treated without having to pay and the community took care of physicians' salaries. Whether meetings between physician and patient occurred in olive groves or courtyard, is open to speculation, but the same principles that promote modern clinics were evident then. Ambulant patients could come to see specialists and the cost did not keep them away. But not all clinics have carried this tradition forward. Today many patients are treated in large, poorly organized hospital clinics notorious for poor facilities and lack of human interest.

When one large city clinic attempted to improve conditions so that the morale of the staff as well as that of the clientele could be improved, some amazing facts were brought to light. Many of the physical improvements in the waiting rooms went unnoticed since the poor, who are the main users of this clinic, are also poorly educated. They are not conditioned to expect convenience along with their health services. It is an established fact that health services are low on the list of wants of ghetto dwellers. They want better income,

better housing, better schools, better police protection, and many other improvements. They want health services only when they need them, and then the most they seem to expect is some improvement in their present ailments.

The morale of the staff was not raised appreciably as a result of this experiment since their efforts were pretty much ignored. Appointment systems do not work unless patients show up when they are expected. Missed appointments discourage the staff and the students, but the students suffer most when they are unable to follow through on their cases. We are only beginning to comprehend the hopelessness and ignorance that has trapped so many of the ghetto dwellers, but it affects every facet of their lives.

The average hospital employs three to four people for each patient. Compare this with an outpatient department that in 1947 recorded 59 outpatient visits per clinic employee at a cost of $2.66 per visit. By 1966 this number had risen to 72 visits for every clinic employee at a cost of $6.93 per visit. This demonstrates the more favorable balance of employees to patients in the outpatient area, and it also demonstrates that this is where productivity can be increased. It is one more reason for concentrating on ambulatory services as a possible solution to the demands for services that are being made on the health industry.

The organization of the industry so far has been almost entirely a matter of chance. It has been based primarily on the physicians' fee-for-service practice, with no definite plan for the placement of hospitals and other health facilities. The consumers had no say in the distribution of the medical care. It was entirely in the hands of the provider. Changing patterns of disease, a rapidly evolving technology, rising costs, a more sophisticated consumer public, new methods of financing, and a population that is changing in its age distribution, all have made the absurdities of the present distribution system apparent.

But this is not all. As charity institutions whose first commodity was mercy, they attracted the homeless, the insecure, the uneducated, and the uneducable as employees in the lower echelon. These people were willing to work for subsistence wages and often less. Their productivity was usually as low as their training, and they were not the cheap source of labor that everyone imagined. Those hospitals that would like to continue to function with this kind of wage scale are being forced by union pressure to pay living wages. This is what is causing rapidly rising costs; in a service industry such as health care institutions, labor is and always will be the biggest item in cost. The only solution is increased productivity, and this increase is more likely to occur in outpatient facilities.

Patterns of patient care have changed as the patterns of disease have changed. Communicable diseases have lost their power to terrorize. Not long ago they were so prevalent and virulent that there were special hospitals for their treatment, and quarantines were routinely placed on homes where communicable diseases were diagnosed. Today's children are unaware of the meaning of quarantine, as they are unaware of the ravages of most childhood diseases. Polio and now measles and mumps have all been conquered except for occasional cases where preventive measures have not been administered. Even tuberculosis, with mass detection techniques and new drugs, is slowly being brought under control. The death rate has fallen, and the length of hospitalization has been shortened.

Chronic diseases, however, have replaced acute diseases as the chief causes of death. In 1900, 40 of every 100,000 of the population died of diphtheria; by 1940 this figure was reduced to 1. There were 210 deaths per 100,000 population caused by pneumonia in 1900; by 1940 there were

70. The tuberculosis death rate dropped from 199 in 1900 to 46 in 1940, but the cancer death rate went from 64 to 210 in the same time period.

Mental illness is of ranking importance, not so much as a killer but as a chronic disease that removes people from the working population. Recent drugs have made remarkable advancements in the treatment of these patients, but, as in the case of tuberculosis, long periods of follow-up are required after discharge from the hospital. Unfortunately, few outpatient facilities are available for the follow-up of these patients, and those facilities that exist are often poorly located.

The emphasis has been on building more hospital beds, not on constructing outpatient facilities. Third-party payers have been particularly guilty of influencing this trend, and the government, through Hill-Burton funds, has pushed construction in the same direction. Add to this the fact that doctors have been slow to gravitate to any kind of group practice, and the reasons for the present hospital-centered health care system are very evident.

This is an era of great change in the health care field. The rising costs of health care are most surely causing much of this change to occur. The government has assumed responsibility for the health care for certain groups, but one segment that is hard hit when it comes to securing health care is moderate-income families with children. At today's prices, medical care is priced almost out of their reach, and they frequently pass up the advantages of early diagnosis and preventive checkups.

For people like these, not poor enough to qualify as indigents and not rich enough to be able to buy medical care, prepaid group practice plans are a godsend. Lessening the financial risks makes it possible for people to take advantage of preventive checkups, and it means better health for the entire community. When figures for maternal and infant deaths, premature births, and fetal deaths are compared, they are far lower in a population that is covered by a prepaid plan than in a population that receives any other kind of medical distribution. Because prepaid plans need large numbers of paticipants and must be well organized if they are to succeed, too few of them are in existence.

Two of the better known organizations are the Kaiser Permanente Foundation on the West Coast and the Health Insurance Plan of Greater New York. The Group Health Association of Washington, D. C., the Group Health Cooperative of Puget Sound, and the Ross-Loos Medical Group of Los Angeles are others. There are some organized in heavily unionized areas such as Detroit, and union members and their families are covered. The exact range of services provided varies with each group, depending, among other things, on whether the group owns its hospitals. The plans do not always cover surgery. That these groups are successful in what they attempt to do is attested to by the fact that the Conference on Group Practice urged the development of more of them.

Other decisive changes within the health care field are likely to occur as a result of action by major university medical schools. They are being urged to expand the scope of their programs to go beyond the period of undergraduate medical education. It is very likely that in the not-too-distant future the isolated practitioner who works apart from professional and university affiliations will go the way of the one-room schoolhouse. In contrast, when doctors graduate from medical school they will take internships and residencies that are supervised by that school and will become members of a continuing education program fostered by their school. Even though the concept has yet to be adopted, it is taken for granted that existing patterns of care may die and fade away as their practitioners die and fade away. The hope of the future of comprehensive medicine rests

with youth. The effort to organize the medical technology and knowledge that becomes broader every day will find its beginnings in the hospital-based outpatient department, preferably one with a university affiliation.

Other factors that are influencing the development of outpatient facilities, some of which have already been mentioned, are (1) a young population,* (2) the population explosion, (3) the rural-to-urban shift, (4) the manpower shortage (this makes it necessary to group physicians to greater advantage), and (5) the technologic revolution, which goes on and on with no end in sight.†

One of the more exciting happenings in technology is the multiphasic screening program that the Kaiser Permanente Foundation is developing in cooperation with the federal government. This screening technique involves the use of a multichannel analyzer that can run 17 tests or more on one blood sample. The results, plus a medical history, EKG, and EEG, show any abnormalities in a short period of time. The mass screening technique detects the sick people in a society so that they can receive prompt treatment. As a health index, it gives a medical profile of an individual or a population.

Of the many kinds of medical care available, surely the most viable is the hospital-based outpatient department and its affiliated hospital. This is not to say that other methods of practice are not important and should be abandoned. On the contrary, there should always be a choice available to the consumer, whether he prefers a

---

*One in every three persons is under 15 years of age. This group has been encouraged to have checkups, and preventive medicine is very important for this group.
†This technologic change in itself creates some of the health industry's problems; e.g., more equipment is needed, labor requirements are changed, new job occupations are required for new techniques, and overall costs are increased.

proprietary clinic, a private physician, or the more high-powered services of a hospital and its outpatient department, particularly if it is university affiliated. In the latter, comprehensive medical care can be practiced at its best. Comprehensive medical care includes complete care from birth through old age, with all specialties represented, including those for acute and chronic diseases, therapy, and rehabilitation. The consuming public wants a minimum of inconvenience and trauma, but at the same time it wants the latest and best in health care that is likely to originate in a dynamic setting.

Why don't hospital-based outpatient departments enjoy this reputation now? Some do. Others suffer from a variety of causes, one being environment. Another is mismanagement or, better still, nonmanagement, for some have literally been left to themselves. The old idea of charity clinics for the poor, with time donated by the physician as he saw fit, has left a stigma on outpatient departments that is hard to erase.*

In the past, staffing of all personnel was poorly managed. The nurses were frequently those who failed to measure up to hospital standards of motivation or ability. The same was true of other employees. Records were sketchy and were completely separate from those of the hospital so that there was no continuity of care. But these things have been changing.

Medical schools for years believed that in order to do satisfactory teaching they must have a supply of indigent patients to "practice" on. They set out in search of low-income areas in which to establish affiliations. The University of Chicago proved that this was not necessarily the

only or even the best method. The university's method proved that students could receive excellent training by examining paying patients under expert supervision. These patients could articulate their symptoms, thereby making diagnosis simpler and more accurate, and they were willing to come back for follow-up visits so that the student could see the results of the treatment.

In a typical hospital outpatient department of a university-affiliated primary comprehensive care system, this pattern of influence is slowly evolving. Hospitals in the area that specialize in eye diseases, children's diseases, rehabilitation, and skin and cancer diseases have gradually become affiliated with the university. There will be still more affiliations in the future.

Often these complexes are in a community setting that leaves much to be desired. In 1960, 236,000 people were living in one such area; their incomes ranged from $1,756 to $5,634 a year, which against today's living index means poverty. There were more than 24,000 persons on public assistance in 1962; 14,036 families and individuals earned less than $3,000 a year.

The health statistics, as might be expected, are fully as depressing as the income figures. The area contained 11.8% of the city's population, but in 1956 it had 23% of the city's reported cases of syphilis, 23% of the city's fatal deaths, 24% of the city's illegitimate births, 19% of the city's premature births, 19% of the city's infant deaths, and 17% of the city's reported cases of active and probably active tuberculosis.

Any health plan for this area would need heavy and continued government financing. This means financing in addition to that provided by the federal government. The city could do much to provide these funds by instituting a prepaid system of medical care on the order of the Memphis Plan.*

*The present trend is to eliminate traditional clinics and to replace this concept with physicians practicing in groups. In this type of practice the patient is seen by appointment by a particular physician. The advent of Title XVIII and Title XIX has encouraged this trend.

*See Hardy, R. C., and Durbin, R. L.: Low income groups can pay their way, Mod. Hosp. **89:**71, Dec. 1957.

Those who could pay some but not all of their medical care would be required to do so. The city would make up the difference between what the person could pay and what was charged; in some cases this would be the entire cost. But everyone would be covered by insurance.

There are many outpatient department users across the country who are already covered by some prepaid insurance. About 50% of the outpatients are covered by Title XVIII and Title XIX; another 25% or 30% are covered by Blue Cross and Blue Shield.* If city governments were to assume responsibility for the indigent groups, prepayment plans would cover most of the population.

To keep such a complex in tune to the community and its needs there must be some communication between the two. This is usually done through the board of trustees, which includes some members from the community. The board should also include members from the medical staff, although this has not been standard practice. Physicians, since they play a prominent role in the business and professional life of such an undertaking, should be represented in the major policy-making decisions. It should result in an effective board because many segments of community business and professional interests are represented. Some members that participate on the hospital board should also be active on the outpatient board.

There will be more overlapping of personnel and equipment between the hospital and the outpatient department. This is one of the advantages of having them in proximity: duplications of costly equipment and personnel will not be necessary. The departments that are vital to this overlapping principle should be conve-niently located to the inpatient and outpatient facilities, including medical records, pharmacy, x-ray, laboratory, emergency room, business office, personnel department, purchasing, and social service. A central billing office can cover both areas with a maximum of efficiency.

One difference between the two facilities that must be kept in mind as personnel are deployed to the two areas is that each area has its own specific needs. The patient in the inpatient facility is horizontal, and there is time for the personnel to get to know him and to chart the best course to recovery. He will stay, as a rule, a matter of days or sometimes weeks and occasionally months. In the outpatient department, however, the patient is vertical and is there for only a matter of hours. He may return for further visits, but these are usually of even shorter duration. To become aware of his needs in this short time, the personnel must be alert, efficient, and "tuned in." They should be pleasant, courteous, interested, and able to adjust to an ever changing set of faces. This calls for highly skilled personnel, for the feeling is always one of hurry. This is in opposition to the traditional method of outpatient staffing.

Guiding this complex organization is a medical advisory board appointed by the executive committee of the medical staff. The members are responsible for all decisions relating to the quality of this care. Administration works closely with them. Each outpatient administrator makes the decisions regarding the outpatient activity, keeping in mind the prevailing philosophy: good patient care. Teaching and research can be accommodated if this comes first. The number of assistants that he needs depends on the volume of visits per day and other features peculiar to the institution, but the overall responsibility will be to coordinate them with the inpatient facility. He must work closely with all the clinics and with the physicians who are in charge.

---

*At present, these patients, after hospitalization, may be seen by a private physician in his private office. In this case they rarely seek care in the large and crowded outpatient clinics.

In some departments a clinic coordinator who is trained in his job and has well-defined duties can make the difference between an institution that functions and one that bogs down. Those who qualify for this position must have a minimum of 2 years of college. The clinic coordinators work closely with the record librarian in checking out charts, in keeping track of them, and in seeing that they are completed and returned to the record room. They also work closely with the physician to see that he meets with the patient and that all available information about the patient is at hand. It is the clinic coordinator who schedules the tests that are ordered, checks on results and sees that they are entered in the charts, and makes certain that the doctors' comments are also entered. These individuals, when properly trained, make the outpatient department "hum." It is incredible how detail work of this nature can bog down a clinic operation, especially one with a work load of 700 visits a day.*

When the operation involves a large volume of visits, it becomes a major task to schedule the resources, the people, the space, and the time. Some system is needed for handling this mass of information. The "Sabre System" has been the answer for American Airlines, which developed the system for covering similar mass scheduling that involves such diverse items as reservations, availability, food preferences, and spare parts. The need is just as strong in the health field for a similar classification, storage, and distribution of information.

The personnel department in such an institution becomes a vital link in the dispensing of quality care as long as its members are reminded that this is the prime objective of the complex. They must also be aware of the differences between the inpatient and outpatient facilities and of

*An excellent prototype can be found in the operation of the University of Chicago's clinics.

the fact that employees differ in their ability to cope with the two work situations. The personnel department cannot be an isolated department; it must be an active, informed part of the organization.

With all this talk of participation and coordination, it becomes apparent that what is needed is a flow of records, services, and patients between the two facilities and, just as important, a flow of information. To achieve this there must be a common objective: good patient care. After that must come communication, cooperation, and an air of freedom in which each individual is permitted to function to his maximum. There is no room for fears and prejudices if the objective is to be reached.

Proprietary clinics are at the other end of the pole. They are composed of individual entrepreneurs who have formed a group for certain advantages. They are not in practice to provide low-cost medical care for the masses. However, the advantages to the patients are considerable. Costly diagnostic equipment and the usual laboratory services are available as well as the specialists who must interpret test results and diagnose. For the patient, they are usually convenient and pleasant, though not inexpensive. For the physician, many troublesome administrative and accounting routines are performed by qualified assistants.

Proprietary clinics are a twentieth-century development and have become more popular in some parts of the country than in others. There are many of them in the Midwest and Far West, but comparatively few in the East. The East is still very partial to a kind of medicine that is dispensed from a corner of a residential home. One wonders what kind of professional contacts are engendered by such a system, what opportunities for consultations and continuing education are encouraged, and what kind of medical records are kept under the circumstances.

One aspect of care that has received some stimulation through Medicare and one that is always discussed in relation to low cost is the home care service. Patients who have recovered from the acute stages of their illnesses can be discharged so that costly hospital beds can be used for other acutely ill patients. The limited supervision that these patients require can theoretically be dispensed in their homes. Perhaps a stay in an extended care facility has preceded this final step. At any rate, in the final stages of a patient's recuperation the services of a nurse, dietitian, social worker, physical therapist, or physician are presumably available upon request. Unfortunately the shortage of manpower in each category makes this a beautiful plan in theory only. Given a choice between the regular hours of an institution and the uncertain conditions they are likely to encounter in home visits, most workers choose to work in institutions. Most doctors adamantly refuse to make any home visits at all, and with good reason. Despite the fact that most home care programs are failures, there are a few that succeed.

An admitting clinic, known as a diagnostic or triage clinic, is a part of most outpatient departments. Here a patient is seen and a quick diagnosis is made so that the patient can be referred immediately to the proper specialty clinic for further study. Otherwise a patient would have to make his own diagnosis and choose his own specialist, something few patients are qualified to do. The diagnostic clinic saves the time of the patient while it cuts down on the extra shuffling necessary by clinic personnel when patients are transferred needlessly from clinic to clinic.

Cancer clinics cannot exist alone but must be operated in conjunction with other specialties such as otolaryngology and gynecology and where surgeons, radiologists, and pathologists are at hand. There is a great need for early detection, treatment, and follow-up of cancer patients despite ever increasing knowledge of this disease. This will probably always be true. The only really simple detection devices that are known are Pap smears and chest x-ray examinations. The outpatient department is the only logical place for such a clinic. Wherever cancer clinics are maintained, high-energy sources such as cobalt reactors or linear reactors are also available, and a cancer registry is maintained for follow-up and disposition of cancer cases. This is especially valuable for teaching purposes.

Drug addiction is rapidly becoming the nation's number-one teen-age problem. More and more younger people are experimenting with marijuana and hashish, "speed" (methamphetamine), LSD, and heroin. The use of these drugs started in colleges and universities, but has now come into use in high schools and junior high schools. The general populace considers drug use a negative thing and legislation has made it a felonious act. Addicts are usually considered a criminal element in our society and face large penal sentences if apprehended and proved guilty. This makes therapy and prevention more difficult. High schools and colleges are attempting to educate students about these drugs and their effects.

It would seem that drug addiction–treatment centers should be established on an ambulatory basis and that these ambulatory centers should gear up to handle drug addictions in a rehabilitative way and also serve as the community's center for practicing both preventive and correctional techniques. Drug addiction is a disease and should be treated by health personnel in a preventative and curative way.

Venereal disease clinics, which are usually financed by the government, are a source of conflict for certain members of the medical profession. These clinics are established for the purpose of providing free care to those who would not otherwise be able to obtain it, but the services are often used by those who can afford to pay. Venereal disease, however, is increasing, especially among the younger members of the population. Detecting and treating venereal disease is the most important consideration, and all victims should be encouraged to seek help.

Speech and hearing clinics are frequently located in the outpatient department since patients, especially during the beginning process of diagnosis and treatment, may need other services available in the outpatient department. These clinics are sometimes funded by government money.

Well-baby clinics have become a standard and reliable feature of health care in this country and are not necessarily limited to outpatient departments, although this service is offered during regularly scheduled times. Many solo-practicing physicians set aside times for well-baby visits so that mixing of sick and well babies in crowded waiting rooms can be avoided. The Public Health Service has for years made well-baby clinics available to many deprived areas. This is a logical outgrowth of this organization's interest in preventive medicine and its necessary preoccupation with the incidence of communicable disease and other statistics.

Ambulatory outpatient care is considered less costly as compared to inpatient hospital care, and that is one of the chief reasons for so many attempts to promote the growth of more facilities devoted to this care. It is, however, not cheap care, and it can be quite costly. There are a number of reasons for this. As has been previously stated, proprietary clinics never promised or attempted to deliver low-cost medical care to the masses. They cater to the paying patient and expect a good return for their efforts. Hospital-based outpatient departments, especially those affiliated with universities, have often carried on costly teaching and research programs that were totally or partially financed by patients' fees. The "Robin Hood" practice has been as prevalent in outpatient departments as it has been in hospitals, and paying patients have been forced to pay

enough to cover the cost of care for those who could pay little or nothing. This era is now reaching its end. With government and third-party payers contracting on a cost basis for constantly increasing numbers of patients, the number of paying patients who can be overcharged is diminishing. The time has arrived when every patient must provide some form of payment, either out of his pocket, through third-party payers, or as one of an indigent group that some government agency is subsidizing.

COMPREHENSIVE AMBULATORY CARE CENTERS

One of the many innovations that the federal government has been encouraging through the Office of Economic Opportunity is neighborhood health clinics. In Case Hospital's area, two neighborhood health centers will provide new health care delivery systems. These two centers are designed to deliver quality care to residents of two well-defined areas. The goal in each area is to combine categorical services into unified delivery of comprehensive health care. The mechanisms selected to achieve the goal are different. One will be a traditional pediatric clinic using established staffing patterns. The other is more experimental in that health aides indigenous to the area will work with general practitioners. There will be a close affiliation with the university hospital for referrals. It constitutes an extension of the university hospital into the community so that those who need health care can be reached and helped. It is necessary to deliver these services with some goals regarding cost and quality. If either of these is too far out of line, the experiment will have to be considered a failure.

Since these clinics will be located in poverty-stricken areas of the city, some serious study will have to be given to the hours when the clinics will be open. Twenty-four hour service is really needed. Evening hours are absolutely essential if working mothers are to be accommodated. It has been customary for people who could not take time during the day to visit the outpatient department to use the emergency room at night. This is a great inconvenience to the hospital, and is one which no emergency room is equipped to handle. Convenient hours for the consuming public are long overdue.

The operation of two centers makes possible the use of each as a test control upon the other. Thus, although providing for delivery of care, organizational differences that permit evaluation of quality, volume, and cost of services rendered can be structured in each. In one setting, vertical department staffing by specialists and allied personnel will provide services in what is essentially the traditional model. Strenuous efforts will be made, however, to deliver personalized and family-oriented services. The pediatrician and the internist will render most of the care, but obstetricians and surgeons will perform their customary roles. A component of the mental health center will function as an integral part of this operation. A vendor system of pharmacy services will be arranged and carefully monitored to determine the effect of involving neighborhood pharmacists with the health care team. Dental services will be provided, and laboratory and x-ray facilities will be located on the site. Patients that require admission or diagnostic and therapeutic services that are not available at the center will be referred to other facilities. Despite dual sponsorship, a single coordinated record system will be used to permit free interchange of data between both hospitals and the other neighborhood center.

In the other center the staffing pattern will follow more innovative lines. To the greatest extent possible, all personnel, licensed professionals, and allied health professionals will be recruited from the neighborhood itself. General practitioners, osteopaths, and others who fit the Millis Com-

mission's description of the "primary care physician" will form the backbone of patient care teams. As personal physicians, they will maintain ongoing contacts with patients and their families. Within each patient care team there will be internists and pediatricians recruited for the specific function of providing consultative help for primary care physicians. This intimate contact will make possible progressive development and promotion for these physicians through this ongoing, built-in mechanism for continuing their education. Optimum utilization of nurses, licensed practical nurses, social workers, and neighborhood workers trained to participate as members of the health team will permit each individual to make maximum utilization of his skills.

At all times, in both centers, conscientious efforts will be made to cooperate with local practicing physicians. They have been invited to refer cases to the centers for consultation, laboratory or x-ray services, and other necessary care. In all instances, reports will be returned to the referring physicians. Also, they will be invited to participate in teaching conferences and teaching programs at the centers. They will, of course, be welcome to follow their patients in the hospital. At both centers, training programs and correlated educational offerings are designed to permit upward mobility in each of several census tracts. This process of recruitment and intensive training and education reflects one approach to the problem of recruitment and utilization of health manpower and initiates cooperation between the academic setting and the private practitioner.

Consultative services, including mental health, will be provided. The dental laboratory will serve both centers. One center, however, will have an inhouse dispensing pharmacy, in contrast to the vendor system employed at the other center. Every facet of pharmaceutical services and cost will be subjected to a thorough assessment to determine the relative merits of each system. Home care services will also be provided. In no way are the neighborhood health centers expected to supplant either the private practitioner or the community hospital. Rather, a continuum of health care, beginning with enlightened self-care and advancing through intensive care, extended care, and rehabilitation, will be needed to make it possible to attend each patient in the setting best suited to his needs and at the least cost.

One outstanding virtue of the Office of Economic Opportunity's program is that it provides the equivalent of prepaid comprehensive group insurance for the target population. The 5-year objective of the program is to train the staffs of both centers and their neighborhood advisory groups to maintain the operation on a prepaid basis even after the contract has expired.

Not money alone, but other forms of support are being mobilized to strengthen the program. The city's department of public health plans to locate some of its service programs in these centers. Where appropriate, joint appointments to the university faculty and health department staff will be made. The city school district, the departments of health and public welfare of the state, the community nursing service, and the county medical society are others who have been invited to participate.

In the future, ambulatory care programs at the clinical teaching location will be of two distinct types: specialty referral centers and comprehensive ambulatory care. Specialty referral centers will follow the general pattern of those common throughout the country today. This type of setting, however, tends to isolate physical and psychologic relationships. Comprehensive care will counteract this tendency by considering all aspects of illness of the patient as well as the interrelationships with his family. This concept recognizes the importance

of highly technical and narrowly focused specialty services. At the same time, it recognizes that most care (preventive, diagnostic, curative, and restorative) may be provided outside of the specialty areas. The purpose of comprehensive care is to create a setting in which "nonspecialty" care may be delivered.

Comprehensive care will be located in the same building complex with specialty referral centers and will act as a source of referral to them. It will provide the major portion of health care services to panels of patients in family units, utilizing multidisciplinary group practice. Physical design, staffing, and organization will be oriented to patient need. It will route the patient through the gamut of health care services, including preventive medicine, hospitalization, extended care, home treatment, and community health services. This setting will also provide teaching and research opportunities.

Services are focused in a team in order to create a truly comprehensive approach. Consultation from specialists and the services of nutritionists, social workers, and dentists will be included. Each of these services will be coordinated in a team effort to handle problems of the individual and his family. Visits will be on an appointment basis, with continuing relationships between the team and the patient. The general flow of patients, then, will be from community health centers and comprehensive care to specialty centers and program floors. Follow-up care will be provided at the least specialized location feasible. The patients' health needs will be matched to a facility designed and staffed for that level of care. This will deemphasize inpatient admission for reasons not fully requiring hospitalization.* Thus pa-

---

*It is believed that in the near future prepayment plans will pay for services in ambulatory programs and will encourage people to use these facilities for the prevention of disease as well as for treatment.

tients admitted to the hospital will be in greater need of the highly skilled personnel and facilities found there, resulting in better utilization of inpatient programs.

Community health centers and comprehensive ambulatory care have the potential to provide for the total health care needs of a specific population. Thus the patient will be able to identify a single geographic area and a single group of physicians for his care. The advantage to the health care team lies in the development of an ongoing relationship between themselves and with their patients.

The concept also includes integration of public health, welfare, and health agency services, which makes it all the more comprehensive. Programs of this type make possible highly efficient delivery of care at several points of need, maximizing the utilization of resources at each point. In developing the concept, the broad overall objective is to find ways in which comprehensive care can be provided economically and efficiently, getting the greatest potential out of all resources. As planners of health facilities become involved, they will need better reporting systems on utilization of various types of facilities. If ambulatory care replaces some need for inpatient facilities, overbuilding of inpatient facilities could result. The effect on inpatient facilities would be underutilization. This also is costly to a community.

The future of health care delivery in this country will be patterned around a system of hospital-affiliated ambulatory service in which all health needs of the patient and his family can be met. Such a system will be comprehensive in the sense that complete care from birth through old age, covering preventive medicine as well as treatment for acute and chronic ailments, therapy, and rehabilitation, will be available with a minimum of inconvenience and trauma. This will result in large ambulatory complexes affiliated with smaller inpatient facilities. Every patient who can

be handled as an ambulant will be seen in the ambulatory area. In rural areas the general practitioner will refer them to larger centers when the services of a specialist are needed.

Despite the need for group practice, their growth is slow in all parts of the country. One of the conferences called in 1967 by Secretary of Health, Education, and Welfare John Gardner was on the group practice of medicine and ways in which it could be promoted. This conference was held at the University of Chicago Center for Continuing Education and included representatives from all areas of the health industry: medical school and dental school representatives, private practitioners, insurance company and prepayment plan representatives, union officials, lawyers, and economists.

Since there is an urgent necessity to do something about the high cost of medical care and the methods of distribution, which are in many situations archaic, some of the recommendations that proceeded from this meeting are worth mentioning, for this is an area of health care that will see much development and expansion within the next few years. There will be other conferences in the future that will bear watching as development occurs and new dimensions and trends are uncovered.

1. The conference recommended that the Hill-Burton Program be expanded to encourage the group practice of medicine. The Hill-Burton Program traditionally limited its support to those outpatient facilities that would dispense free care. Since there are no ways to finance this kind of care, there are few requests for this kind of money. It is hoped that federal money will encourage experimentation with group practices other than the traditional outpatient model of care.

2. At present, some state laws dis-

courage the group practice of medicine. It was recommended that the federal government use its leverage to have these laws changed or, if necessary, to institute a federal licensure.

3. Consumer-sponsored prepaid group practice was very much encouraged, but here again some state laws hinder their development. Positive legislation beneficial to their expansion was recommended. Even the Internal Revenue Service should review and alter the rulings that hinder the group practice of medicine.

4. Some hospitals discriminate against physicians who participate in group practice. It was recommended that reimbursement to such hospitals under Title XVIII be denied them while they practice such discrimination.

5. Since all parties concerned are becoming increasingly aware that poor quality care is costly care, it was recommended that some kind of incentive pay be developed for those groups that meet or exceed high performance criteria. These criteria will need to be developed.

6. It was urged that more emphasis be placed on ambulatory care in the training of health care personnel. Manpower is, of course, the critical ingredient in any expansion of health facilities. Ambulatory care is one area where part-time personnel can be used to advantage. The conference recommended that federal support be given on the graduate level to persons engaged in the scientific management of medical care.

7. The conference expressed the need for public education for the wise use of health manpower. This is a far-fetched recommendation. It is an established fact that the public is not primarily interested in health care or its facilities, manpower, or problems until it has a need to use them; when the need is past, it quickly forgets them.

8. The conference's recommendations regarding financing of group practice included some recommendations directed at existing prepayment and financing plans. These were (1) that a choice between group practice and solo medicine be permitted when plans are established with employee-employer groups, (2) that carrier marketing and administration of both solo and group practice plans be promoted, and (3) that a tie between large-scale prepayment plans and group practice through capitation be promoted. The representatives believed that if these recommendations were followed, participation in group prepayment plans would increase sixfold.

9. The federal government was requested to add further incentives; e.g., (1) provide a subsidy so that major group practice plans can expand their facilities, (2) provide the required capital and operating funds for the creation of new plans, (3) encourage the use of Office of Economic Opportunity neighborhood health center concepts in developing and expanding group practices, (4) combine Title XVIII and Title XIX payments for Medicare beneficiaries who elect to use hospital-based physicians organized as a group practice, and (5) encourage the training of personnel specifically for use in developing new plans. Major insurance companies were encouraged to lend money for group practice and development.

10. One very meaningful suggestion was that the government pull all of its

sources of aid together and make the information available through one outlet. There are many sources of government aid now available to group practice, but they are fragmented and spread through numerous agencies. Anyone seeking help needs a blueprint to find them all. Some are available through the medical assistance program, some through the regional medical programs, some through the Public Health Service, the Department of Health, Education, and Welfare, and also through the planning act Public Law 89-749. What is desperately needed is some direction toward the group practice of medicine by controlling all existing services.

Group practice permits the existence of many specialty clinics, something that is not possible in the solo practice of medicine. These clinics have become standard features of traditional hospital-based outpatient departments.

A significant result of Case Hospital's reorganization was the identification of a more appropriate mechanism for delivering ambulatory care using group-practice guidelines within each program. *It is essential to remember that this discussion involves the ambulatory activities within a program and that these are only a portion of its total, interrelated activities, which also include inpatient care, education, and research.*

The system of operating private practice offices for outpatients who pay usual and customary fees and a clinic for those who are medically indigent is neither socially nor economically defensible, and thus a group-practice type of activity was designed to replace the previous clinic opera-

---

*Based on Springall, W. H.: Group practice in the university teaching setting, Hosp. Admin., Spring 1971.

tion with the cost of its operation reflected in the total practice costs of the physician rather than as a hospital cost.

The existing outpatient building was reorganized to identify ambulatory space related to each program. The physicians in each program were organized in a group. The total system was based on the group-practice principle, although each group has considerable internal flexibility. The hospital provides space and any special services that the physician may wish to utilize at a predetermined charge. There are five basic objectives:

1. *"Group-practice" administrative mechanisms*

Ambulatory practice is conducted as a defined segment of each program. It is the responsibility of each program director to arrange the appropriate staffing of the practice with due recognition to the needs of patients and the teaching and research needs of the institution.

The basic objectives are to assure a high quality of medical care to each patient served by the group and to conduct the care in such a way that it can serve as an optimal model for the education of medical students, interns, and residents who may receive portions of their education in the ambulatory setting. The following criteria serve as guidelines:

a. One or more qualified staff physicians are responsible for each session and supervise the care of each patient. They may delegate certain portions of the care to residents, interns or students whose activities they supervise, accepting basic individual responsibility for the patient.

b. The staff physician who treats a patient submits a charge to the patient. Fees are deposited to the account of his group. If a group consists of full-time or parttime persons engaged for this activity, the fees are deposited in an account created for such purposes and the physician may be paid an appropriate remuneration from the account for his activities.

c. Insofar as possible, the physician who sees a patient follows the patient in order to provide continuity of care. In the event he is unavailable at any time, this responsibility is fulfilled by other staff members of the group.

d. Appointments for patients are made by each group on the basis of its own capabilities. If desired, a central appointment system can be arranged by the several groups collectively and a central reception area can be established.

e. The billing of patients is the responsibility of each group, although a central billing facility can be provided if desired. Such a central facility can, in collaboration with the hospital admission and fiscal offices, facilitate certain determinations of patient eligibility for third-party payments.

f. If a group desires that a patient be transferred to, or seen in consultation by, another specialty group, it arranges an appointment with that group directly. The transferring group remains responsible for the patient's care until the patient has been properly admitted by another group and discharged from its own.

g. Direct costs for the operation of each group are the responsibility of the group. Such direct costs include the following:

(1) A reasonable square-footage rental cost to include amortization of space, heat, light, and reasonable maintenance

(2) Equipment and supplies

(3) Personnel engaged in direct support of the practice activities and any other services provided directly to the support of the group

h. Each group has the responsibility of establishing its professional charges with the understanding that ethical fee schedules will be observed for appropriate patients. In the event that the multiple groups or the institution should contract with any agency for services, any predetermined fee commitments will be honored by each group. However, it is understood that the institution will not enter into such contracts without the prior consultation and agreement with any groups concerned.

i. It is expected that any special services, such as laboratory and x-ray, which are desired shall be sought from institutionally based departments, provided that such are capable of offering an appropriate service. These departments reserve the right to render their own charges to the patient and may refuse to render services without payment, provided that refusal is discussed with the physician responsible for the patient.

j. The members of each group have the authority to determine whether they can serve individual patients. However, the university expects that they shall make such decisions with due recognition of their role as faculty members of an institution that has certain community responsibilities, and the university shall endeavor to assist them in achieving this objective.

k. Patients admitted as inpatients from the group may either continue as the individual patients of the physician initially responsible or may be transferred to the care of another physician as may be decided by each program and provided that such is acceptable to the individual patient.

2. *Improved patient care*

The fact that an individual appointment system is an integral part of the group should significantly contribute to a reduction of the impersonality of the former system and the long waiting periods characteristic of the clinic "block" appointment procedure. Since a specific doctor follows a specific patient from the beginning of his care until discharge or transfer, it is expected that improved quality of efficient medical care will result. The presence of an appointment system also helps the doctor better schedule his own time, since he knows on any one day precisely how many patients he is to see, and when, and where. It allows him to make better use of nurses, secretaries, and other personnel.

3. *Financial benefits*

In the old system, the hospital collected a clinic fee for all clinic outpatients based on their individual ability to pay. The hospital received $4.00 for all Title XIX outpatients. Since the hospital was acting as the "provider" of care, it received no additional monies for laboratory or other such services that physicians ordered, and the physicians were not reimbursed for professional services. Under the group plan, the patient becomes a "private" patient, and the physicians make reasonable charges to Title XIX, which now reimburses the hospital and the physicians.

Billing the patient can be handled in several ways, but the bill always emanates from the physicians. The individual doctor or the group can bill, or the groups can pay the hospital or an outside billing agency to set up a separate and distinct physicians' billing office. The latter seems to be the most economical.

Although under the new plan the hospital no longer receives a basic clinic fee, it does receive periodic payment from each group for the space required and allocated to that group. This rent charge is made at an established, predetermined rate and is adjusted only as the costs of operating the facility (heat, light, maintenance, housekeeping, etc.) vary. In addition, since the hospital is no longer the "provider" of care, it can charge Title XIX for the special services that are provided from departments such as laboratory and pharmacy. The rent

covers the hospital costs of operating the outpatient facility. The monies collected for special services should potentially show a surplus, since self-paying patients and non–cost contract third parties pay charges instead of costs. Many of the outpatients are on Medicare. Here, as with Medicare inpatients, many physicians were not submitting bills. Since billing has been established in each group, collection efforts have been improved considerably.

The financial situation has improved enormously. It has improved the hospital's cash flow position, since "rental" payments are made regularly and income to physicians has risen significantly. The provision of special services, on a unit-cost basis on demand, should continue to stimulate improved service, as the ordering physician is under no obligation to utilize these services located at the hospital if their costs are out of line or their work unsatisfactory.

4. *Better utilization of facilities and equipment*

The tendency for doctors to admit patients to the hospital in order to receive proper reimbursement is discouraged by creating a system in which physicians are reimbursed for services on an outpatient basis.* This improves hospital utilization since those patients admitted to the hospital are actually in need of its facilities and services. It also discourages physicians from limiting their x-ray, laboratory, and other special-service requests because they realize the hospital is not reimbursed for them. They now order as the patient's needs indicate, not as the hospital's financial woes dictate.

5. *Better teaching environment*

Under this plan, each program has an organized group within which care can be delivered as they see fit. This allows a better supervised, more highly organized

---

*This is particularly significant in light of recent Blue Cross emphasis on paying for more services on an ambulatory basis.

teaching environment. The removal of non-emergency cases from the emergency department should improve patient care and the teaching experience as well.

• • •

What next?

Once a viable ambulatory service has been established and excellent ancillary service can be provided, the population group that the center serves could be identified. By using all of the various mechanisms for financing health care, this population could be offered a prepaid package of comprehensive health care. This would mean that people covered under this prepaid program would be able to get all of their care from the center or its satellites at a time that is convenient to them.

A word of caution. Before a health center offers prepaid care, it should be willing and able to deliver what is promised. An empty promise in this regard will cause more problems than one can imagine. To test this approach to organization and delivery or health care, it would be wise to first test it on a smaller population group. Student, faculty, and employee groups of the institution would be a good place to start.

• • •

The success or failure of the systems-and-program approach to organization rests on two key factors. First, the program director must be able to see the total picture of the integration of teaching, service, and research as definitive parts of his program and must rely heavily on the consumer of the end products of these programs to determine the worthiness of the product. Second, the administrative inputs must have available information relating to fiscal and economic results. This then creates a partnership between professionals and administration and eliminates the wall that has been built up in institutions by this conflict. When physicians and administrators know their proper roles in the packaging and delivery of health care, it makes an easier approach to solving joint problems.

In most institutions, physicians have looked to administration for an unlimited source of funds without any accountability on the physician's part for the use of these funds. When uneconomical programs were decided upon by the whims and fancies of the physician, administration was supposed to act in a magical fashion and finance these ventures. With the creation of physician program directors, their activity in creating costs will be identified and measurable. The responsibility for proper funding of programs will be fixed at the program level. In effect the physician director becomes a policy maker, and administration gets into its proper role of implementation and provision of facts about the outcome. This relationship will be strengthened by a recognition of the common objectives of both. In most health care situations the physician has looked upon the institution, particularly the hospital, as a workshop, and he has acted without any knowledge of or accountability for the effects of his decisions. Of course, the key in all of this is the proper development and implementation of a total health information system that gives instant information relating to quality, quantity, and cost.

In the experience of Case Hospital, there is a willingness on the part of the physician to participate in this role. However, the one question most frequently asked is, "Who will handle the administrative details?" It then becomes apparent that the administrator of the systems must provide well-trained and qualified people as an input to the programs. In day-to-day operations this administrative team relates directly to their program directors. In addition to the responsibility for maintaining accreditation of the individual programs and collectively the total entity, they have the responsibility for assuring that legal requirements, personnel welfare, and safety regulations are adhered to. It is only common sense to recognize that the physician is not an administrator; but he is the only one equipped with the experience and knowledge to provide and deliver health care and is thus able to formulate policy relating to its entirety. In contrast, the administrator is the one really equipped to interpret policy and make it a working fact. The administrator's role in relation to the program then becomes one of being knowledgeable of the facts and interpreting these to the program director in order that policy can be formulated. The administrator also serves as the catalyst for molding the partnership between the medical profession and the other professionals of the health care team.

If a single, prime attribute of the administrator could be identified, it would be his ability to interpret policy to each individual of the health care team. It then follows that he must be an expert in communications. The systems administrator responsible for administrative inputs to the programs has the overall responsibility of conveying information relating to the total entity.

Educational programs for program administrators today are lacking. This requires the development of an individual who can understand the science of administration coupled with the art of administration. He needs to familiarize himself with the terminology of medicine, the practice of system analysis, the implementation of government and other regulations, and the mysteries of research grants and program budgeting.

What is needed is the evolution of a truly sophisticated health care administrator. He will know a little about everything but will know very few details about specifics. He must become a delegator to experts with ability. He must be able to interpret policy and then measure results

in order to convey to his program director the outcome of policies and ideas. He will, indeed, be the leader of the health care team in its day-to-day operations. This then places the administration in its proper context and relieves the competitive forces created both by economics and conflict of objectives heretofore evidenced. He will not have to be trained to the extent that he will receive a doctorate, but he will definitely have to have the basic tools of accounting, statistics, marketing research, and an understanding of computer operations. His value in this role will increase as he is able to weld the partnership of the health care team.

The health care administrator of the future will have to avail himself to not only the techniques of the practice of administration but also to the versatility of teaching and research. It would seem ludicrous not to continually allow the financing for this individual to keep abreast of changing times. He will be evaluated on his ability to present alternative courses of action along with both social and economic price tags to program directors in order that proper policy can be effected. In effect he becomes the man behind the scenes. His influence will not be that of false power; rather, his influence will be his ability to accumulate, evaluate, and present the case in a scientific manner. He becomes the hard core of the organizational structure upon which the superstructure rests. His satisfaction will come in his relationships with human beings and his ability to develop human resources and mold them into a functional working organization. His security will rest in his ability to be fair in his interpretation of facts and to relate these in human terms to individuals. His stature will be his acceptance by other members of the health care team and his philosophic influence in directing their activities. No longer can he rely on dramaturgy and charisma to bring him the status symbols of a large office with a multibutton phone and thick carpeting. His organizational ties will be important as long as the organization provides him with new techniques on how to do his job better and emphasizes the human role of administration rather than the political and mechanical techniques. His "bag of tricks" will change from one of cunningness to that of understanding human nature and the broad philosophies concerning the packaging and distribution of health care. His quest will be to better satisfy and reward his fellow human, not only in monetary terms but in social and intellectual values as well.

The spectrum of administration will have at its ultimate those best equipped to interpret social and human needs and to cope with the details. At the other end is the man still accustomed to directing in the philosophy that "It's right because I say it's right." This individual's future is very limited, and his existence in the spectrum is short-lived.

What are the ingredients for accomplishing this program in health care administration? Above all, an acceptance of the philosophy that people are human and want to do what is right. Next, this is coupled with an organizational structure that creates an environment in which their efforts can be used to the maximum and and their satisfactions and gratifications can be realized. Emotions are replaced by empathy; an administrator will not only have to place himself in the other person's position but demonstrate by his action that he understands that position. The negative role, e.g., denying requests for funds because there is no money today, must change to a positive attitude. Let us reason together to get the most from our present resources and enlarge our scope of service so that we may justify and pro-

cure more resources. It is predicted that programs in health care administration will evolve to teach the student basic philosophies of human endeavors and that the tools will be made available to use these resources in a productive way for both the consumer and the provider.

With the use of tools such as program budgeting and sophisticated information systems, inputs will be made available both for short- and long-range decisions. Health care has been noted for the lack of information available with which to measure the outputs qualitatively, and it becomes mandatory in this type of organization that qualitative values be set on the measures that are used. Without these, alternative courses of action cannot be selected and resource use cannot be maximized. Administration in the past has been criticized for its operating in a cloak of secrecy. Under the program-system approach, the operation becomes visual and spectators can rapidly see how decisions are made and measure in a predictable fashion the degrees of success or failure. The public can then understand what it is getting, determine how much it is paying for it, and properly interpret its worthiness.

In today's arena there seems to be a veil of secrecy surrounding health care and its distribution. The government has tried to overcome this by pumping large sums of money into this system in order to cut an unidentifiable problem. Until the public can see and understand what it is that is costing it hard-earned dollars, it has every right and reason to question the effectiveness, the quality, and the cost of the system. In this way the public, who is in fact the consumer, can evaluate the worthiness of the various programs of health care.

PART FOUR

IMPLEMENTATION

To gain orientation and momentum as an integral part of the health sciences center, Case Hospital adopted goals that were compatible with those of the center. These goals are to (1) develop and implement the most effective and efficient programs of patient care and health care services, (2) develop or participate in developing educational programs and clinical settings for the education of all types of health care personnel, and (3) develop or participate in developing research programs and clinical settings for research of health care and its administration.

To attain these goals, further broad objectives were developed.

1. Application of all **systems** to existing and experimental **programs** in the hospital, the health sciences center and its affiliates, and the community.
2. Development of a "Sabre System" for information flow, with primary focus on scheduling all patient activities.
3. Development of the Case Hospital information system. This system will combine with the previously mentioned scheduling system to produce a total information system for all phases of health activities. It will have the potential of tying into regional information networks in the future.
4. Development of the medical staff organization in a manner that compliments the systems approach. This involves three distinct steps: (step 1) organization of service committees; (step 2) organization of nurse-physician committees; and (step 3) organization of operational advisory nurse-physician teams.
5. Development of strong public relations through strengthening of the public relations department.

Progress toward achieving these objectives involves special emphasis on industrial engineering techniques, business and finance, nursing, quality control, and information systems.

chapter seven

INDUSTRIAL ENGINEERING TECHNIQUES

Industrial engineering can be directly related to many operating problems described previously and to the "hope" described by former Secretary of Health, Education, and Welfare John Gardner for a greater supply and better use of manpower.

Wages and benefits for employees represent 65% to 70% of total hospital costs. Is this necessary? No. Hospitals have built in this cost. Much of the cost has become hidden. It has become "the way we have always done it." Medical technology has advanced, but manpower utilization for supporting it in the hospital has not. One does not have to look far to find people doing jobs that they are not adequately trained to do, or much further to find people performing tasks for which they are overtrained. Hospitals do not have adequate training programs, adequate job descriptions, adequate scheduling, or adequate organization for carrying out proper manpower utilization. They lack performance standards and methods of measuring volume, quality, and cost. There is not enough guidance for those who need it, and there is too much guidance for those who do not.

Hospitals are in the habit of employing the least skilled people in society. This means that the ordinary type of training program used by other industries may not be adequate. What is the solution? Put imagination to work! Do not follow "traditional" instructions. Identify patient needs and define jobs to meet those needs. Create job descriptions that satisfy the needs of the job to be done. Recruit people who can be trained. Create the best training programs possible. Demand more, and pay well. Create a flexible organization to work in, an organization in which doctors doctor, nurses nurse, and administrators administer. Demand that a person develop his ability, give him responsibility for applying it, and give him the freedom for its application.

Through the use of industrial engineering methodologies, significant improvements can be made in quantitative and qualitative standards, and correlations between standards and cost can be developed. Coupled with methods improvement and training programs, these techniques support improved management techniques, better supervisory control, improved utilization of personnel, improved quality of care and service, and better methods and procedures.

The Commission for Administrative Services in Hospitals in Los Angeles, California, and the Community Systems Foundation of Ann Arbor, Michigan, have been pioneers in the application of industrial engineering in hospitals. In the foreword to its manual *Work Measurement for Hospitals,* the Commission for Administrative Services in Hospitals states:

The application of the philosophy and techniques of work measurement to hospital work is a natural, although quite recent link in the chain of management engineering progress. These principles and tools, used for many years in industry, have, with some modification, been just as successful when applied to hospital work. This has been a revelation to some experienced hospital people, who had felt that their work, by virtue of its varied nature and emphasis on care and service, could not be measured in the traditional manner. The reason for the success of work measurement programs to the many diverse activities and problems of running a hospital is that the approach is basic and universal. The pattern of thinking, the questions asked, the tests which are applied can be used with benefit wherever work is done.*

Among the tools employed in this type of approach are:

Work measurement. This method establishes an equitable relationship between work performed and manpower used through time- and work-sampling studies. Work measurement is valuable in establishing times for performing work and predicting, before the fact, the personnel hours required. This type of prediction may be used to establish equitable staffing guides.

Staffing guides. This method ensures that units are staffed properly for various levels of production.

Operation controls. This method gives supervision hour-by-hour control of personnel utilization. This improves productivity and results in potential payroll savings. Supervisors know the location of their employees and when they are available for new assignments.

Quality control. This method establishes and measures objective standards of quality. This tool makes reliable information about quality available to employees and management. It serves as an indicator of the effects that manipulation of other factors such as cost and volume have on quality.

Flow control. This method ensures that interlinking sequences between activities are in fact carried out between persons, departments, and systems.

Methods improvement. This method evaluates methods of work and operations so that weaknesses may be identified and improved.

Backlog control. This method measures work backlog. Backlog levels are related to performance and staffing requirements in order to detect the effects of performance fluctuation and predict the need for increased staffing.

Performance evaluation. This method factually evaluates employee and supervisory performance on an ongoing basis. This pinpoints various weaknesses and strengths and allows for correction and commendation.

Training programs. This method makes possible the training and retraining of employees and supervisors in light of the information made available by the other tools discussed. Coupled with these, training programs ensure that skills are matched with jobs.

Reporting system. This method keeps employees and management constantly aware of the information provided by the other tools by providing periodic reports. The reporting system should be designed not only to indicate the past and current status but also to indicate exceptions to the standard on a timely basis.

The following three project descriptions serve to show how a number of these tools are actually applied to operating situations.

*Commission for Administrative Services in Hospitals: Work measurement for hospitals, Los Angeles, 1965, The Commission.

MEDICAL SECRETARY POOL

This project involves the systematic organization of a medical secretarial pool. It begins with a description of the purpose and location of the pool and then proceeds to a consideration of supervisory responsibilities, work load, work flow, staffing, and work accomplished.

The primary purpose of the medical secretarial pool is to handle secretarial work directly concerned with committing to or abstracting from records medical information relating to care rendered to patients on an inpatient or outpatient basis and as further defined in this description. In order to establish an effective program to carry out this purpose, *all* requests from outside sources for medical and related information contained in hospital records and all requests to outside sources for medical and related information contained in their records should flow through the medical secretarial pool.

The functions of the medical secretarial pool should be distinguished from those of a medical records library, whose primary purpose is to assemble, code, file, safekeep, and ensure patient records and related documents and to compile and disseminate statistical and other collective data and information relating to the overall program of patient care.

Because of the interrelated functions of the medical secretarial pool and the medical records library, it is desirable to have them located adjacent to one another. If location and size of work load and staff permit, they may be under the same department head or supervisor.

The medical secretarial pool requires the supervision of a person who has a working knowledge of medical terminology, systems of recording and abstracting medical and related information, and medicolegal procedures and implications. The supervisor's main functions are as follows:

1. Establish and maintain effective working rapport between the medi-

cal secretarial pool and the medical staff and all hospital departments and outside parties with which she must coordinate the activities of her department

2. Effectively handle personnel and work problems of a group of medical secretaries

3. Interpret administrative and professional policy to her staff

4. Develop standards of performance and achieve an even distribution of work loads

5. Assist in the design of forms and filing and check system

6. Review transcriptions and other records for consistency, accuracy, and completeness

7. Conduct in-service training for secretarial and clerical personnel

8. Perform job analyses and prepare procedures

9. Safeguard confidentiality of medical information, and release information in line with organizational policy

10. Prepare the budget for the medical secretarial pool

11. Select equipment best suited to the advancement of the medical secretarial program, taking into consideration efficient utilization of space and personnel time

Work load description

Work performed in the medical secretarial pool will include the following activities.

Transcription. In order of priority, transcription and medical secretarial work are performed in relation to the following:

1. Consultations

   EXAMPLE:
   a. Use "medical report" form for complete transcription.
   b. Indicate whether the patient is an inpatient or clinic patient.
   c. Type the name of the referring physician at the upper left-hand side of the form.

d. Distribute copies as follows:

For inpatients. White copy to the hospital chart; send to floor immediately if patient is still hospitalized. Pale yellow copy to our "temporary" records file for our reference. Pink copy to the attending physician. Gold copy to the consulting physician. Green copy to the attending physician's hospital department head.

For outpatients. White copy to the clinic chart. Pale yellow copy to our "temporary" records file for our reference. Pink copy to the attending physician. Green copy to the attending physician's hospital department head.

2. Referrals
3. Discharge summaries
4. Release of and requests for information
5. Operative reports
6. Progress notes
7. Follow-up notes
8. Conference reports
9. Staff meetings
10. Memorandums
11. Miscellaneous

    a. Correspondence to other physician's private and governmental agencies, etc.
    b. Research papers (for authorized research)
    c. Papers (to be presented at meetings, conferences, etc.)

NOTE: Clear guidelines should be drawn as to which departments will process certain types of work.

EXAMPLE:

Insurance departments. Certain Bureau of Public Assistance cases, life insurance applications, Department of Employment cases, and other cases with possible legal involvement may be handled by the insurance department. If the insurance department sends a form to a physician for completion, with or without a chart, the response may be dictated to the medical secretarial pool. Unless the form or the chart is available to the pool at the time the dictation is transcribed, there may be some confusion as to transcription procedure. The pool should be notified of impending dictation so that it can obtain the patient's correct name, physician, and patient file number if they are not provided in the dictation. This confusion can be decreased by memos forwarded from the insurance department, but this does not always occur, and the dictation must be held until the form is received. Some delay may also occur in the time lapse of chart transfer.

Community services department. Transcription and subsequent copy typing of material identified with the community services department by virtue of budget or content could be done by that department on the basis that community services department action is ultimately required. Considerations for such include delay in the pool in transcription of material from discs because of transporting of discs between departments, increased control of the completion of all transcription from all records, unpredictability of transcription work load for community services department, which results in work scheduling problems, and the possible loss of discs in the courier system. If, however, the medical secretarial pool transcribes rough drafts of dictation for the community services department, there may be merit in sending the transcription to that department for appropriate action since a decision about the distribution of copies must be made and arrangements for duplicating, etc. may also follow. Decisions need to be made on dictation of the following nature: requests for films, résumés of new products, personal research notes, and personal letters to outside physicians or parties. Physicians should be apprised of the procedure and departmental responsibilities involved in order that they may allow adequate time for processing dictation indicated as a community services department's function.

Pathology department. Although there may be arrangements for the completion of clinical pathologic conference reports in the community services department, their transcription and total preparation is often a function of the medical secretarial pool. It is often required that the draft copy be reworked and changed, requiring additional retyping as the pathologists desire. This is very time-consuming. Consideration should be given to assigning the final copy typing to the pathology secretary. Typing of rough drafts may remain a medical secretarial function. The secretarial personnel available in the pathology department should prepare autopsy reports.

Social-medical department. In some instances, forms specify information that must be completed by a social caseworker, and it is sometimes required that the knowledge of a trained social worker in the social-medical department be utilized to effect completion. In many instances the forms are sent directly to physicians, who dictate the answers, thus involving the medical secretarial pool in the job. Completion of these forms should be a medical secretarial pool function. When completion is required by social caseworkers, the chart and form could be forwarded to that department the same as they are to physicians. Telephone calls related to social welfare problems (other than those related to forms) should be transferred to that department.

X-ray department. Secretarial work related to the x-ray department will not normally be handled by the medical secretarial pool.

Billing. Billings for reimbursement of services performed may be made on certain forms or letter responses. The question of which department is to take action on billing functions is worth consideration. If the insurance department forwards forms or responses that are related to third-party attorney inquiries to the medical record librarian, the librarian places the form in the physician's chart box for his dictation.

Stenography. When emergent time requirements or the nature of the work to be done makes machine dictation impractical, stenographic dictation may be permitted at the discretion of the supervisor.

Miscellaneous. Other types of transcription, stenography, or secretarial work (i.e., research, administrative, etc.) may be done when work load permits at the discretion of the supervisor.

Work flow

Dictation. When prenumbered telephone dictation discs are completed, they are removed from the machine by the control clerk. The control clerk scans the record, marking on the corresponding paper index tape or envelope (1) the point at which the dictation begins, (2) the date, (3) the type of dictation (consultations, referrals, etc.), (4) the name of the person dictating, (5) the priority ("stat" cases only), and (6) the point at which dictation ends.

She scans all dictation on the record, enters its number and date in a control record, and gives the record to the supervisor for assignment to a medical secretary.

Release of information. This involves the release of medical and related information contained in the records to outside physicians, agencies, health plan members, etc. upon their request. All telephone and mail requests received for medical and related information contained in the records are screened by the control clerk. Telephone requests include calls seeking such information as the most current date of a child's immunization or the progress made in completion of a welfare applicant's forms. Mail requests seek a variety of information, some of which are not handled by the pool. Requests appropriately handled by the pool will be processed by the control clerk as follows:

1. Set up a control record of the request
2. Ascertain that the proper permits and releases have been signed
3. Obtain the related records
4. Send the request to the appropriate physician and make the related records available to him
5. Receive a reply from the physician (When the physician requests that a portion of the record be abstracted, she receives the abstracting instructions from the physician and abstracts the record or, if necessary, has the supervisor abstract it. When the physician dictates the information to be released, she receives the transcribed dictation from a medical secretary.)
6. Obtain the physician's signature when necessary
7. Mail the information to the requesting party
8. Make copies for inclusion in the chart by the records room
9. Return the record to the record room
10. Make proper entries in the control record

Requests for information. When requests for medical and related information contained in the records of outside physicans, agencies, etc. originate within the organization; all requests to outside parties for medical and related information should originate on a form No. 128020, "Request for Medical Information," and be sent out through the medical secretarial pool.

Staffing

The following staff guide is used to ensure that the medical secretarial pool is properly staffed for the various levels of production.

Title	Number required
Supervisor	1
Medical secretaries	4
Control clerk	1
Filing clerk*	1

Typical job description

Position: Representative job description for medical secretary

Supervisor: Medical record librarian

Primary purpose: (1) To transcribe medical dictation by physicians of discharge summaries, operation reports, and letters, and (2) to process to completion a variety of types of correspondence.

Duties and responsibilities: (1) To operate remote-control dictating equipment, replace dictating discs as they are filled with dictation, and label and/or number dictation strips in sequence so that dictation is transcribed in the order in which it is taken from the recorders; (2) comply with instructions from physicians with regard to material requiring immediate transcription and transmission; (3) transcribe discharge summaries, operations reports, or letters according to the format

---

*If there is sufficient clerical work load in addition to that done by the control clerk, a filing clerk should be used to file and "search" pool records, answer phones, run errands, deliver messages, assist the control clerk during peak work loads, and perform other miscellaneous tasks.

provided, paying special attention to the number of copies required and to whom copies are to be transmitted; (4) as discharge summaries, operation reports, or letters are transcribed, process as determined in detailed procedure, e.g., when a discharge summary is transcribed, pull identification card from physician's file, attach it to transcribed discharge summary, and transmit to medical record librarian; (5) keep dictation strips showing number of minutes of dictation transcribed or otherwise, as directed, maintain work loads; (6) refer to medical dictionary, *Physician's Desk Reference,* medical terminology and anatomy texts, and other references as required to determine correct spelling of dictated terms; (7) transcribe a minimum of 5,000 dictated words a day; and (8) process to completion correspondence as directed in detailed procedure provided for this purpose.

General responsibility: The medical secretary will be provided with detailed work procedures because the material she transcribes is closely related to the functions of the technical analysis of records. Technical supervision will be provided by the medical record librarian. Decisions concerning problems will be determined by the medical record librarian.

Knowledge, skill, and special ability: The position requires (1) knowlege of the language of medicine, i.e., to be able to understand the structure of the human body, how it functions, what disease processes affect it, and signs, symptoms, and test findings of disease processes, so that when she is transcribing technical and difficult dictation of medical terms, and sometimes, poor dictation, her familiarity with the language will make it possible for her to maintain a consistent speed in transcribing; (2) skill in typing and operation of remote-control dictating equipment and, if required, operation of photostating equipment; and (3) ability to transcribe a minimum of 5,000 words a day.

Reporting

The supervisor of this particular pool utilizes the chart in Fig. 7-1 to keep a record of the work performed. Through the use of these charts, reports similar to Fig. 7-2 can be made each month. In submitting the report, the supervisor might comment as follows:

Employee hours continue over budget because of an increased work load and backlog build-up. The training of two new medical secretaries has contributed to the backlog. This should diminish as their work improves. The additional work load consists primarily of physicians' personal letters, for which a charge is now being made by the business office.

This report is simple to tabulate, and

								Comments			
Disc no.	Current	Backlog	Total minutes	Hospital	Clinic	Retype	Redictate	Other	Type: operative report, consultation, etc.
1	X		20	X					Consultation
2	X		10		X		X	Could not understand original disc.	Consultation

J. D. — Employee name Med. Sec. — Title Jan. 18, 1969 — Date

Fig. 7-1. Work load record.

Employee	Days worked	Total minutes of transcription	This month daily average min.	Last month daily average min.
gam (new)	23	577	25.09	61.08*
fed (new)	17	859	50.53	63.92*
mjs	22	1,391	63.23	63.00
tol	19	1,769	93.11	90.09
pjw	22	1,854	84.27	82.31
csp	23	1,564	68.00	69.10
	126	7,014	64.04	71.58

*Statistics for old employee

Estimated backlog:	This month	Last month
	1,500 min.	500 min.

Fig. 7-2. Productivity report.

it gives the supervisor a good guide as to how well her medical secretaries are doing. The total minutes of backlog is an estimate calculated by totaling the length of the dictation for each disc in the backlog, taking into consideration the expected difficulty in transcribing. This is done by the control clerk as the discs are sorted and assigned to the secretaries. The backlog estimate is useful in weighing the need for overtime or additional employees, which in turn can affect long-range planning.

This example has shown a very easy general application of some of the industrial engineering methodology mentioned previously. The second project deals with work measurement and its use in determining the work time involved in performing various tasks.

CONTINUOUS TIME STUDY

The continuous time study reveals the productive work requirements of clinical laboratory technicians. This second project describes how a large community hospital developed a continuous time study that would reveal the nature of work being done by clinical laboratory technicians and the percentages of productive and nonproductive work involved.

The study was developed to determine the amount of time that technicians spend in productive work in specific laboratory units and was applied to a predetermined work period to reveal actual productive time in these units. A further step was to identify specific tasks to reveal the nature of the work being done. Specifically, the purposes were stated as follows:

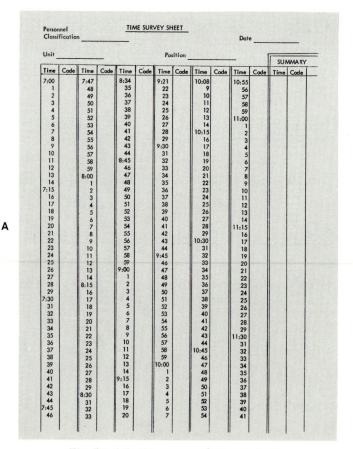

Fig. 7-3, A-C. Time survey sheet (see text).

1. Design a method for estimating the amount of time personnel spend in productive work
2. Design a method for estimating the cost, in terms of personnel time, of producing certain laboratory tests and procedures
3. Apply the method for estimating productive personnel time to a predetermined work period to obtain information about actual productive time
4. Apply the method for estimating the cost, in terms of personnel time, of producing laboratory tests and procedures

During the study, 758.7 hours of actual work among 20 technicians in seven clinical units were observed by student laboratory technicians whose sole assignment during the study was to observe and record laboratory technicians' work.

The students used the following lists of coded activities to record work on the recording sheets shown in Fig. 7-3.

CODE NUMBERS

Bacteriology

1 Urines
2 Stools
3 Miscellaneous swabs
4 Sputum
5 Bronchial washings
6 Nasopharynx, nose, and throat swabs
7 CSF
8 Body fluids

Personnel Classification _____   Date _____

Unit _____   Position _____   SUMMARY

Time	Code	Time	Code	Time	Code	Time	Code	Time	Code	Time	Code	Time	Code
11:42		12:29		1:16		2:03		2:50		3:37			
43		12:30		17		4		51		38			
44		31		18		5		52		39			
11:45		32		19		6		53		40			
46		33		20		7		54		41			
47		34		21		8		55		42			
48		35		22		9		56		43			
49		36		23		10		57		44			
50		37		24		11		58		3:45			
51		38		25		12		59		46			
52		39		26		13		3:00		47			
53		40		27		14		1		48			
54		41		28		2:15		2		49			
55		42		29		16		3		50			
56		43		1:30		17		4		51			
57		44		31		18		5		52			
58		12:45		32		19		6		53			
59		46		33		20		7		54			
12:00		47		34		21		8		55			
1		48		35		22		9		56			
2		49		36		23		10		57			
3		50		37		24		11		58			
4		51		38		25		12		59			
5		52		39		26		13		4:00			
6		53		40		27		14		1			
7		54		41		28		3:15		2			
8		55		42		29		16		3			
9		56		43		2:30		17		4			
10		57		44		31		18		5			
11		58		1:45		32		19		6			
12		59		46		33		20		7			
13		1:00		47		34		21		8			
14		1		48		35		22		9			
12:15		2		49		36		23		10			
16		3		50		37		24		11			
17		4		51		38		25		12			
18		5		52		39		26		13			
19		6		53		40		27		14			
20		7		54		41		28		4:15			
21		8		55		42		29		16			
22		9		56		43		3:30		17			
23		10		57		44		31		18			
24		11		58		2:45		32		19			
25		12		59		46		33		20			
26		13		2:00		47		34		21			
27		14		1		48		35		22			
28		1:15		2		49		36		23			

B

Fig. 7-3, cont'd. For legend see opposite page.

B Sign for OR specimens

C Number and date specimen, card, carbon; check charge slip

D Centrifuge urines, CSF, fluids

E Plate and gram stain

F Read plates and gram stains

G Identification of organisms (transplants)

H Sensitivities

I Preliminaries

J Report culture

K Report sensitivities

L Type up cards and slips

M File cards

N Media in and out of refrigerator, cultures in and out of incubator, CO_2 jars

O A.M. setup

9 Blood cultures

B Number and date specimen, carbon; tag specimen

C Read cultures daily

D Positives, tap, gram stain, plate, identify, sensitivity

E Final check (gram stain and plate)

F Preliminaries

G Report

H Type card and slips

I Collect blood cultures

10 AFB cultures

B Sign for OR specimens

C Number and date specimen, card, carbon, tags, and slides; check charge slip

D Centrifuge urines, gastrics, fluids

E Set up urines, gastrics, grind tissue

F Concentration procedures

G Set up media and slides

H Plate and AFB smear

I Stain AFB smears

J Read cultures weekly

K Read AFB smears

L Identification (smears, transplants)

Fig. 7-3, cont'd. For legend see p. 128.

M Report cultures and smears
N Type cards
11 Fungus cultures
  B Sign for OR specimens
  C Number and date specimen, card, carbon, tags; check charge slip
  D Centrifuge if necessary
  E Plate and wet mount
  F Set up media and slides
  G Read wet mount
  H Read cultures weekly
  I Identification
  J Report wet mounts
  K Report cultures
  L Type cards
12 Parasitology
  B Number and date specimen, card, carbon
  C Ova and parasite wet mounts and search
  D Concentration for ova
  E Search for tapeworm head
  F Occult bloods
  G Microscopics
  H Trypsin
  I Fat
  J Starch
  K Report results
  L Type cards
13 Serology
  B Number and date specimen, card, carbon; tag for tube
  C Centrifuge
  D Aspirate off serum
  E Obtain sheet and type
  F Check sheet, pack, and mail
  G Record report on card
  H Type card
14 Virology
The procedure is essentially same as for serology except for freezing and sending of specimen to state laboratory
15 Nursery formula
  B Number and date specimen; set up card
  C Melt agar
  D Plate
  E Read plates
  F Report results
  G Clean up
16 Media preparation
  A Autoclave
  B Prepare media
17 Glassware
18 Solutions
19 Miscellaneous procedures
  A Urine colony counts

  B Quellungs
  C Cough plates
  D Tellurite plates
  E Tube dilution sensitivities
  F *Leptospira*
  G *Toxoplasma*
  H Serology (*Neisseria gonorrhoeae*)
  I Guinea pigs
  J State laboratory
  K Bone marrow
20 Cytology
  B Centrifuge if necessary
  C Set up jar
  D Set up slides
  E Make smears
  F Deliver to cytology department
21 Morgue
  A Obtain specimens from morgue
  B Plant, identify, etc.
  C Report results
22 Standby time
23 Coffee break
24 Lunch
25 Teaching
26 Learning
27 Personal time
28 General housekeeping
29 Clerical (professional), i.e., writing reports, etc.
30 Clerical (nonprofessional)
31 Clerical and check supplies
32 Special surverys
  A *Escherichia coli*
  B *Staphylococcus*
  C Water
  D Solutions
33 Telephone conversation (within labs)
  A Giving information
  B Obtaining information
  C Referring to another person
34 Telephone conversation (outside labs)
  A Giving information
  B Obtaining information
  C Referring to another person
35 Person-to-person (within labs)
  A Giving information
  B Obtaining information
  C Referring to another person
36 Person-to-person (outside labs)
  A Giving information
  B Obtaining information
  C Referring to another person
37 Interdepartmental errands
38 Pickup and receiving
Chemistry
1 Number specimens
2 Centrifuge specimens

3   Maintenance (nonprofessional) e.g., put glassware away, clean table tops, fill water baths and distilled water jugs, etc.
4   Maintenance (professional), e.g., clean machines and replace worn-out parts
5   Mark tubes
6   Ordering
7   Lunch
8   Coffee break
9   Personal time
10 Standby time (nothing to do)
11 Lab meeting (learning)
12 Actual time obtaining blood from patient
13 Time spent going to and coming from patient on ward
14 Clerical (professional), e.g., calculation of tests
15 Clerical (nonprofessional), e.g., transfer names, results, etc.
16 Research (obtaining professional information, e.g., reading, technique, and statistics
17 Administration (reports)
18 Telephone conversation (within labs)
    A Giving information
    B Obtaining information
    C Referring to another person
19 Telephone conversation (outside labs)
    A Giving information
    B Obtaining information
    C Referring to another person
20 Person-to-person (within labs)
    A Giving information
    B Obtaining information
    C Referring to another person
21 Person-to-person (outside labs)
    A Giving information
    B Obtaining information
    C Referring to another person
    S + Test code number = Solution
    U + Test code number = Urine
    G + Test code number = Gastric
    C CSF
22 Amylase
23 Acetone (serum)
24 Na
25 K
26 Cl
27 CO_2
28 CO_2 (micro)
29 Barbiturates
30 Bilirubin (direct and indirect)
31 Bromide
32 BSP
33 BUN
34 Urea (clearance)

35 Ca
36 Ca (micro)
37 Cephalin-cholesterol flocculation
38 Cholesterol
39 Cholesterol esters
40 Congo red test
41 Creatine
42 Creatinine
43 Creatinine clearance
44 CSF protein
45 CSF colloidal gold
46 Electrophoresis (Hb)
47 Electrophoresis (protein)
48 Fibrinogen
49 Gamma globulin
50 Gastric analysis
51 Glucose
52 Glucose tolerance
53 Glucose (urine)
54 Icterus index
55 Iron (serum)
56 LAP
57 LDH
58 Lipase
59 Phosphorus
60 PBI
61 pH (blood)
62 Porphyrins
63 Phosphatase (acid and alkaline)
64 Salicylates
65 Serotonin
66 Sulfonamide
67 Sweat electrolytes
68 Thymol turbidity
69 Total protein
70 A/G ratio
71 Transaminase (SGOT and SGPT)
72 Uric acid
73 Urinary calculi
74 Xylose tolerance
75 Specimen to go to bioscience
76 Orinase test
77 Diagnex test

Cytology
1   Number specimens
2   Centrifuge specimens
3   Maintenance (nonprofessional), i.e., clean table tops, glassware
4   Maintenance (professional), i.e., clean microscope and aerosol machine
5   Make smears
6   Ordering
7   Fix smears
8   Coffee break
9   Personal time
10 Standby time
11 Time spent obtaining specimens from office

12 Time spent taking slips to office
13 Stain specimens
14 Clerical (professional), i.e., write reports
15 Clerical (nonprofessional), i.e., type cards
16 Research, reading, etc.
17 Making up solutions
18 Refilling staining jars
19 Obtain sputum from patient with aerosol machine
20 Time spent getting machine ready for sputum test
21 Microscopic reading of slides
  A Cervical
  B Miscellaneous
22 File slides
23 Take jars to bacteriology department
24 Mount slides
25 Time spent taking slides to physicians
26 Time spent picking up supplies
27 Time spent taking reports to office
28 Make smears from miscellaneous specimens
29 Telephone conversation (within labs)
  A Giving information
  B Obtaining information
  C Referring to another person
30 Telephone conversation (outside labs)
  A Giving information
  B Obtaining information
  C Referring to another person
31 Person-to-person (within labs)
  A Giving information
  B Obtaining information
  C Referring to another person
32 Person-to-person (outside labs)
  A Giving information
  B Obtaining information
  C Referring to another person

Blood bank
1 Crossmatching
2 Serology
3 Pick up blood
4 Check bank
5 Receive and check delivery of blood
6 Cleaning apparatus
7 Clerical
8 Departmental meetings
9 Lunch
10 Coffee break
11 Standby time
12 Personal
13 Teaching
14 Telephone conversation (within labs)
  A Giving information
  B Obtaining information
  C Referring to another person

15 Telephone conversation (outside labs)
  A Giving information
  B Obtaining information
  C Referring to another person
16 Person-to-person (within labs)
  A Giving information
  B Obtaining information
  C Referring to another person
17 Person-to-person (outside labs)
  A Giving information
  B Obtaining information
  C Referring to another person
18 "Stat" work
19 Give out blood
20 Check supplies
21 Order blood from blood bank

Hematology
1 Heparinized bloods
2 Clotted bloods
3 Slides
4 Blood by finger stick
5 Hematocrits
6 Hemoglobins
7 Counts
8 CSF and other fluids
9 Lee-White
10 RBC fragility (at bedside)
11 RBC fragility (in lab)
12 Bleeding and clotting times
13 Sickle cell preps (at bedside)
14 Sickle cell preps (in lab)
15 Bone marrows
16 Standby time
17 Coffee break
18 Lunch
19 Teaching
20 Lab meetings (learning)
21 Personal time
22 General housekeeping
23 Clerical (professional)
24 Clerical (nonprofessional)
25 Clerical and check supplies
26 Telephone conversation (within labs)
  A Giving information
  B Obtaining information
  C Referring to another person
27 Telephone conversation (outside labs)
  A Giving information
  B Obtaining information
  C Referring to another person
28 Person-to-person (within labs)
  A Giving information
  B Obtaining information
  C Referring to another person
29 Person-to-person (outside labs)
  A Giving information
  B Obtaining information

C Referring to another person
30 Obtain blood specimens from patient
31 Going between lab and patient
32 Administrative time

Histology

1 Placing tissue in paraffin bath (routine)
2 Embedding (routine)
3 Cooling (routine)
4 Labeling blocks (routine)
5 Cutting (routine)
6 Counting blocks
7 Set up instruments, etc. (routine)
8 Drying (routine)
9 Staining (routine)
10 Mounting, cleaning, and labeling (routine)
11 Checking labels
12 Cleaning apparatus, etc.
13 Sorting (gross)
14 Checking (gross)
15 Labeling carriers (gross)
16 Set up equipment (gross)
17 Assist with gross
18 Frozen sections
19 Special stains
20 Autopsy material
21 Preparing solutions
22 "Stat" work
23 Teaching
24 Filing blocks, slides, specimens, etc.
25 Sharpening knives
26 Mechanical maintenance
27 Preparing blocks for numbering
28 Preparing slides with albumin
29 Book work
30 Delivering slides
31 Numbering gross
32 Starting automatic tissue processor
33 Making slide label
34 Telephone conversation (within labs)
   A Giving information
   B Obtaining information
   C Referring to another person
35 Telephone conversation (outside labs)
   A Giving information
   B Obtaining information
   C Referring to another person
36 Person-to-person (within labs)
   A Giving information
   B Obtaining information
   C Referring to another person
37 Person-to-person (outside labs)
   A Giving information
   B Obtaining information
   C Referring to another person
38 Personal time
39 Lunch

40 Standby time
41 Coffee break

Pathology

1 Addis count
2 Albumin (quantitative)
3 Basal metabolic rate
4 Bence Jones protein
5 Benedict's quantitative sugar test
6 Bile
7 Calcium
8 Concentration test
9 Dilution test
10 Fibrindex
11 Partial thromboplastin time (PTT)
12 Prothrombin consumption
13 Prothrombin time
14 Skin tests
15 Thromboplastin generation time
16 Urinalysis (partial)
17 Urinalysis (complete)
18 Urobilinogen (fecal)
19 Urobilinogen (urine)
20 Pregnancy test
21 Centrifuging of specimens
22 Clean up and care of equipment
23 Collection of blood
24 Coffee break
25 Lab conference
26 Lunch
27 Preparation of reagents
28 Standby time
29 PSP test
30 Telephone conversation (within labs)
   A Giving information
   B Obtaining information
   C Referring to another person
31 Telephone conversation (outside labs)
   A Giving information
   B Obtaining information
   C Referring to another person
32 Person-to-person (within labs)
   A Giving information
   B Obtaining information
   C Referring to another person
33 Person-to-person (outside labs)
   A Giving information
   B Obtaining information
   C Referring to another person
34 Removal of specimens and slips to be typed from basket
35 Personal time
36 Obtaining supplies from another department
37 Clerical (writing reports, book entries)
38 Readying of equipment
39 Securing typed slips from office and handing in reports

40 Checking supplies and ordering
41 Maintenance of equipment
42 Research (obtaining professional information)

The time survey sheet (see Fig. 7-3, *A-C*) is designed for use in continuous time observation studies. It may be used by a person observing an employee at work or by the employee himself. Used by the employee, it enables him to record various increments in his daily routine without bothering with a stopwatch. It is quite useful in making long-range growth projections and cost analysis where random sampling studies are not deemed feasible.

To use this sheet it is necessary to develop a code corresponding to the major activities comprising an individual job. These codes are used to record activities since it is obviously easier to record a number than to write a detailed explanation of an activity. As an example, if the code for coffee break is 2 and if the employee takes a coffee break from 10:00 to 10:15, he draws a horizontal line between 9:59 and 10:00 and another horizontal line after 10:15; in the code column he writes the number "2."

Using cytology as an example, where one technician worked from 8 A.M. to noon, and directing our attention to the cytology code list on p. 138 and the recording sheet shown in Fig. 7-4, *A*, it was found that the technician began work at 8 A.M. and engaged in activity No. 11, i.e., obtaining specimens from the office. At 8:03 A.M., 3 minutes later, she began numbering specimens and continued to do so until 8:13 A.M., when she began clerical work. The clerical work required a period of 12 minutes, until 8:25 A.M., at which time the technician switched to staining specimens. Specimen staining continued until 9 A.M., when she took a 7-minute coffee break, and then resumed staining specimens at 9:07 A.M.

Activity codes continued to be recorded opposite corresponding times until the end of the work period, in this case 12 P.M. (Fig. 7-4, *B*). If the work period had extended into the afternoon, the remaining pages of the recording form would have been used. At the end of the work period, the total time for each activity was summarized in the appropriate column on the form. Total times from the summary column were then used to determine the cumulative totals at the end of the study.

For the particular day shown, the technician worked 4 hours; her payroll time shown on the departmental books was also 4 hours, indicating that she was paid 100% of her working time.

At the end of the 7 days, the coded activities were divided into three categories: (1) direct productive time, (2) indirect productive time, and (3) nonproductive time (see chart on p. 138). Comparisons were drawn between each of these categories. Additionally, the time actually worked was compared to payroll time on the departmental books (see chart).

Similar comparison in all of the laboratory units gave the following results.

Bacteriology

In a work period of 77.8 hours actually worked, direct productive time plus indirect productive time equaled 86.8% whereas nonproductive time equaled 13.2%. Since payroll time for the same work period was 88.8% of the time actually worked, direct productive time plus indirect productive time equaled 96.6% of payroll time.

Blood bank

In a work period of 77.8 hours actually worked, direct productive time plus indirect productive time equaled 84.3% whereas nonproductive time equaled 15.7%. Since payroll time for the same work was 92.0% of the time actually worked, direct productive time plus indirect productive time equaled 91.1% of payroll time.

TIME SURVEY SHEET

Personnel Classification **LAB. TECH**

Date **Nov 14, 1968**

Unit **CYTOLOGY**   Position _____

1

SUMMARY

Time	Code	Time	Code	Time	Code	Time	Code	Time	Code	Time	Code	Time	Code
7:00		7:47		8:34		9:21		10:08		10:55			
1		48		35		22		9		56			
2		49		36		23		10		57			
3		50		37		24		11		58			
4		51		38		25		12		59			
5		52		39		26		13		11:00			
6		53		40		27		14		1			
7		54		41		28		10:15		2			
8		55		42		29		16		3			
9		56		43		9:30		17		4			
10		57		44		31		18		5			
11		58		8:45		32		19		6			
12		59		46		33		20	13	7			
13		8:00	11	47		34		21		8			
14		1		48		35		22		9			
7:15		2		49		36		23		10			
16		3	1	50		37		24		11			
17		4		51		38		25		12			
18		5		52		39		26		13			
19		6		53		40		27		14			
20		7		54		41		28		11:15			
21		8		55		42		29		16			
22		9		56		43		10:30		17			
23		10		57		44		31		18			
24		11		58		9:45		32		19			
25		12		59		46		33		20			
26		13	15	9:00	8	47		34		21			
27		14		1		48		35		22			
28		8:15		2		49		36		23			
29		16		3		50		37		24			
7:30		17		4		51		38		25			
31		18		5		52		39		26			
32		19		6		53		40		27			
33		20		7	13	54		41		28			
34		21		8		55		42		29			
35		22		9		56		43		11:30			
36		23		10		57		44		31			
37		24		11		58		10:45		32			
38		25	13	12		59		46		33			
39		26		13		10:00		47		34			
40		27		14		1		48		35			
41		28		9:15		2		49		36			
42		29		16		3		50		37			
43		8:30		17		4		51		38			
44		31		18		5		52		39			
7:45		32		19		6	24	53		40			
46		33		20		7		54		41			

A

Fig. 7-4, **A** and **B**. Time survey sheet for cytology department (see text).

2

Personnel
Classification _____   Date _____

Unit _____   Position _____

Time	Code	Time	Code	Time	Code	Time	Code	Time	Code	Time	Code	Time	Code (SUMMARY)
11:42		12:29		1:16		2:03		2:50		3:37		10	1
43		12:30		17		4		51		38		5	3
44		31		18		5		52		39		7	8
11:45		32		19		6		53		40		5	10
46		33		20		7		54		41		3	11
47		34		21		8		55		42		93	13
48		35		22		9		56		43		6	14
49		36		23		10		57		44		12	15
50		37		24		11		58		3:45		76	21A
51		38		25		12		59		46		14	24
52		39		26		13		3:00		47		4	25
53		40		27		14		1		48		5	31A
54		41		28		2:15		2		49		240 MIN.	
55	10	42		29		16		3		50			
56		43		1:30		17		4		51			
57		44		31		18		5		52			
58		12:45		32		19		6		53			
59	END	46		33		20		7		54			
12:00		47		34		21		8		55			
1		48		35		22		9		56			
2		49		36		23		10		57			
3		50		37		24		11		58			
4		51		38		25		12		59			
5		52		39		26		13		4:00			
6		53		40		27		14		1			
7		54		41		28		3:15		2			
8		55		42		29		16		3			
9		56		43		2:30		17		4			
10		57		44		31		18		5			
11		58		1:45		32		19		6			
12		59		46		33		20		7			
13		1:00		47		34		21		8			
14		1		48		35		22		9			
12:15		2		49		36		23		10			
16		3		50		37		24		11			
17		4		51		38		25		12			
18		5		52		39		26		13			
19		6		53		40		27		14			
20		7		54		41		28		4:15			
21		8		55		42		29		16			
22		9		56		43		3:30		17			
23		10		57		44		31		18			
24		11		58		2:45		32		19			
25		12		59		46		33		20			
26		13		2:00		47		34		21			
27		14		1		48		35		22			
28		1:15		2		49		36		23			

B

Fig. 7-4, cont'd. For legend see opposite page.

CYTOLOGY

Direct productive time*		Indirect productive time—cont'd	
Activity code number	*Total time (minutes)*	*Activity code number*	*Total time (minutes)*
1	61.0	31	
2	20.0	A	35.0
5	0.0	B	0.0
7	0.0	C	0.0
13	374.5		35.0
19	0.0	32	
21		A	0.0
A	312.0	B	0.0
B	63.0	C	0.0
	375.0		0.0
24	67.0	Total minutes	243.5
28	7.0	Total hours:	4.1
Total minutes	904.5		
Total hours:	15.1		

Nonproductive time‡

8	17.0
9	9.0
10	26.0
Total minutes	52.0
Total hours:	0.8

Indirect productive time†

3	41.5
4	0.0
6	0.0
11	19.0
12	0.0
14	35.0
15	47.0
16	0.0
17	11.0
18	15.0
20	0.0
22	10.0
23	4.0
25	14.0
26	0.0
27	0.0
29	
A	0.0
B	0.0
C	0.0
	0.0
30	
A	9.0
B	3.0
C	0.0
	12.0

Actual time on job

	Minutes		Hours
Direct productive time	904.5	=	15.1
Indirect productive time	243.5	=	4.1
Nonproductive time	52.0	=	0.8
Total	1,200.0	=	20.0
When 20.0 hours	100.0% actual time on job		
15.1 direct hours	75.5%		
4.1 indirect hours	20.5%	=	96.0%
0.8 nonproductive hours	4.0%		
	(100.0% of days worked)		

Payroll time for same work period§

20.0 hours	2.5 8-hour days paid
20.0 hours	2.5 8-hour days actually worked
2.5 days worked	100% of 2.5 days paid

*Time spent directly in the production of laboratory tests.
†Time spent indirectly in the production of laboratory tests and all other time working the laboratory unit.
‡Time during which no work was produced.
§Time recorded on the payroll to be paid for in salaries.

Chemistry

In a work period of 170.5 hours actually worked, direct productive time plus indirect productive time equaled 87.4% whereas nonproductive time equaled 12.6%; payroll time for the same work period equaled 98.7% of the time actually worked.

Cytology

In a work period of 20.0 hours actually worked, direct productive time plus indirect productive time equaled 96.0% whereas nonproductive work equaled 4.0%. Since payroll time for the same period was 100.0% of the time actually worked, direct productive time plus indirect productive time equaled 96.0% of payroll time.

Hematology

In a work period of 160.7 hours actually worked, direct productive time plus indirect productive time equaled 80.7% whereas nonproductive time equaled 19.3%. Since payroll time for the same period was 97.0% of the time actually worked, direct productive time plus indirect productive time equaled 83.1% of payroll time.

Histology

In a work period of 96.0 hours actually worked, direct productive time plus indirect productive time equaled 98.7% whereas nonproductive time equaled 1.3%. Since payroll time for the same work period was 85.8% of the time actually worked, direct productive time plus indirect productive time equaled 112.8% of payroll time.

Pathology

In a work period of 91.5 hours actually worked, direct productive time plus indirect productive time equaled 83.4% whereas nonproductive time equaled 16.6%. Since payroll time for the same work period was 118.3% of the time actually worked, direct productive time plus in-

direct productive time equaled 68.2% of payroll time.

• • •

Since separate lists of coded activities were used for each clinical laboratory unit because of individual differences in work and work procedures, an interchange of activities between direct productive time and indirect productive time categories may have occurred. When making general comparisons therefore, it was deemed advisable to combine these two categories as representing all productive work of any type.

Taking a look at all seven units combined and referring to Figs. 7-5 and 7-6, we find that in a work period of 758.7 hours actually worked, direct productive time plus indirect productive time equaled 88.2% whereas nonproductive time equaled 11.8%. Since payroll time for the same work period was 97.2% of the time actually worked, direct productive time plus indirect productive time equaled 90.9% of payroll time. The fact should be noted that although payroll time equaled 97.2% of the time actually worked when the seven units are combined, it ranges from 85.8% in one unit to 118.3% in another, a range of 32.5% when the units are compared individually.

With the realization that productivity fluctuates because of many variables, the results were presented as reliable estimates of productivity that may be applied to any work period. Such applications result in estimates that are reliable as approximations but not as exact projections.

The results of this study may be used for many purposes. The bacteriology department head, for example, might take immediate steps to find out why it is necessary for his employees to spend more time working than they are paid for. It is quite possible that there is too much work load for the staff to handle using existing equipment and procedures. Industrial engineer-

Category	Unit 1 Bacteriology	2 Blood bank	3 Hematology	4 Cytology	5 Pathology	6 Histology	7 Chemistry	8 Average of seven units
Direct productive	63.9 }=86.8	31.2 }=84.3	43.5 }=80.7	75.5 }=96.0	53.7 }=83.4	75.5 }=98.7	60.2 }=87.4	57.7 }=88.2
Indirect productive	22.9	53.1	37.2	20.5	29.7	23.2	27.2	30.5
Nonproductive	13.2	15.7	19.3	4.0	16.6	1.3	12.6	11.8
Total	100.0	100.0	100.0	100.0	100.0	100.0	100.0	100.0

Fig. 7-5. Hours of actual work, designated by category and unit, representing percentage of total time actually worked (see text).

Category	Unit 1 Bacteriology	2 Blood bank	3 Hematology	4 Cytology	5 Pathology	6 Histology	7 Chemistry	8 Average of seven units
Direct productive	71.2 }=96.6	33.7 }=91.1	44.8 }=83.1	75.5 }=96.0	43.9 }=68.2	86.3 }=112.8	61.1 }=88.6	59.5 }=90.0
Indirect productive	25.4	57.4	38.3	20.5	24.3	26.5	27.5	31.4
Nonproductive	14.6	16.9	19.9	4.0	13.5	1.4	12.7	11.9
Total	111.2	108.0	103.0	100.0	81.7	114.2	101.3	102.8

Fig. 7-6. Hours actually worked, designated by category and unit, representing percentage of total payroll time for same work period (see text).

ing, methods improvement, automated equipment, and changes in numbers and job assignments of employees will assist in finding a solution.

Another use might be to employ the study results to project the number of additional employees needed for an increase in work load of a specific nature. Yet another use is constructed by totaling the direct productive time and indirect productive time spent on each specific type of test and adding its allocated share of nonproductive time. This total represents the basic labor cost of the total of that kind of test produced during the study; total cost divided by total tests gives the labor cost per test and establishes the labor increment for pricing the test.

WORK SAMPLING STUDY*

The last project reports a work sampling study conducted by the consulting firm of Ernst & Ernst in a large community hospital in the Southwest.

Hospital costs throughout the country are rising steadily and rapidly, and there is every indication that the trend will continue. Increasing wage rates have resulted in higher labor costs, and advances in medical technology have required the procurement of expensive equipment and facilities. The increase in human life expectancy, prolonging the need for and increasing the incidence of medical care, has further complicated the problem.

Hospital managements have sought a solution that will reduce costs without sacrificing or reducing the standards of patient care. Labor costs are the most susceptible to cost reduction. In most hospitals the expenditures for salaries and wages range from 60% to 75% of the total cost of the entire operation. This cost is usually flexi-

---

*The material in this section (with modification) is from the report of the work sampling study of the Tucson Medical Center conducted by Ernst & Ernst and is used with the organization's permission.

ble, and opportunities for revision and improvements are available as compared to the less flexible expenditures for capital equipment and physical facilities. Labor costs accounted for 71% of the total expenditures for the hospital for the fiscal year 1963.

Labor costs in hospitals have been difficult to measure and evaluate. Activities include nursing, x-ray, maintenance, and housekeeping, varying from simple to complex. Professional and nonprofessional personnel are involved. Improvements in equipment, medicines, and procedures continually create the addition of new duties or the revision of old duties or both. Also, 24-hour availability 7 days a week causes difficult schedule problems.

Work sampling, a comparatively new method of work measurement, can assist in solving this problem of measurement and evaluation. Work sampling has been used successfully for the analyses of the activities of many hospitals and other businesses. It is a practical method of measuring and analyzing activities so that proper personnel utilization can be attained. Specifically, work sampling is a scientific measuring technique based on the statistical law of probability that states that samples taken at random from a large group tend to have the same characteristics and pattern of distribution as the large group. Accumulated data become extremely reliable if a sufficiently large group of samples can be obtained over a representative period of time.

A simple illustration can be used to prove the reliability of the technique. Consider the use of a bowl of 1,000 beads, of which 800 are white and 200 are red. A random selection of 10 beads from the thoroughly mixed bowl in most cases will produce 8 white beads and 2 red, or a ratio close to the actual 4 to 1 ratio. As more selections are made and cumulatively tabulated, results will more closely correspond to the actual 4 to 1 ratio.

In this illustration, the numbers of white beads and red beads are known. To determine these data when only the total number of beads is known, the total is multiplied by the percentages obtained from the random samples. If, for example, random selections show that 90% of the beads are red and 10% are white, it can be concluded that of a total of 1,000 beads, 900 are red and 100 are white.

Hospital activities such as nursing services and housekeeping can be compared to the beads in the bowl. Total hours of activity, like the total beads, can be obtained. If, from random observations, percentages are then determined for productive time and nonproductive time, the total times of these categories can be calculated. A thorough analysis and evaluation can then be made of the entire activity.

The activity of a nursing ward can be used as a particular example. Each worker would be observed at random intervals as working or not working. Working could be subdivided into R.N. work, L.P.N. work, and other work. After a representative number of observations had been obtained, the relative proportion of total time spent in each category would be determined. Results might be as follows:

R.N. work	30%
L.P.N. work	40
Other work	20
Delay (nonproductive)	10
	100%

By extending the total hours of the activity by each percentage, the total time per category could be determined. If 90 total man-hours were expended, then approximately 27 hours were spent on R.N. work, 36 hours on L.P.N. work, 18 hours on other work, and 9 hours represent delay time (nonproductive).

Work sampling was used at the hospital to analyze certain nursing wards to determine if utilization of personnel could be improved. If so, the derived data would serve as a basis to determine if utilization in comparable wards could be improved and to determine staffing needs for the planned intensive care unit.

The nursing wards of the north wing (24 beds) and south wing (41 beds) were studied. All shifts were included, and the time period was extended from 7 A.M. Thursday, November 14 to 7 A.M. Thursday, November 21.

Preparation for work sampling study

The administrative resident and in-service director of the hospital determined the activities to be studied, selected the observers, and estimated the time required for observations. Personnel of the firm of Ernst & Ernst provided general guidance, instruction, and assistance in preparation for the study and summarized and interpreted data obtained.

The objectives of the study of nursing activities were to determine (1) the actual hours worked, identified as to employee classification and level of work performed; (2) the level of work performed, by type of patient; (3) the staffing standards by employee classification and by level of work; and (4) details of nursing activities.

Selection of observers. Registered nurses were selected as observers because they were familiar with the work and would have little difficulty in identifying tasks, and because their participation, rather than that of nonprofessionals or outsiders, would result in greater acceptance of the study results.

The registered nurses selected as observers did not observe the wards in which they usually worked. Seven observers were used, one for each shift of each ward, except for the day shift of the south wing, where two observers were assigned.

All observers received general training and orientation before the start of the first study. The following areas were covered:

1. General objectives and purposes of the study

2. Fundamentals of work sampling
3. Explanations of nursing activities
4. Mechanics of taking the study
5. Importance of accuracy in tallying

Determination of nursing activities. During the study, the observer was required to describe briefly the work being done by each worker. It was important that each observer describe activities accurately so that comparable summarizations would result. Descriptions had to be coded, after the study, for analysis and evaluation.

All work was coded into detailed activities as follows*:

100 Patient care, treatment services, and contacts
101 Ace bandages, application of
102 Ambulation: assisting patient to bed, chair, walking, wheelchair, with or without physical assistance
103 Assisting with patients, miscellaneous: i.e., helping with patients, other personnel, special duty nurses, lab technicians, etc.
104 Bath, bed or complete: preparing unit for, or giving ("giving care to isolation patient" when procedure not identifiable)
105 Bath, partial: setting up for procedure, giving "finishing," preparing for baths, helping with tub or shower baths, "setting up for A.M. care"
106 Bed, occupied, making
107 Bed, unoccupied: patient in or out of room, straightening unoccupied beds, making, etc.
108 Blood pressures, taking
110 Catheterization, catheter care: draining, irrigating, etc.
111 Comfort measures for patient: changing diapers, holding baby or burping, playing with child; making comfortable in bed; putting dry pad under patient; adding blanket, pillows, covers; adjusting bed, bedboards, pillows; closing or opening curtains, adjusting shades
112 Coughing or deep breathing patients in bed: posture, drainage care
113 Croupette, O₂ tent, steam kettle: setting up, preparing, adding water, icing, filling, or emptying; isolette, regulation or operation; nebulized therapy

---

*Activities numbered 101 through 560 cover productive work; the 600 series is used to identify delay, both allowable (lunch, coffee break, etc.) and unallowable (unnecessary talking, idleness, etc.).

120 Doctor, assisting, with patient: drawing blood, treatments, examining, exchange transfusions, applying stockinette, helping with cast, passing tubes, etc.; services for physician
121 Dressings, compresses, hotpacks, irrigation, or wounds; applying tape bandages
125 Enemas: preparing, giving, checking results
126 Escort of patients on unit, miscellaneous: admission; transporting patient from one area of nursing unit or another in bed, wheelchair, or stretcher; discharge
127 Escort of patients to surgery
128 Escort of patients off unit: x-ray and other units or departments (except OR); to morgue with deceased patient
130 Hygiene, patient: giving or assisting with bedpan or urinal, emptying; oral hygiene; wiping baby's nose; care of skin and back, applying lotion to feet
135 Intake and output: collecting, totaling, recording on master sheet, at bedside, place slips at bedside
136 Intravenous: adding fluid or medications; removing subcutaneous I.V.; blood transfusion from patient, discontinuing
137 Intravenous: adjusting, checking, helping to start intravenous fluids, starting
140 Lamp, heat treatments: preparing for and giving perineal care; other heat lamp treatment
141 Miscellaneous services and errands for patients (not connected with treatments): assisting with dress and clothing, shaving, storing patient's luggage; errands for, etc.; repairing toy for patient; wiping patient's face after eating; washing hands after treatment (treatment not identifiable to be otherwise coded)
142 Miscellaneous treatments and procedures for patients: checking on patient's condition; observation at taking heartbeat with stethoscope; giving isolation gown for parents and visitors; procedural admission and/or discharge of patients (not clerical); applying restraints to patient; adjusting traction; applying unguent to baby; placing surgical patient into bed; care of vomiting patient, emesis basin; move from stretcher; irrigate gastric tubes, etc.; incidental treatment activities
145 Positioning patient: turning, exercising in bed, exercising orthopedic patient in bed
146 Positive pressure treatments, intermittent: preparation for, giving
147 Preparing patient for surgery: preps, scrub, or shaving

150 Temperatures, pulse, respirations, vital signs: reading thermometers, preparing to do procedure, recording on slip at bedside, checking for TPRS to be taken
151 Tracheotomy care
152 Treatments: preparing or setting up; obtaining equipment; planning for treatments, especially where treatment classified as miscellaneous or not identified for coding, e.g., "filling basin with ice"
155 Urine specimens, stool, sputum, collection and care of: checking diabetic urines, midstreams, taking to lab
156 Weighing patients, bedscales: assist with, recording in book, weighing babies
157 Weighing patients: finding scales
158 Weighing patients, standing: recording on chart; verbal exchange of information regarding patient or direction of care of patient
160 Clerk, patient-centered contact with personnel
161 Doctor, patient-centered contact with personnel
162 Head nurse or person in charge, patient-centered contact with personnel
163 Miscellaneous, patient-centered contact of personnel: with other department, administration, pharmacy, unknown recipient
164 Nurse's aide, patient-centered contact with personnel
165 Orderly, patient-centered contact with personnel
167 Patient, verbal contact with personnel: talking with, including intercom, reassurance, information, teaching, "charting," amusing patient
168 Registered nurse, patient-centered contact with personnel
170 Rounds, on patients: with doctors, alone, or with personnel, "walking round"
171 Student nurses, patient-centered contact with personnel
172 Supervisors and faculty, patient-centered contact with personnel
173 Visitors, patient-centered contact with personnel
174 Practical nurse, patient-centered contact with personnel
175 Nurse assistant, patient-centered contact with personnel
176 Isolation technique: masking and gowning
177 Handwashing
200 Medications
201 Charting medications: includes signing out narcotics (often not defined by observer and becomes part of Nurses' notes [460])

202 Checking med cards: Kardex, routine
203 Giving medications: oral, injections, instillations, applications
204 Narcotics, counting: checking
205 Ordering medications: including stock drugs, stenciling and writing requisitions (often included in transcribing orders as it is often done concurrently)
206 Preparing medications: oral, s.c., i.m., "pouring," setting up
207 Putting medications away, med cards, stock drugs
208 Transcribing or checking doctor's orders: making out med cards, to Rand, Kardex, etc. (often includes ordering drugs as part of process)

300 Dietary
301 Diets: checking and ordering
302 Feeding patients: feed, juice, water, baby formula; helping with food preparation in unit; positioning patient to eat
     Forcing fluid: gavage, tube feeding included
303 Kitchen, care of: cleaning counters, tables trays, refrigerator; sending dishes to kitchen, etc.
304 Preparing, passing, or delivering food, trays, nourishment: nourishment and coffee to patients, including formula, late trays, removal of trays from cart (late trays)
305 Removal of trays: coffee cups, dietary equipment from rooms, putting away in kitchen
306 Water pitchers: collecting, washing, preparing, and passing out water to patients

400 Clerical, ordering, copying, paper and pencil tasks, telephoning
450 Additions to charts, filing, and stenciling: adding sheets, nurses' notes to charts, setting up new charts, filling in charts, lab slips, filing old charts, stenciling forms for chart, dating
451 Admission and discharge books, entering patients into
452 Assignments, copying, individual: copying from Kardex, writing, checking own assignment, planning own assignment
455 Listing or making out routine lists of orders on patients: TPR, coffee, intake and output, communion, surgery patients, weights, making entries on lists, posting lists for use
456 Mail, messages for patients: sorting and delivery, packages and flowers, writing appointments for patients in person (not phone)
457 Miscellaneous clerical activities: assembling discharge charts; labeling miscellaneous items; clerical work of admissions; Addresso-

graph plates, check; messages and notations to physicians, identification band, preparation; making out Rand cards for new patients or copying (not writing doctor's orders); assembling charts for OR

458 Miscellaneous requisitioning, ordering of patient or unit supplies: related stamping, laboratory, x-ray, solutions, repair of equipment, inventories, checking stock supplies

460 Nurses' notes, charting (often includes recording of medications because done at the same time and cannot be coded separately)

461 Nursing office report: writing patient report for

462 Ordering, CSR: supplies for individual patients

465 Patient's name: stenciling on chart, etc.

466 Permits, operating room: getting signed, witnessing, etc.

467 Messenger service: sending and receiving

468 Recording on chart: TPR, graphing, weights, charting, intake and output, blood pressures, copying temps on temp chart

470 Telephoning, admission or discharge or transfer of patients

471 Telephoning to CSR concerning orders for patient on floor

472 Telephoning doctors, for, to, paging, or taking messages for

473 Telephoning, inquiries about patients from relatives and friends, messages for patients, or making calls for patients

474 Telephoning, miscellaneous: to other departments, making appointments for patients, to obtain services, messages, etc.

480 Valuables, patients', care of

481 Medications, patients', care of

500 Personnel- and unit-centered activities: cleaning and care of equipment

501 Assigning personnel, daily: assigning, planning, and directing personnel, lunch assignments, daily assignments, checking on assignments of personnel

505 Checking and supplying patient and unit areas: checking emergency cart

506 Curbwaiter: loading and unloading (CSR)

507 Equipment: moving and returning, i.e., large or wheeled type

508 Evaluation: preparing, giving, or receiving

510 Floor cleaning: cleaning, wiping-up spills, etc.

515 Linen: putting away

516 Linen handling: getting and supplying, distributing, putting unused linen away from unit, disposal of soiled linen

517 Looking for personnel or keys, returning

520 Medication rooms, care of: cleaning or tidying; care of medication equipment

521 Meetings, conferences, lecture attendance

522 Miscellaneous personnel and unit activities; discussions of problems: with other departments, services, janitorial, housekeeping, dietary, reading memos or informational material, contacts with other departments' personnel, i.e., administrator, student instructors, respondent unknown

525 Nurses' station, care of: report rooms, dusting, cleaning, care of plants, etc.; supply of nursing station paper forms, etc.; putting charts away to clear desk area

526 Ordering, requisitioning supplies for unit from CSR

527 Orientation of personnel: getting or giving, on or off floor, getting physical or shots, personnel health care

530 Patients' charts, checking: reading notes, studying, reading orders, checking chart for charting (usually head nurse), checking list for patient entry for treatment

531 Checking chart or Kardex for specific order, i.e., pain meds, etc. (not transcribing order)

535 Relief duties, calls to other floors: to work or assist (off floor) relieving private duty nurse, in specialty rooms, ICU, etc.; meals (not when assisting physician)

536 Report, routine: giving or receiving, team report

537 Reporting to duty: coming on or going off duty

540 Storing unit supplies from CSR

541 Supply room, solarium: cleaning, storage room

542 Team conferences, meeting: preparation for team conference, evaluation of team conference

543 Terminal care of equipment: removal from units, washing, cleaning; autoclaving, i.e., washbasins, I.V., etc.; disposal of trash; return of equipment (BP cuff); clean bottle warmer

544 Time sheets, preparing for personnel

545 Treatment and examining rooms, specialty treatment rooms: cast room, cleaning and arranging

546 Unit and patient areas: general cleaning and picking up (stripping), cleaning discharge units

547 Utility room, cleaning and care of: care of supplies, straightening shelves

550 Clerk, unit- and personnel-centered contact of

551 Doctors, personnel- and unit-centered contact of

552   Head nurse, unit- and personnel-centered contact of

553   Nurse's aide, unit- and personnel-centered contact of

554   Orderly, personnel- and unit-centered contact of

555   Registered nurse, unit- and personnel-centered contact of

556   Student nurse, unit- and personnel-centered contact of

557   Supervisors, unit- and personnel-centered contact of

558   Practical nurses, unit- and personnel-centered contact of

559   Nurse assistant, unit- and personnel-centered contact of

560   Errands off floor (not patient escort): to clinical lab, moving equipment from the nursing unit area, pharmacy, etc.

600   Miscellaneous and unclassifiable: reading note from patient, nursing activities study, activities related to tagging for, signed list that work completed, workroom

601   Coffee break

602   Personal time

603   Lunch time

604   Standby time

Classification of patients. The charge nurse in each ward predetermined the type of illness and the degree of nursing care necessary for each patient in the ward and assigned to each patient a code representing these data. For example, code G80 relates to a "special care" patient suffering from a "nervous system" disorder as follows:

DEGREE OF CARE

R Intensive care unit

A unit in which there is a concentration of highly skilled personnel and specialized equipment to supplement and reinforce the general health services available in the hospital

Patients who are critically, seriously, or acutely ill and who require constant observation and highly skilled technical nursing care should be admitted or transferred to this unit.

G Special care unit

A unit in which care is given to patients who do not require intensive care but who do require a greater amount of highly skilled nursing care than is found in semiself-care and self-care units

The physical facilities and nursing care found on this unit are similar to those found on most medical-surgical wards of a general hospital.

B Semiself-care unit

A unit in which care is given to patients who are semiambulant and are able to participate in planning and administering their own care

These patients are usually in the recovery or convalescent stage of illness and require varying amounts of nursing care and supervision.

Most patients admitted to this unit are nearing discharge from the hospital and need teaching and emotional support to prepare them for their return home.

Y Self-care unit

A unit in which care is given to patients who are ambulant and physically self-sufficient but who require nursing supervision and/or preparation for diagnostic or therapeutic services not feasible on an outpatient or office basis

O Long-term care unit

A unit in which care is given to patients who are expected to be hospitalized for a prolonged period of time (usually more than 30 days)

Patients admitted to this unit include those who are hospitalized as a result of chronic or terminal illness, patients with multiple fractures who need continued physical assistance, severe burn patients who are past the critical stage but need much nursing attention, and hemiplegic patients who need encouragement and rehabilitation.

An active rehabilitation program is provided, and patients and nurses usually work together in planning and rendering care.

Many of these patients might be adequately cared for in convalescent nursing homes or under a home care program if these facilities are available.

TYPE OF ILLNESS

10   Allergy

15   Blood and lymphatic

20   Cardiovascular

25   Deficiency and metabolic

30   Dental and oral

35   Ear, nose, and throat

40   Endocrine

45   Eye

50   Gastrointestinal

55   Genitourinary

60   Gynecologic and obstetric

65   Infections and parasitic

70   Liver and biliary

75   Musculoskeletal
80   Nervous system
85   Neuropsychiatric
90   Physical and chemical
95   Respiratory
100 Skin and connective tissue

Patient codes, on cards, were on the beds of the patients, and the observer noted the code whenever a worker was in contact with a patient. Codes were kept current for new and transferred patients and for those patients for whom the degree of care was changed. More than one number was used as necessary.

Calculation of number of observations. The number of observations needed for any work-sampling study is determined by the degree of accuracy desired. Obviously, more observations will provide more accuracy, and fewer observations will mean less accuracy; therefore the desired objective is an acceptable level of accuracy without an unreasonably large number of observations.

A practical approach must be used in the choice of the activity used for the determination of the number of needed observations. The use of an activity with a low percentage will mean a great many observations; the use of one with a high percentage will mean comparatively few observations. For these reasons, the practical approach is to select an activity that consisted of from 25% to 40% of the study.

In discussions with the administrative resident and in-service director previous to the study it was determined that the charge and registered nurses account for approximately 33% to 40% of the total charged hours. It was also estimated that aides account for approximately 35% to 40% of the charged hours.

The necessary number of observations was determined from a table of observations required to remain within the confidence limit of 95%, plus or minus 10%, which has been accepted for hospital activities.

After the total number of observations was obtained, it was necessary to determine the length of the study and the average number of workers per shift in order to determine the basic objective: the number of observation rounds per shift. It was determined that 7 consecutive days would be representative of the activities to be studied.

After the first day we computed the charged hours for the charge and registered nurses and aides. In each case, these activities accounted for approximately 37% of the charged hours. This information supported the original estimate of required observations.

Selection of random times. A table of random numbers was used for the selection of the times for the observation rounds. The use of such a table assures complete random selection without bias.

Work sampling form. A copy of the work sampling form used is shown in Fig. 7-7. Separate sheets were used for each observation round of each shift of each ward. Six different colors were used for easy identification of the three shifts for the two wards.

Heading information (ward, shift, date, and observation) of the work sampling forms was inserted at the beginning of each shift before release to the observers. The observer signed the work sampling forms before returning them at the end of the shift.

Studies by all observers were monitored as necessary to assure that correct and comparable data were obtained. The monitoring was done by personnel of Ernst & Ernst with direct assistance from the administrative resident and the in-service director. Continuous supervision was employed during the first day of the study, but thereafter only occasional monitoring was needed, particularly at the beginning and end of each shift.

At the indicated time on the work sampling form, the observer noted the activ-

Work sampling program

Observer ______________ Shift 1 (7-3) ☐ Date ______

North wing ☐ 1 Shift 2 (3-11) ☐ Time ______ AM PM

South wing ☐ 2 Shift 3 (11-7) ☐ Page ______

	Brief description of what was being done	Do not write in this space	Patient color and code	Level of work								
				Charge nurse 1	R.N. 2	L.P.N. 3	N.A. 4	Clerk 5	Aide 6	Orderly 7	Nonnursing work 8	Nonwork 9
1 Charge nurse												
2 R.N.												
2 R.N.												
2 R.N.												
3 L.P.N.												
4 N.A.												
4 N.A.												
5 Clerk												
6 Aide												
6 Aide												
6 Aide												
6 Aide												
6 Aide												
6 Aide												
7 Orderly												
8 Other (describe)												
Remarks:												

Fig. 7-7. Work sampling form. (From Ernst & Ernst: Report of the work sampling study of the Tucson Medical Center, Tucson, Ariz., Nov. 1963.)

ities of each worker in the ward. On the horizontal line for the employee classification of the worker observed, the observer wrote a brief description of what was being done. The observer then checked the vertical column for the level of work performed. If patient contact of any kind was observed, the patient code (letter and number) was recorded in the proper column.

There was an accounting for all workers charged to the ward. If some were missing, the supervisor of the ward was consulted and the activity of the missing worker was determined at that time or at the next observation round. Observations had to be as instantaneous as possible. Every effort was made to avoid anticipation or bias by the observers.

Accuracy and thoroughness by the observer was stressed continually, as the success of any work sampling study is directly dependent on the reliability of the information obtained. The observer recorded all pertinent data in the "remarks" area whenever there were any questions, which were later resolved with the assistance of the monitors.

The actual hours spent in each job clas-

sification were determined from the actual daily hours reported by the observers. This information was checked by the monitors by reference to personnel and time records. The hours of employees that were part-time, late, early leave, etc. were taken into consideration. The amount of patient hours, by type of patient, was accumulated by the observers and checked by the monitors. Actual hours by job classification and type of patient were summarized for the week from the daily information accumulated.

Data obtained from study

Tables 7-1 and 7-2 compare the hours charged to the activity to the actual hours of work (and nonwork) determined from the work-sampling study. This was done by level of work and for each shift of both wards.

Charged hours were obtained through normal timekeeping procedures for each day of the study. The actual hours shown are the hours for the level of work, i.e., R.N. work, L.P.N. work, etc., regardless of who performed the activity. Clerical work, for example, was done by almost everyone

Table 7-1. Comparison of charged hours and actual hours by level of work*

Level of work	North wing (7 days)								
	Days			Evenings			Nights		
	Charged hours	Actual hours	Actual hours with allowance	Charged hours	Actual hours	Actual hours with allowance	Charged hours	Actual hours	Actual hours with allowance
C.N.	57	39.1	43	57	49.5	54	39	3.9	4
R.N.	113	101.3	111	47	42.9	47	23	51.1	56
L.P.N.	32	18.0	20						
N.A.				56	36.4	40		1.5	2
Clerk	53	51.6	56	47	40.4	44		9.8	11
Aide	136	137.9	151	128	94.0	103	57	29.0	32
Orderly	1	3.0	3					1.5	2
Nonnursing		4.0	4		15.7	16		3.9	4
Nonwork		37.1	4		56.1	32		18.2	9
Total	392	392.0	392	335	335.0	336	119	118.9	120

*Modified from Ernst & Ernst: Report of the work sampling study of the Tucson Medical Center, Tucson, Ariz., Nov. 1963.

in the wards. An allowance for lunch and coffee breaks (50 minutes for every 8 hours) was added to the actual hours of the work sampling study so that an equitable comparison could be made with charged hours.

Nonnursing work is work that normally would be performed by other than nursing services personnel. In this study this included housekeeping, laundry, kitchen, and similar functions.

Nonwork under "actual hours" (vertical column) includes unnecessary delays such as talking and idleness and necessary delays such as lunch, coffee breaks, and personal time. Nonwork under "actual hours with allowance" (vertical column) includes only unnecessary delays.

In addition to knowing how much R.N. work and L.P.N. work, etc. is being done, it is also important to know who is doing it. This information is shown in Tables 7-3 and 7-4. Data are again summarized for each shift of both wards. Actual hours (without the allowances for lunch, coffee breaks, personal time, etc.) were used so that productive hours could be analyzed separately from delay hours.

As an example of the information available from Tables 7-3 and 7-4 of the 101.3 actual hours of R.N. work in north wing on the day shift, 9.0 were performed by the charge nurse and 92.3 were performed by registered nurses.

It is possible to determine how employees in each classification spend their time by reading the vertical column for each classification. For example, during the week of the study, clerks on the day shift of north wing spent 44.6 hours on clerical work, 1.0 hours on aide work, 1.5 hours on nonnursing work, and 6.0 hours on nonwork.

The analysis of the nonwork in each employee classification can be very informative. By subtracting from the individual totals the allowable delay time for lunch, etc. (a standard 50 minutes for each 8 hours), the amount of unallowable delay time can be determined.

Tables 7-3 and 7-4 analyze time as to how it is spent and by whom, but they do not measure or evaluate patient contact time. For example, it is possible for one registered nurse to be 100% productive, yet spend very little time with the patients,

Table 7-2. Comparison of charged hours and actual hours by level of work*

	South wing (7 days)								
	Days			Evenings			Nights		
Level of work	Charged hours	Actual hours	Actual hours with allowance	Charged hours	Actual hours	Actual hours with allowance	Charged hours	Actual hours	Actual hours with allowance
C.N.	56	45.4	50	57	25.7	28	51	3.5	4
R.N.	193	169.0	185	122	119.1	130	69	98.5	108
L.P.N.				40	34.4	38			
N.A.	104	90.7	99		1.0	1	24	16.6	18
Clerk	56	59.3	65	56	37.8	41		32.2	35
Aide	231	222.8	244	200	173.3	190	151	97.5	107
Orderly	23	16.0	18	57	25.2	28	1	2.0	2
Nonnursing		3.5	4		8.2	8		8.0	8
Nonwork		56.3			107.5	68		37.7	14
Total	663	663.0	665	532	532.2	532	296	296.0	296

*Modified from Ernst & Ernst: Report of the work sampling study of the Tucson Medical Center, Tucson, Ariz., Nov. 1963.

whereas a second nurse may be less productive and devote much more time to the patients. This important information, necessary for the complete analysis of any nursing activity, is provided in Tables 7-5 and 7-6. Data are summarized by shift for both wards. Available patient hours were determined from the daily log kept for each ward, and partial hospital stays were considered in the calculations.

The following information can be obtained from these figures:

1. Total hours of patient contact for the week.

Table 7-3. Distribution of work sampling actual hours by employee classification and distribution of employee classification by level of work*

Level of work	Charged hours	Actual hours	North wing (7 days) Employee classification						
			C.N.	R.N.	L.P.N.	N.A.	Clerk	Aide	Orderly
Days									
C.N.	57	39.1	38.6	.5					
R.N.	113	101.3	9.0	92.3					
L.P.N.	32	18.0	3.0	1.0	14.0				
N.A.									
Clerk	53	51.6	.5	6.0		.5	44.6		
Aide	136	137.9	2.5	1.5	11.0		1.0	121.9	
Orderly	1	3.0							3.0
Nonnursing		4.0				.5	1.5	2.0	
Nonwork		37.1	2.5	10.0	6.5		6.0	12.1	
Total	392	392.0	56.1	111.3	32.0	.5	53.1	136.0	3.0
Evenings									
C.N.	57	49.5	47.5	2.0					
R.N.	47	42.9	1.5	41.4					
L.P.N.									
N.A.	56	36.4				35.9	.5		
Clerk	47	40.4	2.0	1.0			36.9	.5	
Aide	128	94.0				9.6	1.5	82.9	
Orderly									
Nonnursing		15.7		.5		1.0	.5	13.7	
Nonwork		56.1	5.6	1.5		10.1	6.6	32.3	
Total	335	335.0	56.6	46.4		56.6	46.0	129.4	
Nights									
C.N.	39	3.9	2.9	1.0					
R.N.	23	51.1	44.7	6.4					
L.P.N.									
N.A.		1.5					1.5		
Clerk		9.8	.5				9.3		
Aide	57	29.0	1.0				28.0		
Orderly		1.5							1.5
Nonnursing		3.9					3.9		
Nonwork		18.2	5.9				12.3		
Total	119	118.9	55.0	7.4			55.0		1.5

*Modified from Ernst & Ernst: Report of the work sampling study of the Tucson Medical Center, Tucson, Ariz., Nov. 1963.

2. Distribution by level of work
3. Distribution by type of patient
4. Actual patient hours by type of patient for the week
5. Total hours of nonpatient contact
6. Percentages of patient contact time

Recommendations

A. Eventually eliminate one aide on evening shift of north wing ward. Tables 7-1 and 7-2 indicate this conclusion. The data in Table 7-1 for the evening shift show that the nonnursing hours and the nonwork

Table 7-4. Distribution of work sampling actual hours by employee classification and distribution of employee classification by level of work*

Level of work	Charged hours	Actual hours	Employee classification						
			C.N.	R.N.	L.P.N.	N.A.	Clerk	Aide	Orderly
South wing (7 days)									
Days									
C.N.	56	45.4	45.4						
R.N.	193	169.0	2.0	164.0	3.0				
L.P.N.									
N.A.	104	90.7		3.0		86.7		1.0	
Clerk	56	59.3	3.5	4.0			50.8	1.0	
Aide	231	222.8		3.5		8.5		207.3	3.5
Orderly	23	16.0							16.0
Nonnursing		3.5	1.0			.5	.5	1.5	
Nonwork		56.3	4.0	14.4		8.0	4.5	18.9	6.5
Total	663	663.0	55.9	188.9	3.0	103.7	55.8	229.7	26.0
Evenings									
C.N.	57	25.7	25.7						
R.N.	122	119.1	23.2	94.4				1.5	
L.P.N.	40	34.4	2.4	2.4	29.1			.5	
N.A.		1.0				1.0			
Clerk	56	37.8		2.4		.5	34.9		
Aide	200	173.3	1.4	2.9	5.8		1.0	162.2	
Orderly	57	25.2						.9	24.3
Nonnursing		8.2						8.2	
Nonwork		107.5	1.9	22.3	3.9		17.4	37.8	24.2
Total	532	532.2	54.6	124.4	38.8	.5	54.3	211.1	48.5
Nights									
C.N.	51	3.5	3.5						
R.N.	69	98.5	46.2	52.3					
L.P.N.									
N.A.	24	16.6				16.6			
Clerk		32.2	4.0	2.5		2.0		23.7	
Aide	151	97.5	2.0	.5		1.5		93.5	
Orderly	1	2.0				.5			1.5
Nonnursing		8.0						8.0	
Nonwork		37.7	2.5	4.0		3.5		27.7	
Total	296	296.0	58.2	59.3		24.1		152.9	1.5

*Modified from Ernst & Ernst: Report of the work sampling study of the Tucson Medical Center, Tucson, Ariz., Nov. 1963.

Table 7-5. Distribution of patient contact hours by type of patient and by level of work[*]

North wing (7 days)

Level of work	Days — Type of patient						Evenings — Type of patient						Nights — Type of patient					
	Intensive care	Special care	Long-term care	Semi-self care	Self-care	Total	Intensive care	Special care	Long-term care	Semi-self care	Self-care	Total	Intensive care	Special care	Long-term care	Semi-self care	Self-care	Total
C.N.	1.5	3.5		2.0	.5	7.5	3.0	4.6		3.5	4.1	15.2		.5				.5
R.N.	2.5	10.0		4.0	2.5	19.0		5.6		5.0	3.5	14.1	3.4	6.4		2.9		12.7
L.P.N.		10.0		1.5		11.5												
N.A.							5.6	13.6		5.6		24.8		.5		1.0		1.5
Clerk		.5		1.0		1.5												
Aide	3.5	32.1		22.0	3.0	60.6	.5	22.7		16.7	9.1	49.0	2.0	16.2		1.5	1.0	20.7
Orderly														1.5				1.5
Total	7.5	56.1	—	30.5	6.0	100.1	9.1	46.5	—	30.8	16.7	103.1	5.4	25.1	—	5.4	1.0	36.9
Available patient hours	30	432		428	163	1,053	25	432		434	195	1,086	32	454		438	200	1,124
Noncontact hours						291.9						231.9						82.1
Patient contact (%)						25.5						30.8						31.0

[*]Modified from Ernst & Ernst: Report of the work sampling study of the Tucson Medical Center, Tucson, Ariz., Nov. 1963.

Table 7-6. Distribution of patient contact hours by type of patient and by level of work*

South wing (7 days)

Level of work	Days — Type of patient						Evenings — Type of patient						Nights — Type of patient					
	Intensive care	Special care	Long-term care	Semi-self care	Self care	Total	Intensive care	Special care	Long-term care	Semi-self care	Self care	Total	Intensive care	Special care	Long-term care	Semi-self care	Self care	Total
C.N.	4.5	7.5		2.5		14.5	1.9	1.4	.5	3.9	.5	8.2						
R.N.	18.9	21.9		18.9	2.5	62.2	4.4	6.8	1.0	3.4		15.6	11.1	10.6	1.0	6.6	3.0	32.3
L.P.N.	14.0	27.9		16.0	.5	58.4	5.3	7.3	.5	1.9	.5	15.5	5.5	3.5	.5	2.0		11.5
N.A.																		
Clerk							.5			.5		1.0						
Aide	5.0	49.3		57.3	6.0	117.6	9.7	29.0	8.7	14.0	1.9	63.3	17.6	27.6	6.5	4.5	.5	56.7
Orderly	1.0	8.0			1.5	10.5	1.9	.5		2.9		5.3				1.0	.5	1.5
Total	43.4	114.6		94.7	10.5	263.2	23.7	45.0	10.7	26.6	2.9	108.9	34.2	41.7	8.0	14.1	4.0	102.0
Available patient hours	110	684	56	768	199	1,817	109	728	56	760	189	1,842	125	755	56	773	184	1,893
Noncontact hours						399.8						423.1						194.0
Patient contact (%)						39.7						20.5						34.5

*Modified from Ernst & Ernst: Report of the work sampling study of the Tucson Medical Center, Tucson, Ariz., Nov. 1963.

hours for the week (16 hours and 32 hours) are high in comparison with other shifts. The total of this unnecessary time (48 hours) could be corrected by eliminating one person.

Further analysis of the same figure discloses only 103 hours of actual aide work compared to 128 hours charged. Although this difference in time does not equal a full person, the aide work that would remain after the aide reduction could be handled by the nursing assistant who has excess time.

Analysis of Table 7-3 supports the recommendation that an aide should be eliminated. Of the 15.7 hours of nonnursing work, 13.7 were spent by aides. Also, the total of 83.4 productive hours normally permits about 8 hours of nonwork. Subtraction of these 8 hours from the 32.3 hours of both allowable and unallowable delays indicates that 24 hours can be eliminated.

This exhibit also supports the contention that the nursing assistant can take on aide duties remaining after reduction of one aide. The nursing assistant is already doing some aide work, and although 10.1 hours were spent on nonwork, only about 4 hours are necessary for lunch, etc.

B. Eventually eliminate one orderly on evening shift of south wing ward. Table 7-2 shows 68 hours of nonwork (after deduction of allowances for lunch, coffee breaks, etc.) during the week for the evening shift.

Although 57 hours were charged for orderly work, only 28 hours of such work were required. By eliminating one orderly the excess orderly work could be absorbed by the clerk, as only 41 hours of clerical work are required, compared to 56 hours charged.

Table 7-4 again verifies the recommendation. Half the total time of the orderly (24.2 hours of 48.5) was spent on nonwork; normally, nonwork time would be about 2 hours. Also, the clerks spent 17.4 hours on nonwork instead of a normal 4 hours.

C. Replace one aide with one clerk on night shift of south wing ward. Table 7-2 shows 35 actual hours (with allowances) of clerk work for the week with no hours charged. It also shows 107 actual hours of aide work, but with 151 hours charged. Table 7-4 shows that most of the clerk work is being done by aides. This situation would be corrected by implementing our recommendation.

D. Eventually eliminate one nursing assistant or registered nurse on day shift of south wing ward. Table 7-6 indicates that the amount of patient contact hours for the week by the day shift is abnormally high in comparison with other shifts in this wing. Patient contact hours on the day shift are almost 2.5 times greater than on the evening shift (263.2 versus 108.9); normally, they should be approximately equal, as time spent on extra meals, baths, etc. on the day shift is usually offset on the evening shift by a greater number of visitors and by the natural irritability of the patient at bedtime. The north wing ward (Table 7-5) appears to maintain a normal patient-contact relationship between day and other shifts as 100.1 hours were spent in patient contact by the day shift as compared to 103.1 hours spent by the evening shift.

A direct comparison of the south wing ward day shift with the day shift of north wing ward also discloses that the number of patient-contact hours for the day shift of the south wing ward appears excessive. Comparison is possible because the patient mix in the two wards is surprisingly similar; for each ward, about 80% of the patients are in the special care and semiself-care categories; about 15% of the patients in north wing ward are self-care, whereas the figure for south wing ward is about 11%, and for the intensive care patient, it is 6% for south wingward versus 3% for north wing ward. The remainder of the patients in the south wing ward required long-term care.

The comparison of the two wards indi-

Table 7-7. Staffing standards (hours per patient day by level of work and degree of patient care)*

Level of work	Intensive care			Special care			Semiself-care			Self-care		
	Days	Eve-nings	Nights	Days	Eve-nings	Nights	Days	Eve-nings	Nights	Days	Eve-nings	Nights
R.N.	3.85	2.46	2.58	1.27	.74	.52	.84	.48	.18	.41	.57	.16
Aide	2.22	2.20	1.90	1.31	.87	.49	1.03	.52	.10	.42	.56	.08

*Modified from Ernst & Ernst: Report of the work sampling study of the Tucson Medical Center, Tucson, Ariz., Nov. 1963.

cates that, if 100.1 hours of patient contact are required for 1,053 available patient hours in north wing, then about 180 hours, instead of 263, would be needed for the 1,817 available patient hours in south wing (Table 7-6).

It appears that the excessive time is incurred by either the registered nurses or the nursing assistants. On the day shift a total of 120.6 hours was so spent by these two groups, whereas the evening shift of the same ward shows a total of only 31.1 hours.

On the day shift of north wing (Table 7-5), where there were a little more than half as many available patient hours (1,053 compared to 1,817), only 30.5 hours were spent in patient contact by comparable personnel in both groups.

E. Train personnel on evening shift of south wing ward to devote more time to direct patient care. The implementation of recommendation "D" for the day shift in the south wing should reduce the time devoted to patient care without sacrifice of quality. However, it appears that a different change is necessary for the evening shift, as the percent of patient-contact time 20.5%) was abnormally low in comparison with all shifts of both wards. It is suggested that available personnel be trained to devote more time to patient care.

F. Use developed standards for general analysis and staffing needs of planned intensive care unit. Staffing standards were prepared and are presented in Table 7-7. These standards are general and should

be used only as overall guides. Adjustments were made in the data used, based upon our prior recommendations.

Nonpatient contact time was computed by subtracting patient contact hours (Tables 7-5 and 7-6) from the actual hours with allowances (Tables 7-1 and 7-2). Non–patient contact time by level of work and type of patient was allocated, based upon the patient-contact time. The computed non–patient contact time was added to the patient-contact time to arrive at the total hours by level of work by type of patient.

The available patient hours (Table 7-5 and 7-6) were converted to patient days of type of patient. The number of patient days was divided into the total hours by level of work by type of patient to compute the standard hours per patient day by level of work by type of patient.

The data was computed for all levels of work, but only R.N. and aide results are presented since these activities represent over 75% of the total study. More extensive studies should be made if the administration is interested in additional staffing standards. Standards for the long-term patient were omitted since there was only one patient included in the study.

Adjustments were made in the data used, based upon our prior recommendations. As a result, the submitted standards will be exacting, yet practical and realistic. The standards cover the allowances for 10 patients in the shift for 8 hours.

Industrial engineering tools used in this

way are an invaluable management aide—they are not a panacea.

Case Hospital is currently exploring ways of installing these methodologies within its framework of systems and programs. It is particularly interested in exploiting the many advantages to be gained by using these tools without the restrictions of traditional departmental barriers. Since the departments grouped in each system share many similar functional and organizing interests, industrial engineering can be applied on a system rather than a departmental basis. This should result in greater effectiveness than has been experienced when application has been made to departments as single units (although even there the results have been good).

chapter eight
BUSINESS AND FINANCE

For some time Case Hospital has been faced with serious financial problems. An analysis of the potential sources of financing lends insight to this problem. Sources of funds to cover costs include:

1. The patient himself
2. Third-party payer, i.e., government or private insurance company
3. Research grants
4. Teaching monies
5. Profit sector of present hospital services, e.g., the laboratory
6. Deficit financing, i.e., all costs unrecoverable through services are designated as educational costs and are passed on to the university for funding

At various times all have played their part. The most significant single source in both total dollars contributed and number of cases has been the third-party payer. It is for this reason that a shift in this category, from reimbursement on the basis of charges to reimbursement on the basis of costs, has had such a profound effect on current patterns of hospital financing. There has already been a trend in this direction, and it seems clear that this will become the basis for all reimbursement formulas in the not-too-distant future.

For example, in January of 1967 and 1968 there were 89.7% and 90.4% of patient days, respectively, under some form of third-party coverage. At present 50.7% of these are on a cost-reimbursement basis, and this figure will jump to 80.7% if the indication of a Blue Cross switch to cost is substantiated. In operational terms this means an increasingly reduced opportunity for variable pricing of services. Financial losses can only then be made up through the solicitations of funds from outside sources, and these seem to be diminishing.

As previously noted, the doctor is the decision maker who initiates the major portion of hospital costs. It is appropriate then that accountability be assigned to this individual for the financial control of costs.

Pursuing the implications of this suggestion, we end up with the organizational pattern projected for the new hospital: a program floor concept directed by a physician as the program director. The objectives are to bring medical and patient care services as much as possible to the patient rather than vice versa; to encourage physician interdisciplinary cooperation; to stimulate better nursing through specialization; and to promote good management by decentralizing it to the local level, where the nurse and doctor, by working closer together, can achieve more efficient/effective service and educational results.

What does this shift mean in terms of the function and philosophy of the traditional hospital model? The traditional model is divided into systems, which are brokers of resources and programs that consume resources in the delivery of care, teaching, and research. Philosophically, particularly in the case of Case Hospital, it involves moving from a community hospital approach to a clinical teaching laboratory approach. This has significant operational ramifications that must be considered.

1. Packaged programs of care, teaching, and research, with accountable directors, will be identified.
2. Specific and distinct costing becomes feasible on the basis of priced resources supplied to given programs.
3. A division between programs and resources as inputs to these programs is achieved. This fits precisely into the presently established systems and programs organizational approach.
4. The administrator is no longer forced into the inappropriate position of interpreting medical program needs. This is given to the expert, the physician, who then simultaneously assumes the financial responsibility of his programs as well. Thus he has the final voice in the utilization of "bought" resources and in the allocation of assigned beds. Any interchange of these will be at his pleasure. He is held accountable for program definition, resource utilization, quality evaluation, and budgeting and financial control.
5. The totality of this approach offers a system whereby resource inputs may be priced out through a systems approach into programs of care as distinct entities with identifiable aims and functions. This presents a viable opportunity to manage medical costs, to price them out to service, education, or research areas as appropriate, and to secure the means of support. This can be done in inpatient, outpatient, and emergency areas.

First, this will encourage program utilization of only those beds it can finance. Beds that cannot be financed by the program to which they are assigned may be leased to other programs or put out of service if experience shows that they are not needed. Second, it will increase control and accountability. It will improve the efficiency of the use of manpower for which the programs themselves are accountable. It means more immediate control of expenditures at the point where the need for resources is experienced. And third, it will be a significant step toward the achievement of the program floor concept, with improved patient care, increased nursing specialization, and closer medical-nursing affiliation as the ultimate objective. The result would be a better team approach to teaching and delivery of health care.

To solidify a sound business and financial base for systems and programs, a *cost and income control program* was undertaken. This was a systematic revamping of the accounting and financial system to bring it in line with the systems and programs organization. The following outline gives the major points of emphasis.

COST AND INCOME CONTROL PROGRAM

I. *Objectives*: The major objectives of the cost and income control program were to
  A. Provide information for negotiating contractural obligations for service
  B. Provide information for management decisions relating to cost control and evaluation of rate schedules
  C. Provide information relating to annual accountability for all cost incurred and income produced both internally and externally
II. *Phases:* Seven distinct phases were identified for the program
  A. Identification of cost centers
    1. Define objective of identifying cost centers

The objective of identifying cost centers is to determine and report expenditures in direct relationship to given areas of accountability for both direct and indirect expenditures. Accountability includes responsibility for controlling direct costs and for establishing a basis for reporting indirect costs.

2. Define a cost center

A cost center is a given area of responsibility in which expenditures occur and for which accountability is assigned.

3. List all existing cost centers
4. Determine and add new cost centers
5. Determine direct cost centers
    a. Direct cost centers are defined in terms of
        (1) Direct costs
        (2) Indirect costs
        (3) Cost centers to be reallocated to each direct cost center as it is defined
        (4) Formalize and review planned direct cost centers
    b. A review of each direct cost center is made in order to
        (1) Determine what direct costs are now being charged against it
        (2) Determine what direct costs should be charged against it but are not being so charged
        (3) Determine what direct cost services are to be charged against it
        (4) Determine what indirect costs are to be charged against it
        (5) Formalize and review planned charges against direct cost centers
6. Determine which cost centers should be distributed monthly
7. List indirect cost centers

8. Establish asset accounts
9. Outline recommended changes
10. Design and document systems
11. Design and document new forms
12. Develop program and schedule for implementation

B. Grouping of cost centers
    1. Review definitions of each cost center
    2. Prepare a schedule for grouping like cost centers

C. Identification of income-producing centers
    1. Define objective of identifying income-producing centers

    The objective of identifying income-producing centers is to determine services produced and to ensure control of charges for those services rendered against sources of income.

    2. Define an income-producing center

    An income-producing center is a given area of responsibility in which services are produced or which acts as an agent for producing services, resulting in charges against sources of income.

    3. List all ancillary income-producing centers
    4. Determine charges in each ancillary income-producing center
    5. Review in detail each ancillary income-producing center
        a. Review as a system of rendering charges in order to determine current methods of documenting charges and releasing them to the billing section
            (1) Establish flow chart for the current system for creating charges for all income-producing services
                (a) Establish supple-

mentary time schedule

(b) Establish flow-chart standards

(c) Flow chart

(2) Define current controls for ensuring that all income-producing services are billed for

6. List all miscellaneous income-producing centers

7. Define charges in each miscellaneous income-producing center

8. Review in detail each miscellaneous income-producing center

a. Review as a system of rendering charges to determine current methods of documenting charges and releasing them to the billing section

(1) Establish flow chart for the current system for creating charges for all income-producing services

(a) Establish supplementary time schedule

(b) Establish flow-chart standards

(c) Flow chart

(2) Define controls for ensuring that all income-producing services are billed for

9. Determine additional income-producing centers required

10. Outline recommended changes

11. Design and document new systems

12. Design and document new forms

13. Develop program and schedule for implementation

D. Development of unit measures and dollar values

1. Define objective of developing

unit measures and dollar values

The objective of developing unit measures and dollar values is to provide management and operating supervisors with financial and statistical information.

2. Define a unit of measure

A unit of measure is a specific, quantitative statistic assigned to each cost center or department.

3. List cost centers and the corresponding unit(s) of measure applicable

4. Identify the source of the unit(s) of measure for each cost center

5. Review and revise units of measure as approved

6. Design and document new systems, procedures, and forms with appropriate testing

7. Develop program and schedule for implementation

E. Development of a cost step-down method

F. Development of performance budgets

G. Development of a program budget system

PERFORMANCE AND PROGRAM BUDGETING*

One of the highlights of the cost and income control program is performance and program budgeting at the operating level, which is reviewed here because of its pivotal nature in the organization.

Income and expense pots, line object budgets, sweeping policy discounts, and credit losses are not only outmoded but are also a financial management hindrance.

---

*From Durbin, R. L., Springall, W. H., and High, C. P.: Manual for hospital performance and program budgeting at the operating level, Philadelphia, 1967, Temple University Hospital. The figures and statistics in this section are hypothetical and should not be assumed to reflect current economic or work-load values.

Current emphasis is on quality and reasonable cost. Changes in socioeconomics, with increased involvement of local, state, and federal governments, necessitate improved budgetary programs and cost accounting. A new organizational and administrative approach has been established. This approach sees the organization as an aggregate of resources grouped into systems and channeled into programs of health care. The process of budgeting set forth here parallels that approach. It is designed to be thoroughly interwoven with the organization and its administration. In this view, the budget is a means of guiding the appropriation of resources so that they may be placed in perspective to the competing demands made upon them. It serves to coordinate resources and extend organizational goals throughout operations.

Organization is changed to emphasize function, the activities and projects, rather than each itemized means of production. Methods of budgetary programming, performance budgeting, and step-down cost accounting fit this type of organization well. In the arrangement of systems and programs, each has a budgetary program emphasizing its function. These budget programs are summaries built from the aggregate of cost center budgets that project the policies and expectations of systems, programs, and the organization.

Each cost center has a performance budget oriented toward current performance and the means of accomplishment, based on past and current operations. In order to build performance budgets and periodically measure expectations, performance classifications related to productivity and methods of analyzing them must be devised. Classifications such as these are statistically related to productivity and cost. By calculating base classifications and costs, packages of care can be priced. Pricing of this kind is contingent upon a cost step-down accounting method that can identify both the direct and indirect cost of operating each cost center and is in line with the costing methods required by the federal and state governments.

Purpose

The purpose is to establish an effective method of budgeting at the operational level. Performance and program budgeting techniques are used. Such techniques draw managers to a deliberate evaluation of the purposes for which expenditures are made. This process will assist management in forecasting the quantity and cost of services. And, as a control tool, it will establish a standard for measuring volume and cost of performance in individual cost centers. The budgeting process will provide a device for establishing goals and objectives within individual areas of responsibility and a means of measuring effectiveness in obtaining those goals. The organization stresses involvement of administrators and managers. Involvement in actual budget preparation stimulates cost consciousness better than any other means available to management.

Scope

Scope is directed toward preparation of the expense segment of the operating budget with its component parts, the salaries and wages performance budget and the supplies and expense performance budget. The equipment budget and the renovation budget (which comprise the capital budget) are included because of the importance of involving people at the operating level in their planning. These are the areas of expense for which personnel at this level are held accountable.

Objectives

The fundamental objectives of budgeting are **planning, coordinating,** and **controlling.** Planning involves identifying the objectives of the organization. It requires an identification of the resources needed to meet the objectives and formulation of policy related to obtaining and using them. The budget is a statement of this policy in financial terms.

Coordination involves carrying out policy by obtaining budgeted resources and using them efficiently and effectively.

Control entails assuring that the operational tasks that use resources are performed effectively and efficiently.

Planning, coordinating, and controlling at the operational level require intelligent estimates of the following:

1. The volumes and types of service to be rendered
2. The number of personnel required to provide service, and the resulting cost
3. The number and types of supplies and expenses required to provide service, and the resulting cost

Requirements

Minimum requirements for sound budgetary procedures include the following.

Sound organizational structure. The synergistic organizational structure, with its systems and programs, is discussed in Chapters 4, 5, and 6.

A classified and uniform system of accounts. A chart of accounts similar to the *Uniform Chart of Accounts and Definitions for Hospitals,* published by the American Hospital Association, must be adopted. This will establish uniform account identification and definition of terms throughout the organization and its budgetary process. Only on this basis will meaningful and consistent results be obtained for reporting and controlling.

Adequate statistical data. The quality control system maintains the most accurate compilation of statistics and should be the sole source of statistical data.

Defined budget periods. For purposes of demonstration the budget year will coincide with the fiscal year—July 1 through June 30. Examples are based on monthly figures within the fiscal year.

Reporting system. Monthly reports should be prepared for key administrative personnel. Cost centers should be given copies of sections related to their particular areas of responsibility. Discussions between administrators and department heads about variances over and under budget provide an indispensable aid to good management.

Budgeting process

The initial step in the budgeting process must be identification of performance classifications. Performance classifications are intended to measure volume and accomplishment. In this way, the aggregate of means or isolated activities are related to organizational goals. These are tangible things done; and this leads us to a word of caution: performance classifications do not, in and of themselves, measure quality. They are tangible evidence of production to which quantity, cost, and quality must be further related.

Performance classifications will be referred to as **units of measure.** At the cost center level, units of measure relate directly to work performance units. They are intended to assist the supervisor in budgeting for and controlling resources needed for operational outputs. Each input will have to be defined as a relative value unit (R.V.U.) With this identification, quantity, quality, and cost can be measured.

SYSTEM, COST CENTER, AND CODE	UNITS OF MEASURE
Executive and administrative system (061)	R.V.U.'s
Administration 061-01	R.V.U.'s
Comptroller 061-02	R.V.U.'s
Medical director and chief of staff 061-03	R.V.U.'s
Public relations 061-04	R.V.U.'s
Medical services and departments 061-05	R.V.U.'s
Volunteers 061-06	R.V.U.'s

SYSTEM, COST CENTER, AND CODE	UNITS OF MEASURE
Gift shop 061-07	R.V.U.'s
Private offices 061-08	R.V.U.'s
Fixed charges 061-11	R.V.U.'s
Quality control system (062)	R.V.U.'s
Duplicating 062-01	Job hours
Telephone operators 062-02	Extensions
Mailroom 062-03	Message units
Information desk 062-04	Inpatient days
Medical records 062-05	Charts processed; incomplete charts
Admissions 062-06	Admissions
Systems and procedures 062-07	R.V.U.'s
Admissions and information OPD 062-08	R.V.U.'s
Personnel and education system (063)	R.V.U.'s
Personnel 063-01	F.T.E.'s*
In-service training 063-02	F.T.E.'s
Employee benefits 063-03	F.T.E.'s
Business system (064)	R.V.U.'s
Inpatient business office 064-01	R.V.U.'s
Outpatient business office 064-02	R.V.U.'s
Emergency business office 064-03	Emergency visits
Record clerks 064-04	Records
Security and medicolegal system (065)	R.V.U.'s
Security 065-01	Assigned hours
Insurances 065-02	R.V.U.'s
Harbison lot 065-03	Parking spaces
Transportation, logistics, and supply system (066)	R.V.U.'s
Purchasing 066-01	Invoices
Storeroom 066-02	Invoices
Laundry 066-03	Pounds of clean laundry
Sewing room 066-04	Pieces
Dietary 066-05	Total meals
Cafeteria 066-08	Meals served
Total inpatients 066-05	Meals served
Total students 066-08	Meals served
Snack bar 066-06	Transactions
Doctors' dining room 066-07	Meals served
Special events 066-05	Meals served
Central supply 066-10	R.V.U.'s
Environmental services system (067)	R.V.U.'s
Plant operations 067-01	Square feet
Maintentance 067-02	Square feet
Properties 067-04 thru 10, 14, 15 16	Square feet
Housekeeping 067-11	Assigned hours
Elevator operators 067-12	Assigned hours
Boiler plant 067-13	Pounds of steam
Patient care system (068)	R.V.U.'s
Nursing administration 068-01	R.V.U.'s
Recovery room 068-02	Patients
Intensive care unit 068-03	Inpatient days
Bronchoesophagology 068-04	Procedures
Cardiovascular 068-05	Patient days
Nurses' registry 068-06	R.V.U.'s
Operating room 068-07	Operating minutes
Delivery room 068-08	Deliveries

*Full-time equivalents

SYSTEM, COST CENTER, AND CODE	UNITS OF MEASURE	SYSTEM, COST CENTER, AND CODE	UNITS OF MEASURE
Nursery		3 B	
068-09	Nursery days	068-17	Patient days
OPD nursing and clinic		3 MS	
068-10	Visits	068-17	Patient days
Emergency department		3 MN	
068-11	Visits	068-17	Patient days
Physical medicine and		4 B	
rehabilitation		068-17	Patient days
068-13	Procedures	4 M	
School of practical nursing		068-17	Patient days
068-14	Hours of	5 M	
	instruction	068-17	Patient days
Central supply		Men's orthopedics	
068-16	R.V.U.'s	068-17	Patient days
Dermatology clinic		Women's orthopedics	
068-18	Visits	068-17	Patient days
School of nursing education		Professional service	
068-50	Hours of	departments system (069)	R.V.U.'s
	instruction	Clinic coordinator	
Student health		069-00	Outpatient visits
068-51	Visits	Clinic service area	
Jones residence		069-01	Outpatient visits
068-52	Square feet	Dental clinic	
Social work		069-02	Visits
068-55	Hours of service	Tumor clinic	
2 PP		069-03	Visits
068-17	Patient days	Psychiatry clinic	
3 PP		069-04	Visits
068-17	Patient days	Community mental health	
4 PP		clinic 069-05	Visits
068-17	Patient days	Audiology	
5 PP		069-06	Visits
068-17	Patient days	E.N.T. clinic	
6 PP		069-07	Visits
068-17	Patient days	Dermatology clinic	
7 PP		069-08	Visits
068-17	Patient days	Allergy clinic	
8 PP		069-09	Visits
068-17	Patient days	Pharmacy	
9 PP		069-10	R.V.U.'s
068-17	Patient days	X-ray diagnosis	
10 PP		069-11	Films
068-17	Patient days	X-ray therapy	
1 B		069-12	Portals
068-17	Patient days	X-ray nuclear	
2 B		069-13	Procedures
068-17	Patient days	X-ray engineers	
2 A		069-14	R.V.U.'s
068-17	Patient days	Physical medicine and	
2 MS		rehabilitation	
068-17	Patient days	069-15	Procedures
2 MN		Inhalation therapy	
068-17	Patient days	069-16	Minutes of
3 A			service
068-17	Patient days	Pulmonary function	
		069-17	Procedures

SYSTEM, COST CENTER, AND CODE	UNITS OF MEASURE
Anesthesiology	
069-18	Minutes of service
Gastroenterology	
069-19	Procedures
EEG	
069-20	Examinations
EKG	
069-26	Examinations
Cardiac catheterization	
069-22	Procedures
Heart surgery	
069-23	Procedure minutes
Anesthesia workroom	
069-24	Procedures
Bronchoesophagology	
069-25	Procedure minutes
Heart station	
069-26	Examinations
Emergency department	
069-27	Visits
Private OPD lab	
069-28	Tests; R.V.U.'s
Cardiology	
069-29	Tests; R.V.U.'s
Blood bank	
069-30	Tests; R.V.U.'s
Chemistry lab	
069-31	Tests; R.V.U.'s
Endocrinology lab	
069-32	Tests; R.V.U.'s
Hematology lab	
069-33	Tests; R.V.U.'s
Microbiology lab	
069-34	Tests; R.V.U.'s
Pathology lab	
069-35	Tests; R.V.U.'s
Rheumatology lab	
069-36	Tests; R.V.U.'s
Laboratory coordinator	
069-37	Tests (total) R.V.U.'s
Cytology lab	
069-38	Tests; R.V.U.'s
Parasitology lab	
069-39	Tests; R.V.U.'s
Serology lab	
069-40	Tests; R.V.U.'s
Mycology lab	
069-41	Tests; R.V.U.'s
Virology lab	
069-42	Tests; R.V.U.'s

At the systems level, inpatient days and outpatient visits are equated through the use of a relative value unit. Budgeting at the systems level is on the basis of relative value units that relate to the overall goals of the hospital. They are established to assist management in allocating resources among competing demands. In programs, patient days or ambulatory visits are used as units of measure.

The second is the accumulation of statistical data reflecting the volume of performance. Historical data of the volume of service should be accumulated. Table 8-1 shows the number of patient days and the average percentage of occupancy on a nursing unit.

Volume statistics are used for making budgetary predictions of the volume of service for the new budget. Through correctly analyzing historical data by units, services, and percentages of occupancy and relating them to current trends, reasonably accurate estimates can be made for each quarter of the year. Prior to preparation of the final estimate of performance, administration should be consulted on the possible influence of factors such as internal expansion and economic conditions in the community. Changes in these factors should be reflected in the final estimates whenever possible.

Taking the historical information along with future predictions of demands and conditions into consideration, the budget performance report should be prepared as shown in Fig. 8-1.

Budgeted performance is developed for each cost center and is used to establish a position for the salaries and wages expense budget and the supplies and expense budget. These budgets present expenses related to units of measure. It is therefore extremely important that a great deal of time and consideration be given to the preparation of this report because such a large portion of the total budget is based upon its projections.

Once budgeted performance reports have

Table 8-1. Volume of performance

| | Floor number 1 | | | | | | | |
| | First quarter | | Second quarter | | Third quarter | | Fourth quarter | |
Year	Patient days	Occupancy (%)	Patient days	Occupancy (%)	Patient days	Occupancy (%)	Patient days	Occupancy (%)
1	1,837	67	1,823	68	1,553	56	1,519	55
2	1,738	63	2,040	76	2,382	55	3,015	41
3	3,913	53	3,708	53	3,605	50	2,656	37
4	3,440	48	3,852	55	3,098	43	3,398	47
5	3,716	52	4,261	61	3,417	48	2,939	41
Budget this year	3,732	52	4,026	58	3,229	45	3,588	50

| | First quarter | | | Second quarter | | | |
Nursing floors	Available beds	Occupancy %	Budgeted patient days	Available beds	Occupancy %	Budgeted patient days	Available beds
1	7176	52	3732	7020	58	4026	7176
2	5336	76	4055	5220	76	3967	5336
3	9200	40	3680	9000	33	2970	9200
4	1288	55	708	1260	55	685	1288
5	2484	87	2161	2430	89	2139	720
6	3680	87	3202	3600	89	3168	3689
7	2208	90	1987	2160	93	1986	2225
8	2208	90	1987	2160	93	1986	2206
9	2208	90	1987	2160	93	1986	2208
10	3864	90	3478	3780	93	3476	3864
11	3680	92	3386	3600	95	3382	3680
12	3312	90	2981	3240	92	2948	3312
13	3312	90	2981	3240	96	3076	3312
Totals	49956	73	36325	48870	73	35795	48192

Fig. 8-1. Budgeted performance report.

been completed, the expense segment of the operating budget may be begun. The old-line object budget emphasized the means of producing an end product; paper and secretarial time were seen as means of accomplishing a typewritten report. The performance budget transfers the emphasis from the means—which are things that are bought—to accomplishment—the typewritten report. Therefore, instead of budgeting for "X" reams of paper, the secretary, and the typewriter, the performance budget budgets for the 600 typewritten reports that experience has shown can be produced by the means of the paper, the secretary, and the typewriter.

Performance budgeting relates cost to units of measure. This is done through a coding system that relates costs to cost centers and a series of budget worksheets that relate cost to units of measure. Several of the cost centers within the patient care system are shown in the following example. Each is assigned an identifying code.

COST CENTER CODES
Patient care system

Cost center	Code
Nursing administration	068-01
Floor nursing	068-17
Outpatient nursing	068-10
Operating room	068-07
Delivery room	068-08
Social work	068-55

OBJECT CLASSIFICATION CODE

A typical object classification code would appear as follows:

1—068—01—375

1—Identifies the operating fund
068—Identifies the patient care system
01—Identifies the nursing administration cost center
375—Identifies office supplies

Thus expenses such as the following may be charged directly against the cost center that incurred them:

Salaries, wages, and fees
Employee health and welfare benefits
Consumable supplies (office supplies [375])
Replacement for minor nondepreciable equipment
Purchased services
General expenses
Depreciation
General insurance expense
Charges from service departments

Expenses for each cost center should be studied historically. Having done this, performance expenses may be set up in two segments: salaries and wages performance budget and supplies and expense performance budget.

Salaries and wages make up the largest portion of total operating costs. This category accounts for approximately 65% to 75% of the total. For this reason it is imperative to attach great importance to the preparation of this part of the budget. Cost centers should complete the personnel budget forms as illustrated in Figs. 8-2 and 8-3. Future expansion of the organization or cost centers must be considered at this time. Allowances must be made for additional positions that may be created during the year. Salary increases either by job classification or individual must also be considered.

The personnel budget requires that supervisors make detailed advance planning to assure accurate personnel cost estimates. The report should be completed well in advance of the beginning of the fiscal year.

Review and discussion should take place among supervisors and administrators, and approval should be obtained at all levels. This approval gives administration the information necessary to evaluate and control personnel cost. Personnel costs are related to units of measure in order to determine the personnel cost per unit. Fig. 8-2, for example, shows that 14,575 patient days are budgeted for nursing floor number one. The salaries and wages are budgeted at $133,233. Therefore the budgeted personnel cost per patient day it $9.14.

Once the personnel worksheets have been completed, they may be summarized on the personnel summary sheet shown in Fig. 8-3. This summary will be used by departments containing multiple cost centers and also by the systems and programs.

The supplies and expense portion of the performance budget represents 30% to 35% of the total. Historical data for a reasonable period should be developed for each cost center and identified on the basis of cost per performance unit. Cost centers should complete the supplies and expenses, contracts, equipment, and renovation worksheets illustrated in Figs. 8-4 to 8-10. Future expansion of the organization or cost centers must be considered as it was for salaries and wages. An adequate review at all levels must be accomplished.

Supplies and expenses costs are related to units of measure to determine the supplies and expenses cost per unit. Fig. 8-4 shows that 14,575 patient days are budgeted for nursing floor number one. The supplies and expenses are budgeted at $34,832. Therefore the resulting cost per patient day is $2.39.

A listing of contracts for outside service is included in the cost. It is reported in summary form on the summary of contracts sheet (Fig. 8-6) for use by management and the purchasing department.

When the supplies and expenses worksheets have been completed for all cost centers, they may be summarized in the

Text continued on p. 178.

BUDGET YEAR 19 67-68 — PERSONNEL WORKSHEET

COST CENTER Code: 068-21 SYSTEM Name: ____ Nursing Name: Floor #1

UNIT of MEASURE: Patient	Days
EXPENSES PREVIOUS YEAR	110,710.
UNITS PREVIOUS YEAR	14,333
UNIT COST	7.72

ADJUSTMENT to UNIT COST		
UNIT COST	133,233	7.72
ADJUSTMENT	14,575	1.42
ADJUSTED UNIT COST		9.14

JUSTIFICATION for ADJUSTMENT
1. Increase in authorized positions
2. Increase for all Salary groups of $25. per Bi-Weekly payroll effective 7/1/67

CODE	NAME	CURRENT Amount	eff date	SCHEDULED w	v	TOTAL	JUL	AUG	SEP	OCT	NOV	DEC	JAN	FEB	MAR	APR	MAY	JUN
121	M. Jones	250.	1/60	2,080.	160	7,150.	550.	825.	550.	550.	550.	550.	825.	550.	550.	550.	550.	550.
121	J. Burton	250.	1/60	2,080.	160	7,150.	550.	825.	550.	550.	550.	550.	825.	550.	550.	550.	550.	550.
121	P. Weis	250.	1/60	2,080.	160	7,150.	550.	825.	550.	550.	550.	550.	825.	550.	550.	550.	550.	550.
122	H. Mason	225.	3/61	2,080.	80	6,500.	500.	750.	500.	500.	500.	500.	750.	500.	500.	500.	500.	500.
122	G. Wells	225.	3/61	2,080.	80	6,500.	500.	750.	500.	500.	500.	500.	750.	500.	500.	500.	500.	500.
122	A. Watts	200.	7/63	2,080.	80	5,850.	450.	675.	450.	450.	450.	450.	675.	450.	450.	450.	450.	450.
122	B. Smith	175.	8/64	2,080.	80	5,200.	400.	600.	400.	400.	400.	400.	600.	400.	400.	400.	400.	400.
122	R. Molin	175.	7/64	2,080.	80	5,200.	400.	600.	400.	400.	400.	400.	600.	400.	400.	400.	400.	400.
122.	L. Mathis	175.	10/64	2,080.	80	5,200.	400.	600.	400.	400.	400.	400.	600.	400.	400.	400.	400.	400.
123	M. Wilson	175.	12/60	2,080.	160	5,200.	400.	600.	400.	400.	400.	400.	600.	400.	400.	400.	400.	400.
123	J. Conwell	150.	5/63	2,080.	80	4,550.	350.	525.	350.	350.	350.	350.	525.	350.	350.	350.	350.	350.
123	E. Murray	125.	7/64	2,080.	80	3,900.	300.	450.	300.	300.	300.	300.	450.	300.	300.	300.	300.	300.
124	A. Mark	150.	8/63	2,080.	80	4,550.	350.	525.	350.	350.	350.	350.	525.	350.	350.	350.	350.	350.
124	L. James	150.	11/63	2,080.	80	4,550.	350.	525.	350.	350.	350.	350.	525.	350.	350.	350.	350.	350.
***	Sub-total from Form #10781			***														
	TOTAL CURRENT			50,752.	2000	115,185	8,860	13,292	8,860	8,860	8,860	8,860	13,293	8,860	8,860	8,860	8,860	8,860
	OTHER																	
	PREMIUM PAY	1,000.	-----			2,444.	188.	282.	188.	188.	188.	188.	282.	188.	188.	188.	188.	188.
	VACATION COVERAGE	2,000.	-----			4,520.	904	904				904	904					904
	HOLIDAY COVERAGE	1,000.	-----			2,444.			407		407	407	409			407	407	
	ON CALL or OTHER	3,824.	-----			8,640.	720.	720.	720.	720.	720.	720.	720.	720.	720.	720.	720.	720.
	TOTAL OTHER	7,824.				18,048.	1,812	1,906	1,315	908	1,315	2,219	2,315	908	908	1,315	1,315	1,812
	TOTAL BUDGET	58,576.			2000	133,233.	10,672	15,198	10,175	9,768	10,175	11,079	15,608	9,768	9,768	10,175	10,175	10,672

Form # 10780

Fig. 8-2. Personnel worksheet.

BUDGET YEAR 1967-68 COST CENTER CODE: 068 SYSTEM: Name: Patient Care System

PERSONNEL SUMMARY

COST CENTER	SCHEDULED WORK HRS.	TOTAL * PERSONNEL BUDGET	MONTHS											
			JUL	AUG	SEP	OCT	NOV	DEC	JAN	FEB	MAR	APR	MAY	JUN
068-21	58,576	133,233.	10,672.	15,198.	10,175.	9,768.	10,175.	11,079.	15,608.	9,768.	10,175.	10,175.	10,175.	10,175.
068-22	64,104	144,234.	12,981.	14,424.	11,539.	10,096.	11,539.	12,981.	14,423.	10,096.	11,539.	11,539.	11,539.	12,981.
068-23	51,992	116,982.	10,528.	11,697.	9,359.	8,189.	9,359.	10,528.	11,698.	8,189.	8,189.	9,359.	9,359.	10,528.
068-24	9,692	21,807.	1,963.	2,180.	1,745.	1,526.	1,745.	1,963.	2,180.	1,526.	1,526.	1,745.	1,745.	1,745.
068-25	18,640	41,940.	4,409.	4,831.	3,989.	3,569.	3,989.	4,409.	4,831.	3,570.	3,570.	3,989.	784.	-------
068-26	51,680	116,280.	10,465.	11,629.	9,302.	8,140.	9,302.	10,465.	11,628.	8,140.	8,140.	9,302.	9,302.	10,465.
068-27	31,964	71,919.	6,473.	7,191.	5,754.	5,034.	5,754.	6,473.	7,191.	5,034.	5,034.	5,754.	5,754.	6,473.
068-28	31,964	71,919.	6,473.	7,191.	5,754.	5,034.	5,754.	6,473.	7,191.	5,034.	5,034.	5,754.	5,754.	6,473.
068-29	31,964	71,919.	6,473.	7,191.	5,754.	5,034.	5,754.	6,473.	7,191.	5,034.	5,034.	5,754.	5,754.	6,473.
068-30	55,948	125,883.	11,329.	12,588.	10,071.	8,812.	10,071.	11,329.	12,588.	8,812.	8,812.	10,071.	10,071.	11,329.
068-31	53,716	120,861.	10,877.	12,087.	9,669.	8,460.	9,669.	10,877.	12,087.	8,460.	8,460.	9,669.	9,669.	10,877.
068-32	47,564	107,019.	9,632.	10,701.	8,562.	7,491.	8,562.	9,632.	10,701.	7,491.	7,491.	8,562.	8,562.	9,632.
068-33	50,724	114,129.	10,272.	11,413.	9,130.	7,989.	9,130.	10,272.	11,413.	7,989.	7,989.	9,130.	9,130.	10,272.
TOTAL	558,528	1,258,125.	112,547.	128,321.	100,803.	89,142.	100,803.	112,954.	128,730.	89,143.	89,143.	100,803.	97,598.	108,138.

* This Column summarizes all Personnel Costs listed on Form # 10780 (Personnel Worksheet)

Form # 10782

Fig. 8-3. Personnel summary.

BUDGET YEAR 19 67-68

COST CENTER Code # 068-21   Name: Nursing Floor #1
SYSTEM Name: Patient Care System

SUPPLIES & EXPENSES WORKSHEET

Unit of Measure: Patient Days

ADJUSTMENT to UNIT COST		JUSTIFICATION for ADJUSTMENT
UNIT COST	2.17	Estimated price increases for coming year of approximately 10%.
ADJUSTMENT	.22	
ADJUSTED UNIT COST	2.39	

EXPENSES PREVIOUS YEAR	$31,103.
UNITS PREVIOUS YEAR	14,333
UNIT COST	2.17

MONTHS

	TOTAL	JUL	AUG	SEP	OCT	NOV	DEC	JAN	FEB	MAR	APR	MAY	JUN
UNIT – BUDGET YEAR	14,575	1,244	1,244	1,244	1,342	1,342	1,342	1,077	1,076	1,076	1,196	1,196	1,196
UNIT COST	2.39	2.39	2.39	2.39	2.39	2.39	2.39	2.39	2.39	2.39	2.39	2.39	2.39
SUPPLIES & EXPENSE BUDGET	34,832.	2,973.	2,973.	2,973.	3,207.	3,207.	3,207.	2,574.	2,572.	2,572.	2,858.	2,858.	2,858.
CONTRACTS													
IBM TYPEWRITERS (4)	144.							144.					
ABC CONTRACT	4,080.	340.	340.	340.	340.	340.	340.	340.	340.	340.	340.	340.	340.
TOTAL CONTRACTS **	4,224.	340.	340.	340.	340.	340.	340.	484.	340.	340.	340.	340.	340.
BUDGET 19 67-68	34,832.	2,973.	2,973.	2,973.	3,207.	3,207.	3,207.	2,574.	2,572.	2,572.	2,858.	2,858.	2,858.

** Totals included in Supplies and Expenses Budget.

Form # 10783

Fig. 8-4. Supplies and expenses worksheet.

BUDGET YEAR 19 67-68

COST CENTER Code # 068   Name: Nursing floors

SYSTEM Name: Patient Care System

SUPPLIES & EXPENSES SUMMARY *

COST CENTER	TOTAL	MONTHS											
		JUL	AUG	SEP	OCT	NOV	DEC	JAN	FEB	MAR	APR	MAY	JUN
068-21	34,832.	2,973.	2,973.	2,973.	3,207.	3,207.	3,207.	2,574.	2,572.	2,572.	2,858.	2,858.	2,858.
068-22	38,302.	3,192.	3,192.	3,192.	3,192.	3,192.	3,192.	3,191.	3,192.	3,191.	3,191.	3,192.	3,192.
068-23	31,065.	2,589.	2,589.	2,589.	2,589.	2,589.	2,589.	2,589.	2,589.	2,589.	2,588.	2,588.	2,588.
068-24	5,791.	483.	483.	482.	483.	482.	483.	482.	483.	482.	483.	482.	483.
068-25	11,137.	1,114.	1,114.	1,114.	1,114.	1,114.	1,114.	1,114.	1,114.	1,000.	1,000.	225.	----
068-26	31,008.	2,584.	2,584.	2,584.	2,584.	2,584.	2,584.	2,584.	2,584.	2,584.	2,584.	2,584.	2,584.
068-27	19,178.	1,599.	1,598.	1,598.	1,598.	1,598.	1,598.	1,598.	1,598.	1,598.	1,598.	1,598.	1,598.
068-28	19,178.	1,599.	1,598.	1,598.	1,598.	1,598.	1,598.	1,598.	1,598.	1,598.	1,598.	1,598.	1,598.
068-29	19,178.	1,599.	1,598.	1,598.	1,598.	1,598.	1,598.	1,598.	1,598.	1,598.	1,598.	1,598.	1,598.
068-30	33,569.	2,797.	2,797.	2,798.	2,798.	2,798.	2,798.	2,798.	2,797.	2,797.	2,797.	2,797.	2,797.
068-31	32,230.	2,686.	2,686.	2,686.	2,686.	2,686.	2,686.	2,686.	2,686.	2,686.	2,686.	2,685.	2,685.
068-32	28,538.	2,379.	2,379.	2,378.	2,378.	2,378.	2,378.	2,378.	2,378.	2,378.	2,378.	2,378.	2,378.
068-33	30,434.	2,537.	2,537.	2,536.	2,536.	2,536.	2,536.	2,536.	2,536.	2,536.	2,536.	2,536.	2,536.
TOTAL	334,440.	28,131.	28,126.	28,126.	28,361.	28,360.	28,361.	27,729.	27,725.	27,610.	27,895.	27,119.	26,895.
BUDGET 19 67-68	334,440.	28,131.	28,126.	28,126.	28,361.	28,360.	28,361.	27,729.	27,725.	27,610.	27,895.	27,119.	26,895.

* For Multiple Cost Centers

Form #10785

Fig. 8-5. Supplies and expenses summary.

BUDGET YEAR 1967-68

COST CENTER Code # 068   Name: Nursing floors
SYSTEM: Name: Patient Care System

SUMMARY of CONTRACTS *

COST CENTER	TOTAL	MONTHS											
		JUL	AUG	SEP	OCT	NOV	DEC	JAN	FEB	MAR	APR	MAY	JUN
068-21	4,224.	340.	340.	340.	340.	340.	340.	484.	340.	340.	340.	340.	340.
068-22	5,120.	400.	420.	420.	460.	280.	200.	600.	740.	400.	400.	400.	400.
068-23	3,000.	250.	250.	250.	250.	250.	250.	250.	250.	250.	250.	250.	250.
068-24	1,000.	83.	83.	84.	83.	83.	84.	83.	83.	84.	83.	83.	84.
068-25	500.	-----	-----	-----	500.	-----	-----	-----	-----	-----	-----	-----	-----
068-26	4,224.	340.	340.	340.	340.	340.	340.	484.	340.	340.	340.	340.	340.
068-27	60.	-----	-----	-----	-----	-----	60.	-----	-----	-----	-----	-----	-----
068-28	60.	-----	-----	-----	-----	-----	60.	-----	-----	-----	-----	-----	-----
068-29	60.	-----	-----	-----	-----	-----	60.	-----	-----	-----	-----	-----	-----
068-30	5,120.	400.	420.	420.	460.	280.	200.	600.	740.	400.	400.	400.	400.
068-31	3,000.	250.	250.	250.	250.	250.	250.	250.	250.	250.	250.	250.	250.
068-32	-----	-----	-----	-----	-----	-----	-----	-----	-----				
068-33	-----	-----	-----	-----	-----	-----	-----	-----	-----				
TOTAL CONTRACTS	26,368.	2,063.	2,103.	2,104.	2,683.	1,823.	1,844.	2,751.	2,743.	2,064.	2,063.	2,063.	2,063.

note: information purpose -- Summary of Contracts

* For Multiple Cost Centers

Form # 10784

Fig. 8-6. Summary of contracts.

EQUIPMENT WORKSHEET

COST CENTER Code: 068-21 Name: Nursing Floor #1
SYSTEM Name: Patient Care System

BUDGET YEAR 1967-68

PRIORITY and DESCRIPTION	No. of Items	Additions	Improvement	Replacements	estimated cost		CASH REQUIREMENTS by MONTHS											
					each	total	JUL	AUG	SEP	OCT	NOV	DEC	JAN	FEB	MAR	APR	MAY	JUN
T.V. MONITOR for PATIENT ROOMS	24	x			500.	12,000.	3,000.			3,000.			3,000.			3,000.		
ADDRESS-O-GRAPH MACHINE	1			x	50.	50.					50.							
DESK	1			x	50.	50.		50.										
TOTAL						12,100.	3,000.	50.		3,000.	50.		3,000.			3,000.		

Form #10786

Fig. 8-7. Equipment worksheet.

BUDGET YEAR 1967-68 EQUIPMENT SUMMARY * COST CENTER Code #068 Name: _____
SYSTEM Name: Patient Care System

COST CENTERS	No. of items	Additions	Improvements	Replacements	estimated cost each	estimated cost total	JUL	AUG	SEP	OCT	NOV	DEC	JAN	FEB	MAR	APR	MAY	JUN
																		CASH REQUIREMENTS BY MONTHS
068-21	---	---	---	---	---	12,100.	3,000.	50.	---	3,000.	50.		3,000.			3,000.		
068-22	---	---	---	---	---	3,000.			3,000.			100.						
068-23	---	---	---	---	---	100.												
068-24	---	---	---	---	---	---												
068-25	---	---	---	---	---	---												
068-26	---	---	---	---	---	8,000.		2,000.			2,000.			4,000.				
068-27	---	---	---	---	---	---												
068-28	---	---	---	---	---	---												
068-29	---	---	---	---	---	---												
068-30	---	---	---	---	---	10,000.												10,000
068-31	---	---	---	---	---	300.											300.	
068-32	---	---	---	---	---	300.											300.	
068-33	---	---	---	---	---	500.									500.			
TOTAL						34,300.	3,000.	2,050.	3,000.	3,000.	2,050.	100.	3,000.	4,000.	500.	3,000.	600.	10,000.

* For Multiple Cost Centers

Form #10787

Fig. 8-8. Equipment summary.

BUDGET YEAR 19 _67-68_					COST CENTER Code # 068-21 Name: Nursing floor #1														
RENOVATIONS WORKSHEET					SYSTEM Name: Patient Care System														
PRIORITY and DESCRIPTION	No. of Items	Additions	Improvements	Replacements	estimated cost		CASH REQUIREMENTS by MONTHS												
					each	total	JUL	AUG	SEP	OCT	NOV	DEC	JAN	FEB	MAR	APR	MAY	JUN
CHANGE SERVICE ACCOMODATIONS to SEMI-PRIVATE on 2 MAIN SOUTH		×				5,000.											5,000.	

Form # 10788

Fig. 8-9. Renovations worksheet.

BUDGET YEAR 19 67-68

* RENOVATIONS SUMMARY

COST CENTER Code # 068   Name:

SYSTEM Name: Patient Care System

COST CENTERS	No. of Items	Additions	Improvements	Replacements	estimated cost		CASH REQUIREMENTS by MONTHS											
					each	total	JUL	AUG	SEP	OCT	NOV	DEC	JAN	FEB	MAR	APR	MAY	JUN
068–21			×			5,000.											5,000.	
068–22				×		500.		500.										
068–23		×				6,000.									6,000.			
068–24						----												
068–25			×			10,000.												10,000
068–26						------												
068–27						------												
068–28						------												
068–29						------												
068–30			×			8,000.				8,000.								
068–31						------												
068–32						------												
068–33						------												
TOTAL						29,500.		500.		8,000.					6,000.		5,000.	10,000

Form # 10789

* For Multiple Cost Centers

Fig. 8-10. Renovations summary.

supplies and expenses summary sheet illustrated in Fig. 8-5. This summary will be used by departments containing multiple cost centers and also by the systems and programs.

Figs. 8-7 to 8-10 present the equipment worksheet, equipment summary, renovations worksheet, and renovations summary. As was the case with supplies and expenses and contracts, these forms are completed by cost centers, and summary forms are again used by departments with multiple cost centers and systems and programs.

Having assisted the cost centers in completing their *performance* budgets, the systems and programs are now prepared to set up *program* budgets. Although the mechanics are somewhat the same, the purpose of a program budget is different from that of a performance budget.

By way of comparison:

A performance budget process is task oriented—A program budget process is planning oriented

A performance budget process is designed to guide operations—A program budget process is designed to guide policy formulation

A performance budget measures the effectiveness of given ways of operating—A program budget measures the effectiveness among alternative ways of operating

A performance budget focuses on expenditure details—A program budget focuses on expenditure aggregates

A performance budget process utilizes accounting analysis—A program budget process utilizes systems analysis

A performance budget process views work as an end in itself—A program budget process views work as translating resources into end products

The system and the program, as an aggregate of cost centers, is responsible for the performance of each, but its larger responsibility is the aggregate. Hence cost reflected in the program budget is a broad, general summary and is not detailed in terms of specific performance activities.

The program budget for systems relates cost to relative value units that adjust for the mix of inpatient days and outpatient visits and are thus a useful tool for higher level administration in working toward the total budget. As a focal point of translation between operating cost centers and the total organization, the program budget becomes the framework within which service goals are related to activities and units of measure.

For purposes of demonstration, the dollar value of 1 R.V.U. is established at $20. Historical analysis shows that the aggregate direct-operating cost of an inpatient day is $44, the cost of a nursery day is $22, the cost of an outpatient occasion of service is $14, and the cost of an emergency visit is $18. These are direct costs. Indirect costs are taken into consideration in cost finding. Adjusting these costs to relative value units by dividing by $20, the relative value of an inpatient day is 2.23; of a nursery day, 1.10; of an outpatient occasion of service, 0.69; and of an emergency visit, 0.92.

Administration estimates 232,101 inpatient days, 17,230 nursery days, 191,000 outpatient occasions of service, and 45,568 emergency visits for the coming budgetary year. By multiplying the days and visits by their relative value

Inpatient	517,000 R.V.U.'s
Nursery	19,000
Outpatient	131,460
Emergency	39,908
Total	707,368 R.V.U.'s

all systems are asked to budget on the basis of 707,368 R.V.U.'s.

The program budget for programs relates cost to inpatient days or ambulatory visits.

All cost centers have now completed personnel worksheets (Fig. 8-2), and departments with multiple cost centers have completed the personnel summary (Fig. 8-3). As illustrated in Fig. 8-11, salaries and wages costs for all cost centers in each system and program are summarized using the personnel summary sheet. The information entered in this summary should have already been approved at the several administrative levels and thus represents

BUDGET YEAR 19 67-68

PERSONNEL SUMMARY

COST CENTER CODE: 068 Name:
SYSTEM Name: Patient Care System

COST CENTER	SCHEDULED WORK HRS.	TOTAL * PERSONNEL	JUL	AUG	SEP	OCT	NOV	DEC	JAN	FEB	MAR	APR	MAY	JUN
068-01		20,280.	1,560.	2,340.	1,560.	1,560.	1,560.	1,560.	2,340.	1,560.	1,560.	1,560.	1,560.	1,560.
068-02		11,520.	720.	2,160.	720.	720.	720.	720.	2,160.	720.	720.	720.	720.	720.
068-03		22,100.	1,700.	2,550.	1,700.	1,700.	1,700.	1,700.	2,550.	1,700.	1,700.	1,700.	1,700.	1,700.
068-04		23,400.	1,800.	2,700.	1,800.	1,800.	1,800.	1,800.	2,700.	1,800.	1,800.	1,800.	1,800.	1,800.
068-05		31,200.	2,400.	3,600.	2,400.	2,400.	2,400.	2,400.	3,600.	2,400.	2,400.	2,400.	2,400.	2,400.
068-06		9,880.	760.	1,140.	760.	760.	760.	760.	1,140.	760.	760.	760.	760.	760.
068-07		31,200.	2,400.	3,600.	2,400.	2,400.	2,400.	3,600.	2,400.	2,400.	2,400.	2,400.	2,400.	2,400.
068-08		15,600.	1,200.	1,800.	1,200.	1,200.	1,200.	1,200.	1,800.	1,200.	1,200.	1,200.	1,200.	1,200.
068-09		14,300.	1,100.	1,650.	1,100.	1,100.	1,100.	1,100.	1,650.	1,100.	1,100.	1,100.	1,100.	1,100.
068-10		26,000.	2,000.	3,000.	2,000.	2,000.	2,000.	2,000.	3,000.	2,000.	2,000.	2,000.	2,000.	2,000.
068-11		15,600.	1,200.	1,800.	1,200.	1,200.	1,200.	1,200.	1,800.	1,200.	1,200.	1,200.	1,200.	1,200.
068-21														
TO	(SEE COST CENTER SUMMARY for DETAIL)													
068-33	558,528.	1,258,125.	112,547.	128,321.	100,803.	89,142.	100,803.	112,954.	128,730.	89,143.	89,143.	100,803.	97,598.	108,138.
TOTAL		1,497,205.	129,387.	154,661.	117,643.	105,982.	117,643.	129,794.	155,070.	105,983.	105,983.	117,643.	114,438.	124,978.

MONTHS

* This column summarizes all Personnel Costs Listed on Form #10781

Form #10782

Fig. 8-11. Personnel summary.

the formal budget request of the cost centers as an aggregate.

Using the systems summary represented in Fig. 8-12, the total salaries and wages cost of the systems is related to relative value units. According to Fig. 8-12, the total budgeted salaries and wages cost is $1,479,205. By dividing $1,479,205 by 707,368 R.V.U.'s, a personnel cost of $2.09 per R.V.U. is established.

All cost centers have complete supplies and expense worksheets (Fig. 8-4), and departments with multiple cost centers have completed the supplies and expense summary (Fig. 8-5). As illustrated in Fig. 8-13, supplies and expense costs for all cost centers in each system and program are summarized using the supplies and expense summary sheet. The information entered in this summary should also have been approved at the several administrative levels and thus represents the formal budget request of the cost centers as an aggregate.

Using the systems summary presented in Fig. 8-12, the total supplies and expenses cost is related to relative value units. The total supplies and expense cost shown in Fig. 8-12 is $486,840. By dividing this by 707,368 R.V.U.'s, a supplies and expenses cost of 69 cents per R.V.U. is established.

A listing of contracts for outside services has been included in the cost center (Fig. 8-4), and these costs have been included in the systems summary of supplies and expenses. As demonstrated in Fig. 8-14, at the systems level all contracts are listed on the summary of contracts sheet, and the total is transferred to the systems summary shown in Fig. 8-12. Both the listing and the summary will be used for coordinating the hospital operating budget. Beyond that, the listing will be used by administration and purchasing in evaluation and coordinating contracts. Contracts for programs should be negotiated through systems.

Equipment and renovations budgets have been submitted by cost centers (Figs. 8-7 to 8-10) and are summarized at the systems

and programs level on the equipment summary sheet (Fig. 8-15) and the renovations summary sheet (Fig. 8-16). The totals of these summaries are transferred to the summary sheet (Fig. 8-12) and complete its preparation.

Once the complete budget has been approved and put into effect, feedback is required. Fig. 8-17, *A*, shows the form in which actual cost experience is reported at the systems and cost center levels. This information is the basis upon which controls are established to carry out organizational policy within budgetary guidelines. A similar analysis is established for programs reflecting a reallocation of cost from systems to the programs that use their services (Fig. 8-17, *B*). This is the mechanism for pricing programs as packages of care according to the input resources used.

At this point the process of budgeting for performance at the operational level and for programs at the systems and programs level is complete (Fig. 8-17, *C*). The cost centers are represented by the performance budgets. The systems and programs are represented by system and program summaries. These summaries conclude this phase of the total hospital budgeting process. They contain the information necessary for higher levels of administration to evaluate the allocation of total hospital resources.

Continuation of the budgeting process to its conclusion is described in three additional phases: **operating budget, capital budget,** and **cash flow budget.**

The first proceeds with the finalization of cost budgeting. Then it develops the companion segment, the revenue budget, and proceeds to weigh the implications of both.

The second summarizes capital requirements.

The third establishes cash flow budget as a policy and control mechanism for managing financial affairs.

•   •   •

Text continued on p. 189.

BUDGET YEAR 1967-68

SYSTEM SUMMARY

SYSTEM: Patient Care System   068

PERSONNEL

SUPPLIES and EXPENSE

UNIT of MEASURE: Relative Value Unit		UNIT of MEASURE: Relative Value Unit
EXPENSES BUDGET YEAR	1,479,205.	EXPENSES BUDGET YEAR	486,840.
UNITS BUDGET YEAR	707,368.	UNITS BUDGET YEAR	707,368.
UNIT COST	2.09	UNIT COST	.69

MONTHS

EXPENSES	TOTAL	JUL	AUG	SEP	OCT	NOV	DEC	JAN	FEB	MAR	APR	MAY	JUN
S. and W.	1,479,205.	129,387.	154,661.	117,643.	105,982.	117,643.	129,794.	155,070.	105,983.	105,983.	117,643.	114,438.	124,978.
S. and E.	486,840.	40,831.	40,828.	40,826.	41,061.	41,060.	41,061.	40,429.	40,425.	40,120.	40,595.	39,819.	39,595.
TOTAL	1,966,045.	170,218.	195,489.	158,469.	147,043.	158,703.	170,855.	195,499.	146,408.	146,293.	158,238.	154,257.	164,573.

OTHER

	TOTAL	JUL	AUG	SEP	OCT	NOV	DEC	JAN	FEB	MAR	APR	MAY	JUN
CONTRACTS**	34,298.	2,653.	2,827.	2,754.	3,273.	2,413.	3,434.	3,341.	3,833.	2,654.	2,653.	2,653.	2,654.
RENOVATION	35,800.	-----	500.	-----	8,000.	1,000.	5,000.	-----	300.	6,000.	-----	5,000.	10,000.
EQUIPMENT	36,900.	3,000.	2,050.	3,600.	3,000.	2,050.	500.	3,000.	4,800.	700.	2,000.	700.	10,500.

** Included in Supplies and Expense Budget.

	TOTAL	JUL	AUG	SEP	OCT	NOV	DEC	JAN	FEB	MAR	APR	MAY	JUN
BUDGET	1,966,045.	170,218.	195,489.	158,469.	147,043.	158,703.	170,855.	195,499.	146,408.	146,293.	158,238.	154,257.	164,573.

Form #10790

Fig. 8-12. Systems summary.

BUDGET YEAR 67–68   COST CENTER CODE # 068   Name:
Patient Care System

SUPPLIES & EXPENSES SUMMARY *

COST CENTER	TOTAL	JUL	AUG	SEP	OCT	NOV	DEC	JAN	FEB	MAR	APR	MAY	JUN
068-01	14,400.	1,200.	1,200.	1,200.	1,200.	1,200.	1,200.	1,200.	1,200.	1,200.	1,200.	1,200.	1,200.
068-02	6,000.	500.	500.	500.	500.	500.	500.	500.	500.	500.	500.	500.	500.
068-03	15,600.	1,300.	1,300.	1,300.	1,300.	1,300.	1,300.	1,300.	1,300.	1,300.	1,300.	1,300.	1,300.
068-04	3,600.	300.	300.	300.	300.	300.	300.	300.	300.	300.	300.	300.	300.
068-05	24,000.	2,000.	2,000.	2,000.	2,000.	2,000.	2,000.	2,000.	2,000.	2,000.	2,000.	2,000.	2,000.
068-06	2,400.	200.	200.	200.	200.	200.	200.	200.	200.	200.	200.	200.	200.
068-07	72,000.	6,000.	6,000.	6,000.	6,000.	6,000.	6,000.	6,000.	6,000.	6,000.	6,000.	6,000.	6,000.
068-08	3,000.	250.	250.	250.	250.	250.	250.	250.	250.	250.	250.	250.	250.
068-09	2,400.	200.	200.	200.	200.	200.	200.	200.	200.	200.	200.	200.	200.
068-10	6,000.	500.	500.	500.	500.	500.	500.	500.	500.	500.	500.	500.	500.
068-11	3,000.	250.	250.	250.	250.	250.	250.	250.	250.	250.	250.	250.	250.
068-21 to 068-33	334,440.	28,131.	28,128.	28,126.	28,361.	28,360.	28,361.	27,729.	27,725.	27,610.	27,895.	27,119.	26,895.
TOTAL	486,840.	40,831.	40,828.	40,826.	41,061.	41,060.	41,061.	40,429.	40,425.	40,310.	40,595.	38,819.	39,595.
BUDGET 1967–68	486,840.	40,831.	40,828.	40,826.	41,061.	41,060.	41,061.	40,429.	40,425.	40,310.	40,595.	38,819.	39,595.

* For Multiple Cost Centers

Form #10785

Fig. 8-13. Supplies and expenses summary.

BUDGET YEAR 1967-68   SUMMARY of CONTRACTS *   COST CENTER Code #068 Name: SYSTEM: Name: Patient Care System

COST CENTER	TOTAL	MONTHS											
		JUL	AUG	SEP	OCT	NOV	DEC	JAN	FEB	MAR	APR	MAY	JUN
068-01	144.		144.										
068-02	----												
068-03	----												
068-04	4,224.	340.	340.	340.	340.	340.	340.	340.	340.	340.	340.	340.	340.
068-05	60.			60.									
068-06	500.								500.				
068-07	----												
068-08	----												
068-09	3,000.	250.	250.	250.	250.	250.	250.	250.	250.	250.	250.	250.	250.
068-10	----												
068-11	----												
068-21 to 068-33	26,368.	2,063.	2,103.	2,104.	2,683.	1,823.	1,844.	2,751.	2,743.	2,064.	2,063.	2,063.	2,064.
** TOTAL CONTRACTS	34,298.	2,653.	2,827.	2,754.	3,273.	2,413.	3,434.	3,341.	3,833.	2,654.	2,653.	2,653.	2,654.

** This is for information -- Summary of all costs for System

* For Multiple Cost Centers

Form #10784

Fig. 8-14. Summary of contracts.

BUDGET YEAR 1967–68   * **EQUIPMENT SUMMARY**   COST CENTER CODE # 068   Name: SYSTEM Name: Patient Care System

COST CENTERS	No. of Items	Additions	Improvements	Replacements	each	Total	JUL	AUG	SEP	OCT	NOV	DEC	JAN	FEB	MAR	APR	MAY	JUN
					estimated cost						CASH	REQUIREMENTS	BY	MONTHS				
068-01						600.			600.									
068-02						---												
068-03						400.						400.						
068-04						---												
068-05						---												
068-06						---												
068-07						800.								800.				
068-08						---												
068-09						200.									200.			
068-10						100.											100.	
068-11						500.												500.
068-21 to 068-33						34,300.	3,000.	2,050.	3,000.	3,000.	2,050.	100.	3,000.	4,000.	500.	3,000.	600.	10,000.
TOTAL						36,900.	3,000.	2,050.	3,600.	3,000.	2,050.	500.	3,000.	4,800.	700.	3,000.	700.	10,500.

* For Multiple Cost Centers

Form #10787

Fig. 8-15. Equipment summary.

BUDGET YEAR 1967-68 * RENOVATIONS SUMMARY COST CENTER Code# 068 Name:
SYSTEM Name: Patient Care System

COST CENTERS	No. of Items	Additions	Improvements	Replacements	estimated cost each	estimated cost total	JUL	AUG	SEP	OCT	NOV	DEC	JAN	FEB	MAR	APR	MAY	JUN
068-01						----												
068-02						----												
068-03						----												
068-04						5,000.						5,000.						
068-05						----												
068-06						300.								300.				
068-07						----												
068-08						----												
068-09						----												
068-10						1,000.					1,000.							
068-11						----												
068-21 to 068-33	----	--	--	--	----	29,500.		500.		8,000					6,000.		5,000.	10,000.
TOTAL	----	--	--	--	----	35,800.	---	500.	---	8,000	1,000.	5,000.	---	300.	6,000.	---	5,000.	10,000.

* For Multiple Cost Centers

Form #10789

Fig. 8-16. Renovations summary.

ANALYSIS of COST CENTERS by SYSTEMS

DESCRIPTIVE DATA	CURRENT MONTH						YEAR to DATE					
	ACTUAL		BUDGET		VARIANCE over (under)		ACTUAL		BUDGET		VARIANCE over (under)	
	TOTAL $	C/U*	TOTAL $	C/U*	TOTAL $	C/U*	TOTAL $	C/U*	TOTAL $	C/U*	TOTAL $	C/U*
PATIENT CARE SYSTEM												
Nursing Administration												
Salary and Wages	21,948.	7.72	21,333.	7.72	615.	---	43,498.	7.65	42,645.	7.72	853.	(.05)
Supplies and Expenses	6,742.	2.37	5,994.	2.17	748.	.20	13,594.	2.39	11,987.	2.17	1,607.	.22
Total	28,690.		27,327.		1,363.		57,092.		54,632.		2,460.	
Recovery Room												
Salary and Wages	21,621.	7.60	22,621.	8.19	(1,000.)	(.59)	43,242.	7.60	45,242.	3.19	(2,000.)	(.59)
Supplies and Expenses	8,762.	3.08	9,777.	3.54	(1,015.)	(.46)	17,524.	3.08	19,555.	3.54	(2,031.)	(.46)
Total	30,383.		32,398.		(2,015.)		60,766.		64,797.		(4,031.)	
Nursing Floors Floor #1												
Salary and Wages	26,352.	9.27	25,245.	9.14	1,107.	.13	52,704.	9.27	50,487.	9.14	2,215.	.13
Supplies and Wages	5,896.	2.07	6,601.	2.39	(705.)	(.32)	11,792.	2.07	13,202.	2.39	(1,410.)	(.32)
Total	32,248.		31,846.		402.		64,496.		63,691.		805.	

* Cost per Unit

Fig. 8-17, A-C. Reporting form (see text).

ANALYSIS of COST CENTERS by SYSTEMS as of: _____

DESCRIPTIVE DATA	CURRENT MONTH ACTUAL TOTAL $	C/U	BUDGET TOTAL $	C/U	VARIANCE over (under) TOTAL $	C/U	YEAR to DATE ACTUAL TOTAL $	C/U	BUDGET TOTAL $	C/U	VARIANCE over (under) TOTAL $	C/U
SUMMARY												
ADMINISTRATIVE and EXECUTIVE	126,105.	2.14	120,956.	2.05	5,149.	.09	223,526.	1.90	241,912.	2.05	(18,386.)	(.15)
QUALITY CONTROL	32,550.	.55	33,945.	.58	(1,395.)	(.03)	63,662.	.54	67,890.	.58	(4,228.)	(.04)
PERSONNEL and EDUCATION	65,903.	1.12	45,531.	.77	20,372.	.35	133,688.	1.13	91,062.	.77	42,626.	.36
BUSINESS SYSTEMS	43,989.	.75	52,678.	.89	(8,689.)	(.14)	83,750.	.71	105,356.	.89	(21,606.)	(.18)
SECURITY, MEDICAL, LEGAL	10,903.	.19	9,261.	.16	1,642.	.03	22,989.	.19	18,522.	.16	4,467.	.03
TRANSPORTATION, LOGISTICS, SUPPLY	162,572.	2.76	156,098.	2.65	6,474.	.11	318,066.	2.70	312,196.	2.65	5,870.	.05
ENVIRONMENTAL SERVICE SYSTEM	189,354.	3.22	163,012.	2.77	26,342.	.45	384,628.	3.26	326,042.	2.77	58,604.	.49
PATIENT CARE SYSTEM	265,876.	4.52	303,732.	5.15	(37,856.)	(.63)	538,542.	4.57	607,464.	5.15	(68,922.)	(.58)
PROFESSIONAL SERVICE SYSTEM	362,730.	6.16	278,886.	4.73	83,844.	1.43	677,490.	5.75	557,772.	4.73	119,718.	1.02
TOTAL	1,259,982.		1,164,099.		95,883.		2,446,341.		2,328,198.		118,143.	

* Cost per Unit

Fig. 8-17, cont'd. For legend see opposite page.

ANALYSIS of COST CENTERS by SYSTEMS

DESCRIPTIVE DATA	CURRENT MONTH						YEAR to DATE					
	ACTUAL		BUDGET		VARIANCE over (under)		ACTUAL		BUDGET		VARIANCE over (under)	
	TOTAL $	C/U*	TOTAL $	C/U*	TOTAL $	C/U*	TOTAL $	C/U*	TOTAL $	C/U*	TOTAL $	C/U*
GROSS HOSPITAL EXPENSES												
SALARIES and WAGES	847,712.	14.41	841,160.	14.27	6,552.	.13	1,808,940.	15.31	1,682,320.	14.27	126,620.	1.07
SUPPLIES and EXPENSES	412,270.	7.00	322,939.	5.48	89,331.	1.52	637,401.	5.41	645,878.	5.48	(8,477.)	(.07)
TOTAL	1,259,982.		1,164,099.		95,883.		2,446,341.		2,328,198.		118,143.	

* Cost per Unit

Fig. 8-17, cont'd. For legend see p. 186.

The value of the systems and programs organization is probably most vividly demonstrated in the performance and program budgeting process. It forms a matrix for the entire organization in all of its angular relationships and in its three major administrative processes: planning, coordinating, and control. Further relief is given when the aggregate of systems and programs are seen as an organizational system concerned with goal determination and goal achievement through resource acquisition and disposition. In this framework, budgeting becomes an impetus to planning, coordinating, and controlling and in turn becomes a process for their implementation.

To implement any idea, one must be able to somehow measure the expectations against the performance. The case study has used as its basic evaluator program and performance budgeting techniques. This will identify profit centers.

In health institutions, profit has to be examined in its broadest sense, i.e., the maximum return on resources used both in economic and social units. In Case Hospital the implementation was started by the identification of areas within the hospital for inpatient care—this being the units, beds measurable in patient days—and in the outpatient area by floor and examining rooms, with the utilization measure in both visits and occasion of service.

The term *profit center* does not mean the elimination of income and cost centers but implies that the focus and control is on the positive and negative differences of these two identifiable centers. To finance health care in its totality, the program receives units from the system in order to carry out its purpose in relation to teaching, research, and service. The measurable unit within the program can be identified as the number of patients received and treated, number of students educated, and dollar amount of research done. The one overriding unit in the program is identified as a health care unit. Every unit within this package must be financed.

The source of the financing is important to the overall programs but is not necessarily important to each individual program. In accountability terms the program manager must have a solvent program. This solvency is evaluated by the number of reimbursed units versus the number of nonreimbursed units, and the scope of the program is determined by the ability to balance this equation.

The Case Hospital study has attempted to define the areas or resources in terms of mandatory values available in the total complex. These sources are monies from patients cared for and services rendered, teaching allocations by the political subdivisions, the profit made on hospital services, the profit or excesses made on the practices of physicians' services at charges versus the cost of providing these services, gifts, and unspecified donations to the pool, either from endowments or gifts that are available to the pool.

Based on the earnings and the worthwhileness of the various programs, these revenues are made available to the individual program manager for use and accountability. One other source available is the identification of deficits and proper funding of these by the legislative bodies. One of the things this type of accountability rapidly points out is the lack of adequate financing, particularly on the part of city and state governments to provide for the cost of patients they have accepted responsibility for. This type of financing is not unique to health centers since the federal government has used this approach in financing the operation of the government for many years.

The program managers collectively act as a legislative body to determine the worthiness of individual programs and exchange their own resultant resources dependent on their own sincerity in the belief that the total is greater than the sum of the individual parts. It has become necessary in financing endeavors to receive cost from sources for all the activities of the endeavor. With cost contracts reimbursing the large percentage of the patient population in a hospital, it is no longer possible to overcharge a paying segment of the population to cover cost incurred in the non-paying portion of the population. This has resulted in the decline of variable pricing of hospital services that heretofore allowed for the care of large indigent populations at the expense of the larger paying population. With the emphasis now on cost contracts to pay only the cost of care for their recipients, other third-party and private contractors wish to pay at the same rate of cost as the federal government pays for its services.

Again, this points out the role of the hospital as being not that of a banker but that of a broker providing the services only to those who can afford at least the cost of the services. Large medical centers located in low-income areas are the first to experience this radical change in financing, i.e., more of the population is protected by some form or other of a private insurance plan paying the provider costs. All hopsitals will recognize the inadequacies of the cost reimbursement and will be forced to develop new means for financing current operations and allowing for new and modern equipment in order to advance. Unless the funding of depreciation is done on the basis of current cost rather than historical cost, replacement of depreciating funds will not be possible.

Contributions from the paying public will be adversely affected as changes in the tax laws adversely affect their gifts. County, city, and state hospitals, and those voluntary hospitals in states where they have the practice of floating bonds for hospital construction will be in the best position for replacing and expanding their facilities.

It would seem that in order to accommodate all of the public it becomes mandatory that an agency or commission representing the public be formed to act as a measure against piecemealing of the financ-

ing of the health care institution. This agency must be quasi-public and must be as free of pressures as possible. It must relate to both the public and private sector and measure the promises of health care to the public against the needs and performance of the providing agencies.

At the present time Blue Cross seems best able to meet this demanding role. However, it must free itself of its close relationship to the individual hospitals and act in the interest of its public rather than be prejudiced of the needs of its provider of health care. Whether this can happen will be dependent on the acceptability on the part of the government or private enterprise. However, without this broad-spectrum look at financing, the total system is not practical because it will be underfinanced.

A parallel problem is the availability of cash to meet current operations. This means that third-party contractors and paying patients will either have to advance payments for anticipated care received or make prepayment before the service has been rendered. One possible way to eliminate this would be to contract for a large portion of the populace's care and prorate payments over the year. However, this would mean contracting with the providers on an annual basis for a certain percentage of the population and prepaying this. In order to control hospital costs, incentives have been mentioned. In order to increase efficiency and encourage best utilization of hospital facilities, it is indeed facetious to hold hospital boards or hospital administrators responsible for this efficiency.

The physician, by his omissions and commissions, is the only one directly able to influence and control health care expenditures, so any system will have to include the management role of the doctor. However, along with this need will come the need to identify the quality, quantity, price, and proper place of health care services. As long as this is left without tangible measuring devices, it is only a matter of opinion as to what is good, what is efficient, and what is bad. It would seem that in order to approach the problem of total health care for the entire population at this time it is important to look at how the public and private sectors can begin to pool their resources to reach this objective and measure and implement total resources available for delivery of health care. A negative income tax plan in which premiums for health care insurance are deductible items of expense and subsidies are made for the purchase of private health care insurance through government participation should be examined. The continuance of present methods in allowing certain sectors to pay at varying rates in certain markets can only lead to the collapse of the total packages. Physician managers must become imaginative in making the package of health care psychologically, economically, and physically acceptable. Services like those of a cafeteria will need to become available where the consumer can pick out the bits and pieces of the total package he thinks he needs and not be confused by too much being offered at one time.

It would seem that the program concept allows for the activity of specific objectives that are trying to be accomplished. It appears that, by the use of system inputs, highest quality can be obtained. The concept emphasizes accountability and feasibility, particularly in means of financing. The program concept is always subject to review by its consumers, and nonproductive programs in both economical and social terms can be eliminated without a total collapse of the entity. However, program managers must be physicians who will set the overall objectives and policies to be implemented by administrators. Physicians have not been known for their administrative talent, and therefore they should recognize their own inadequacies and delegate those details to administrators who are trained to cope with all elements of the program, be they teaching, research, or service. There should be identifiable programs that relate to various ways and means of providing their objectives to all segments of a population. It does very little good for a hospital to announce that it will provide health care to its community when it is not able to operate its own outpatient department at the convenience of the community.

Two basic problems are (1) how to quantify inputs and to identify output units that reflect program objectives, and (2) how to identify cost and measurement of cost units. Once this has been done, responsibility centers for efficiencies of inputs through system administrators can be accomplished, and accountability for maximum utilization of aggregate inputs at the program level can be maintained. In this fashion, trade-offs through use of "pay-off tables" can be established in the systems level for maximum efficiency, and alternative courses of action can be identified in the program levels for adequate decision making.

Before performance budgeting can be established, it becomes imperative that unit values that include both direct and indirect costs translated into units of performance be assessed and that program accountability for identifiable output units reflecting the program's objectives be established. This then gives performance measurements at the systems level of input and accountability at the program director's post.

Programs reflecting output should be identifiable and reflect program goals, such as patient days in hospitals, and performance units should be able to be measured in terms of the smallest identifiable unit of input.

chapter nine
NURSING

A project is currently being designed to experiment with patterns of nursing care and utilization of nursing personnel. It is believed that registered nurses and other nursing personnel can be used more efficiently in creating programs of care on the patient unit that are of better quality, use personnel in a more efficient and professional manner, and are less costly in terms of underutilization of personnel potential. These new programs can be brought about by making maximum use of new concepts of patient care, equipment, technology, and building design; by reworking the nursing organizational structure and the staffing and supervisory patterns; and by developing the full potential of the personnel, using sound in-service training programs when necessary.

For many years there has been little consistent correlation between the abilities and potential abilities of nursing personnel and their job assignments and work patterns. The development of jobs seems to have been the simple result of immediate reaction to cries of personnel shortages and other pressures of the moment, with little perception of a logical plan or a future pattern.

Think for a moment of the common complaint of a shortage of nurses in our hospitals. The yardstick most frequently used to define this shortage has been the ab-

sence of registered nurses giving direct patient care at the patients' bedsides. Is this sufficient evidence of a shortage? Is it an acceptable method of defining a shortage? Must a registered nurse be at every patient's bedside? Indeed, what is needed at a patient's bedside? What tasks need to be done there? Who should do them? The answers to these questions define the pattern of patient care for a particular patient. It is essential then that these answers be sought out if more effective and efficient patterns of patient care are to be developed. Only in this way can an appropriate framework of activity performance be constructed. This type of unstructured, objective, and analytic approach shifts the emphasis away from a refined account of what nursing now *is* to a projection of what it *should and could become.* If progressive development occurs, it will be largely the result of such deliberations.

Following this approach, a broad picture of what the professional nurse is has been derived. A professional nurse is:

One who helps to develop comprehensive programs of delivering patient care

One who supervises programs of delivering patient care

One who participates in physically delivering patient care when the complexity and acuity of the case so demands

With this as the base, certain extensions follow. Analysis of nursing tasks to be done suggests the team nursing concept as an effective and efficient delivery system. In turn this indicates the need for instituting a variation of the unit manager concept to assume responsibility for all supportive nonnursing functions.

The aim throughout is the placement of individual talents and abilities at that place and time where they can be maximally utilized. The result is the development of personnel potential, which increases individual satisfaction. Ultimately this will effect a change in the total program. It is anticipated that this change will be in the direction of increased efficiency and effectiveness of total operation.

Nursing personnel are currently performing activities that do not require a proficiency in rendering nursing care, provided that they are needed. They should be relieved of these nonnursing responsibilities and activities so that they may spend their time in patient care. Furthermore, the needs of today's patients, the changing composition of care, the academic backgrounds and commensurate attitudes and competencies of registered nurses, the shortage of these nurses, and the schooling and ability of auxiliary nursing personnel, all point to the fact that the registered nurse may no longer be needed at every patient's bedside.

Auxiliary nursing personnel, aided by automation, may be able to perform most of the activities currently assigned to registered nurses for many patients. Their potential to do this should be explored, developed, and utilized.

The role of the registered nurse should be redefined. The role of a more professional nurse should be developed. The professional nurse is needed to develop comprehensive programs of nursing care, to supervise that care, and to render care to the acutely ill patient. She should be placed in a position that requires her full potential and should be assigned responsibilities and activities that require her greatest proficiency.

To the end of pursuing these possibilities, studies and pilot programs should be conducted that use definitive means of exploring more efficient and effective nursing personnel utilization and manpower development.

The primary emphasis of such studies should be to explore ways of maximizing efficient and effective use of nursing personnel while at the same time maintaining or improving upon current quality of care and dollar cost.

Prerequisite to such a study is a factual demonstration of the existing utilization of personnel, quality of care, and dollar cost. This prerequisite establishes the base against which the results of alternative systems studied can be measured. It may be accomplished through personnel utilization studies.

Part of the study of the existing situation should be a complete listing of all personnel activities that occur or should occur on the nursing unit. Once the base is established, these activities may be examined, regrouped, shifted, eliminated, or added to, and alternative systems of personnel utilization can be explored.

One possible alternative is the use of ward managers to assume those responsibilities and activities that are questionable nursing personnel assignments. The following is a discussion of ward management and nurse utilization.

WARD MANAGEMENT

To fully appreciate the complexity involved in the management of a patient unit, one needs to look back over the history of medicine, nursing, and hospitals in the United States and to follow them forward in their focus upon the patient units.

Prior to 1850 the person who directed ward activities was in most cases either the owner of the building that housed the hospital or an appointed delegate of some charitable person or group. She would go about doing and having done as she saw fit, with little thought to organization or method. The sick were simply "seen to." A woman became a nurse by being present, seeing, and doing.

During the Crimean War, Florence Nightingale embarked on a career of setting straight the need for sanity and organization in nursing practice and in hospitals. Her work came at a time when Crawford Long's work with ether as an anesthetic, Pasteur's experiments with bacteria, Bergmann's introduction of steam sterilization, and other scientific explorations were paving the way for great advances in medical practice. Hospitals began to grow and organize, producing a need for better nursing education and practice.

Traditionally, nurses had been educated through apprentice training in hospitals. The case method, in which nurses engaged in whatever nursing and nonnursing activities were necessary for the proper attention to their patients, was common. As the new era took shape, hospitals began to take a close look at their methods of nursing education; and concurrently nonhospital schools of nursing were opened. As "school-trained" nurses graduated, they did not go into bedside nursing but rather went either into nursing schools as teachers or into hospitals as teachers and supervisors, and thus a new level of hospital supervisory nurse emerged.

With these advances came a demand for more careful organization of nursing practice. Where once a single matron or head nurse had supervised all nursing activities, a broader hierarchy began to form. Head ward nurses were appointed under the direction of the nursing supervisor or director. Under the supervision of the head ward nurse, the student nurse gave bedside care with the aid of nonnursing personnel. All engaged in both nursing and nonnursing activities; care remained on the case basis. Thus established, this pattern remained structurally unchanged through the early years of the twentieth century.

In 1905 the Council on Medical Education and Hospitals of the American Medical Association was formed; in 1907 the Association of Hospital Superintendents changed its name to the American Hospital Association; in 1911 the American Nurses' Association was founded; and in 1925 the Committee on the Grading of Nursing Schools was initiated. Medical practice advanced, nursing practice advanced, hospitals kept pace, and patient care improved. The advances in medicine, nursing, hospitals, and patient care brought a demand for more nurses.

During the 1920s a real shortage of trained nurses became greatly apparent for the first time, and an increasing number of nonnursing persons found their way into patient care by serving as aides and orderlies. Although these people were functionally oriented, the overall pattern of staffing for the case method continued.

At this point, when nursing and hospitals might have been considering a revision in the existing pattern of nurse staffing and practice in order to accommodate the nurse shortage, the Great Depression of the 1930s struck. Severe economic conditions resulted in low bed occupancy, increased charity load, and decreased income from endowments and other sources. The economic strain caused many hospitals to close and made it difficult for most others to operate.

The impact of the Goldmark Report (published in 1923) on nursing education continued to promote changes throughout the Depression, however. By 1940 nursing education was graduating better qualified nurses, who engaged in patient care along with student nurses, aides, and orderlies.

December 7, 1941 . . . Pearl Harbor . . . World War II. The expansion of the armed forces drew thousands of nurses out of the civilian hospital force into the service. Left with inadequate staffs for patient care, hospitals had no choice but to enlist the aid of untrained auxiliary workers. These workers became proficient and were recognized as being a new class of hospital nursing personnel.

During the war, advances in medical technology introduced an abundance of new medical and related technicians and specialists into the hospitals. New drugs, medical, surgical, and therapeutic treatment plans, complicated equipment, and a vast array of new knowledge became available to medical practice. At the same time the American public became aware that hospitals now offered services important to their welfare. Prepayment plans made hospitalization available to many who had gone without it in the past. Inpatient occupancy and the need for more nurses increased.

Nurses and the patient unit suddenly became the hub of a complexity of medical care. Retaining their responsibility for seeing that nursing care tasks were performed properly but also remaining in short supply, nurses were given additional administrative, teaching, and leadership responsibilities. They became leaders of teams that combined student nurses, practical nurses, aides, and orderlies. Nursing duties became specialized because managerial functions had been added and because patient care had become specialized. The patient unit was a new entity. A new system of management and patient care had emerged. A vivid hierarchal structure of staffing among head nurses, staff nurses, student nurses, practical nurses, ward clerks, aides, and orderlies had arisen around the *team method* of patient care.

As the demand for more patient care grew and, at the same time, as more administrative duties, both nursing and nonnursing, were given to the staff nurse, it became necessary to add more personnel to the nursing team and to appoint a *team leader*. The team leader was responsible for the care of the patients assigned to her team and spent most of her time directing and coordinating its activities. Only when unusual or difficult problems arose did she spend more time with the patient than was required by the administration of medications and a quick periodic check of the patient's condition.

At this point, nurses were responsible for the complete administration of the patient unit. This included nursing activities related directly to patient care and nursing administration and to nonnursing activities such as the requisitioning of supplies. The resulting absence of registered nurses at the patient's bedside (which has been the primary indicator used to identify a nursing shortage) increased abruptly. This, coupled with new views toward patient care, caused some hospitals to begin experimenting with the *ward manager* system on the patient unit as a means of relieving nurses of nonnursing duties and returning them to patient care.

The ward manager system varies greatly from one hospital to another and may even be referred to by a different name, but there is one basic similarity: a person, usually called a ward manager, is employed to relieve nurses of nonnursing responsibilities. The ward manager, under certain organizational structures, also gives hospital administration direct representation on the patient unit.

New York Hospital, New York City

In 1948 a pavilion manager system was established at New York Hospital.[1] The system involved the use of a nonnurse assistant pavilion manager assigned as assistant to the head nurse on the patient unit. The duties of the assistant pavilion manager were as follows:

1. Make out a daily work list for patient traffic
2. Note which patients have tests scheduled and what specimens need to be collected for the laboratory

3. See that orders for tests and specimens are carried out
4. Check all stock supplies and requisition replacements
5. Check in delivered supplies
6. Check discharged patients for appointments and any necessary instructions
7. Inspect operative and treatment permits for signatures
8. Meet new patients on admission, assign their beds, and orient them to the floor
9. Relieve the ward clerk during her lunch hour
10. Supervise auxiliary workers and check to be certain that their work is completed
11. Attempt to answer questions for the procession of doctors, patients, nurses, and visitors

The pavilion manager was directly responsible to the head nurse on the unit since it was believed that the head nurse should be responsible for all phases of patient care.

Salary range was established between that of the staff nurse and the assistant head nurse.

Memorial Center for Cancer and Allied Diseases, New York City

Another early experiment with ward managers was conducted at Memorial Center for Cancer and Allied Diseases in 1951.

To relieve nurses of all nonnursing responsibilities, a floor manager directly responsible to hospital administration was employed to manage all nonnursing services and the general operation of the unit.

The floor manager was given direct contact with the patient. Upon admission of a new patient, the admitting office contacted the floor manager, who greeted the patient, took him to his room, explained visiting hour regulations and other hospital routines, and introduced him to his fellow patients.

The service responsibilities of the floor manager were as follows:

1. If [the patient's] signal bell is not working, she has it fixed.
2. She sees that his room is kept clean and orderly.
3. She has his mail and flowers delivered to him.

4. When a patient is discharged, she has his unit cleaned and prepared for another patient.
5. She maintains the floor's standards of equipment and supplies.
6. She supervises the general housekeeping and maintenance of the entire division.*

The system was originally established as an experiment on one unit in September 1951. By March 1952 there were three floor managers covering one floor each, from 7:00 A.M. until 11:00 P.M., 7 days a week.

Spohn Hospital, Corpus Christi, Texas

From experiments with the ward manager system at Spohn Hospital in 1952 it was revealed that a floor manager could relieve the nurse of 50% of her nonnurse responsibilities.[2]

Among the duties of the floor manager were the following:

1. Check each room for cleaning before a new patient arrives
2. Order new light fixtures, etc.
3. Arrange for a fresh, more attractive color scheme when a room needs repainting
4. Call for a magazine or a pack of cigarettes from the drugstore for a patient
5. Listen to a patient's troubles and complaints
6. Order, check, and distribute supplies
7. Maintain order in rooms and corridors
8. Deliver new patients to their rooms and notify the head nurse of their arrival

Sinai Hospital of Baltimore, Inc., Baltimore, Maryland

Supported in part by research funds from the National Institutes of Health and in cooperation with the Division of Nursing Resources of the Public Health Service, Sinai Hospital of Baltimore, Inc., undertook an experiment in ward management from March 1956 to March 1957. By June 1964 the floor manager pattern had been expanded to include all nursing units of the 430-bed hospital.

The experiment was based upon the hypothesis that "a floor-manager pattern

---

*From Nonnursing managers for hospital divisions, Amer. J. Nurs. **52**:323, March 1952.

for the nursing units, if conceived and administered according to sound principles of hospital administration, will improve patient care."[3] The premises and objectives were as follows:

PREMISE	OBJECTIVES
1. Mature women without benefit of advanced education or lengthy programs of professional training have the capacity to assume, with safety and efficiency, many of the non-nursing and non-professional duties and responsibilities performed by nurses and dietitions.	1. To relieve nurses and dietitians of as many non-nursing and non-professional duties and responsibilities as can be safely passed on to other personnel who require less preparation and training.
2. Specialization in the performance of many of the menial and semi-skilled non-nursing and non-professional procedures of the nursing unit is unnecessary, uneconomical and undesirable in the interest of good patient care.	2. To reduce specialization in the performance of the menial and semi-skilled non-nursing and non-professional procedures of the nursing unit.
3. Maximum supervision of non-professionals at the point of direct service to patients, and at reasonable cost, may be obtained by the combination of supervisory rules.	3. To obtain maximum supervision of non-professionals at the point of direct service to patients.
4. The complexity of the nursing unit compels a realignment of duties and responsibilities according to a pattern conducive to increased efficiency in management and to simplicity in comprehension of lines of authority and channels of communication.	4. To increase the effectiveness and to strengthen the position of the head nurse by simplifying the organizational channels and administrative machinery through which she administers her unit.*

*From Gladstein, S., Prasated, G., and Thorne, M. N.: A floor-manager pattern for the nursing unit, Baltimore, 1959, Sinai Hospital of Baltimore, Inc., p. 10.

The floor manager, who was directly responsible to the floor management department, was made responsible for the coordination and supervision of most nonnursing and nonprofessional activities on the patient unit, including:

1. Housekeeping
2. Preparation and serving of meal trays
3. Requisitioning and control of supplies and linen
4. Care of equipment
5. Messenger service
6. Supervision of maids

By introducing the floor manager onto the unit, the head nurse was given one person to whom she could turn with most of the problems and needs that did not involve direct patient care or professional training. Dietitians were relieved of many nonprofessional duties, and problems of overspecialization among semiskilled workers functioning in patient areas were modified.

To be considered for the job, an applicant must have graduated from high school and be a woman between the ages of 25 and 50. Certain other aptitudes were specified.

The organizational pattern of the hospital was adjusted to accommodate the floor manager system by establishing a floor management department. The department operated with the same independence as any other hospital department, being responsible for the training of its new employees and for providing coverage 7 days a week.

Working from 7:00 A.M. until 11:30 P.M., a period that corresponds to the day and evening shifts of nursing, the floor manager was given charge of from three to six maids, who prepared and served meal trays, washed dishes, cleaned floor bathrooms, utility rooms, nurses' stations, and all other rooms and patient areas, made beds, ran errands, and performed other duties assigned by the floor manager.

Salt Lake County General Hospital, Salt Lake City, Utah

A floor manager program was initiated on one patient unit at Salt Lake County General Hospital during June 1958.

Under the supervision of the assistant hospital director, the floor manager served as a representative of hospital administration and certain hospital departments (housekeeping, laundry, maintenance, central service, storeroom, and ordering supplies from pharmacy) on the patient unit. She had neither direct supervision over personnel nor direct patient contact.

The responsibilities of the floor manager, through area supervision, included:

1. Continued inspection of all areas and equipment of nursing stations to which assigned
2. Initiating action of Housekeeping and Maintenance departments to ensure maintenance of safety, functional and esthetic standards established with the Nursing Service supervisory personnel involved
3. Supervising maintenance of all supply levels and procurement systems of Central Service, Pharmacy, Laundry, and Storeroom or other agencies according to requirements established with Nursing Service
4. Supervising budget development and implementation, safety program, personnel policy interpretation and development and other administrative programs with personnel of the nursing stations to which she is assigned.*

By November 1959 there was one floor manager covering two surgery units (64 beds) and the emergency room (approximately 2,000 visits per month); one covering two medical floors (57 beds) and pediatrics (32 beds); and a third covering three geriatric floors (96 beds). These floor man-

agers were recruited from within the hospital. One was formerly a ward clerk, one was a nurse's aide, and the third had been a clerk in pharmacy; all three women were between the ages of 35 and 50.

Floor managers were on the job 8 hours a day, 5 days a week. Hourly and daily schedules of activity were made up for each floor manager. Suggestion books were placed on each nursing station so that anyone could leave a message for the manager at any time.

Douglas C. Carpenter, Jr. evaluated the program as follows:

In the early development of the program, the head nurses were a little slow to relinquish some of their responsibilities. Also, the ward clerks who had been ordering supplies were somewhat hesitant to give up this activity; some of the department heads expressed concern that the floor manager may become a tool of Nursing which had the backing of Administration. The floor manager at this early stage felt the Nursing personnel looked upon her as a spy of Administration. But as the program progressed, these problems gradually disappeared although there still remains some remnants. There are a few problems that continue to recur from time to time and appear to be inherent in the program, namely: (1) attempts may be made by the head nurse to bypass Nursing channels in getting her problems, which are basically nursing problems, direct to Administration through the floor manager. (2) Department heads may have "axes to grind" and they may try to enlist the support of the floor manager. (3) The floor manager and head nurse must be able to maintain good rapport, yet sometimes the relationship may be strained when there are major disagreements between them. (4) Many times the floor manager may be caught between Administration or any of the other departments on one side of an issue and nursing service or the head nurse on the other side. Nursing personnel may attempt to come directly to the floor manager with her problems which should be channeled through the head nurse and the head nurse may interpret this as a threat to her.*

*From Carpenter, D. C., Jr.: The floor manager, unpublished journal paper presented to the class and faculty of the Department of Hospital Administration, Washington University School of Medicine, St. Louis, Nov. 4, 1959.
Carpenter was one of the original pioneers of unit management in his training of the initial complement of floor managers for the nine units at Salt Lake County General Hospital.

*From Carpenter, D. C., Jr.: The floor manager, unpublished journal paper presented to the class and faculty of the Department of Hospital Administration, Washington University School of Medicine, St. Louis, Nov. 4, 1959, pp. 21-22.

Time and practice seemed to overcome most of the initial difficulties experienced in the program. Nurses accepted the floor managers and felt that they were instrumental in raising the quality of patient care. Other departments felt that they had a direct representative on the patient unit.

Representing hospital administration, the floor manager was able to assist in many administrative functions that were of immediate importance to patient care and at the same time to keep the assistant hospital director abreast of unit activities.

Qualifications for the position included certain specified aptitudes in addition to a high school education, at least 2 years of college-level training, and a minimum of 2 years' experience in some coordinating capacity.

University Hospital, University of Kentucky Medical Center, Lexington, Kentucky

On April 24, 1962 University Hospital, University of Kentucky Medical Center, began operation. It did so with a fully incorporated *division steward* system, which corresponds in some degree to ward and floor manager systems in other hospitals.

The organizational and administrative patterns at University Hospital are somewhat different from those found in most hospitals, and therefore a partial description of these patterns must accompany a description of the division steward system.

The general medical and surgical inpatients units have approximately 59 intermediate care acute beds and a 6-bed intensive care unit. All of this is under the immediate supervision of an assistant director in the department of nursing services whose nonnursing functions are those usually assigned to the head nurse and supervisor.

Under the assistant director there is a division steward whose duties include the following:

1. Select, train, and supervise the unit clerks and unit aides assigned to the division

2. Represent the assistant director to other hospital departments such as pharmacy, central supply, and housekeeping
3. Make and maintain a schedule of appointments for patients to other hospital departments such as x-ray and physical therapy and assist the team leader in meeting the patient's appointment schedules
4. Make appointments for patients to OPD following discharge from the hospital
5. Assist the nursing staff in relaying messages concerning the patient's conditions to relatives and friends
6. Maintain standard of equipment and supply on the division
7. Receive, store, and make proper disposition of mail
8. Make daily rounds to each patient's room to check the patient's identification bracelet and bed card and to check for maintenance needs
9. Assist in division budget administration and maintain statistical records required in its preparation
10. Represent the assistant director to division personnel on matters relating to personnel policies and payroll
11. Keep time and other payroll records
12. Perform other duties as delegated by the assistant director

In the office of the director of nursing services there is a department steward who carries the same general responsibilities as the division steward except that he deals with these matters on the departmental level.

Organizationally, the division steward comes under the direct administrative jurisdiction of the assistant director in charge of the patient unit, but much of the training and day-to-day coordination of administrative activity takes place between the department steward and the division steward. The coordination extends to periodic meetings of division stewards, which are held by the department steward.

The hospital is generally pleased with the program and has no particular plans to make any changes in it. The one major problem encountered arises from the fact that since the relationship between the division steward and the assistant director is new, the assistant director must delegate functions and responsibilities on the basis of patterns with which she is not familiar.

Teaching Hospital and Clinics, The J. Hillis Miller Health Center, University of Florida, Gainesville, Florida

The Teaching Hospital and Clinics were opened in 1958 with a unit manager system designed to entirely relieve nurses and nursing service of nonnursing responsibilities. The system places the entire responsibility of nonnursing ward management upon hospital administration, which in turn supervises the ward managers.

The ward manager's responsibilities include the following:

1. Assist in the administration and coordination of all services within the hospital as they affect each patient on the unit
2. Assist in preparation of budgets and allocation of funds
3. Direct procurement and maintenance of supplies and equipment
4. Direct and supervise ward clerks and couriers
5. Cooperate with nursing staff, medical staff, and administration in formulating policies that pertain to the unit
6. Represent administration within the unit, and act as liason between administration, the patient, and each of the services
7. Maintain contact with patients relating to administrative detail

This system is perhaps the most completely analyzed, the best documented, and the most widely publicized.[4-11] It also seems to have gone further toward evaluating organizational relationships and the effects of this particular system upon nursing personnel utilization as well as interpersonal relationships on the patient unit. The most important feature to be recognized in reviewing this project is that, from its inception, it embodied substantial planning and philosophy formulation in order to establish a corporate coordination of medical care, nursing care, and management throughout the entire hospital organization.

In 1964 the system was operating well. In that year the position of assistant in administration was established to coordinate the activities of all patient floor unit managers, and a department of operation research, headed by an industrial engineer with a Ph.D. degree, was formed to assist in evaluating the program.

• • •

It is unfortunate that three decades ago the concept of hospital administration was not well enough advanced to show that many of the activities and responsibilities being pushed upon nurses should not be nursing responsibilities. The management of nonnursing activities should be the responsibility of a person well equipped to manage hospital care as a professional manager.

What takes place on a patient unit is a program of patient care composed of medical care, nursing care, and hospital care. The proper rendering of each is a professional matter; the coordination of the three into a comprehensive program of overall patient care is the responsibility of the hospital administrator.

The responsibilities for nursing care and hospital care on the patient unit have traditionally been combined. As experience with the ward management system accumulated, the need to develop the management of hospital care as a professional activity in its own right—a latent need in the beginning—became recognized as a legitimate need to be treated on its own merit, in addition to the need to relieve nurses of responsibility to it and return them to the patient's bedside.

The evolution of these two areas of differing professional expertise has caused considerable difficulty and confusion in developing the ward manager concept and lends equal difficulty in evaluating it. One therefore needs to separate discussion of the two and to evaluate ward management on its ability to accomplish a professionalization of the management of hospital care and on its ability to free nurses of the responsibility for hospital care. Implications for nursing professionalization and organization are discussed in the next section.

A ward management system, then, when adequately developed and implemented, presents:

1. Opportunity for direct administrative contact with the management of hospital care on the patient unit, enabling administration to develop effective programs of patient care according to sound administrative and management principles
2. Opportunity to develop the management of hospital care on the patient unit into a body of professional activity
3. Opportunity to develop effective methods of adjusting and orienting the patient in the hospital environment
4. Opportunity for effectively coordinating, on the patient unit, the many services and activities that support medical and nursing care according to sound administrative and management principles
5. Opportunity to relieve nurses of hospital care responsibilities for which they are not generally well equipped by virtue of professional education or experience, thus making available more nursing time for nursing care and the professionalization of the nurse

Most of the problems (discounting the complaint that ward management has not, itself, returned the nurse to the patient's bedside *or* professionalized her) that have arisen with the operation of the system stem from the fact of change, the weaknesses in a new organizational structure and function, the abuse of a new organizational structure and function, or a combination of these.

Three basic patterns of organizational structure and function have been used. All divide, to varying degree, responsibilities for nursing and hospital care on the patient unit; all leave the head nurse, or her equivalent, responsible to nursing; one makes the ward manager responsible to nursing; one makes him responsible directly to hospital administration; one makes him responsible to a new department of ward management.

The present system of care on the patient unit, which is noted for status, professional, and departmental frictions and for diverse and elusive interpretations of patient care, is redesigned to include still another departmental or subdepartmental entity. A new entity brings with it new frictions, loyalties, and ideas about patient care. The introduction of such a new entity into the system can benefit the ultimate purpose of a more unified and effective program of patient care, but not without careful nurturing during its inception and implementation.

One cannot emphasize too strongly that, if a ward management system is used, it is not, in and of itself, a solution as to how to use nursing personnel time more efficiently or effectively. It does remove some phases of inefficient use and makes more nursing personnel time available for use in a different way. How to use the additional time is a separate question.

PROFESSIONAL NURSING

The ward management system has proved to be an effective mechanism for "freeing" the nurse from hospital care.

However, is the making *available* of more nursing time for direct patient care a substantial goal in its own right?

Has the resulting extra nursing time effectively returned the professional nurse to the patient's bedside?

Has anyone developed a reliable means of measuring and evaluating the quality of nursing care?

The shortage of nurses at the patient's bedside has been identified with "poor" patient care. Does an increased number of hours spent in direct patient care ensure "good" or "better" patient care?

What is nursing care?

With these questions satisfied, will we find that the nurse still belongs at every patient's bedside?

Collectively, these questions exemplify the confusion that shrouds nursing practice and professionalization. As the ward manager system "freed" nurses of the responsibility for management, the free time helped to define the nursing problem, but magnified rather than solved it.

Few hospitals have undertaken an orderly evaluation of their nursing practice and professionalization through the use of sound research principles; this must be done before satisfactory solutions can be arrived at.

Nursing care involves what the nurse learns in school and in practice, what the public expects, and what the hospital and the physicians require.

Many research projects have been undertaken to define and establish standards and measurements of nursing care. Two general approaches have been most frequent: (1) approaches by educators, theorist, and researchers outside the hospital organization to establish definitions, standards, and measurement that may be applied to hospitals collectively, and (2) approaches by hospital departments of nursing and/or administration to establish definitions, standards, and measurements based on preexisting conditions in that hospital and primarily related to goals established within the department of nursing.

In an earlier chapter the hospital was defined as being a formal social organization charged with the responsibility of promoting and maintaining health and treating illness within the community, and of functioning internally to discharge the responsibility through programs of care, of which socialization and protection are a part. To fulfill this responsibility, the hospital organization takes on bureaucratic characteristics, and these characteristics interfere with the exercise of nursing activities at the point where care is rendered. This happens because patients *are not* members of the hospital organization, do not share many of its internal values, and cannot, today, be expected to fit well into its bureaucratic system. On the other hand, nurses *are* a part of the organization, are expected to share its values, and are expected to fit into and adhere to its system. Conflict therefore results. Two approaches may be considered.

First, the graduate nurse is more than simply a technician; she has a good mind and is capable of making operational decisions. Perhaps her position in the organization should be one in which she internalizes organizational values but remains flexible enough to adjust to the patient and interact effectively with him.

Second, using Goffman's concept of spontaneous involvement, "When an individual becomes engaged in an activity, whether shared or not, it is possible for him to become caught up by it, carried away by it, engrossed in it—to be, as we say, spontaneously involved in it."[12] If the hospital can produce a high degree of spontaneous involvement by the patient in its organization at the same time that the nurse is adjusting to him, a more effective interaction will result. This spontaneous involvement requires that each, the hospital and the patient, share the other's values. This is a companion idea to that of socialization in the foregoing definition of the hospital, and must take place largely after the patient is hospitalized.

The point at which the nurse interacts with the patient is on the patient unit, usually at the bedside. What interaction is appropriate is the subject of professionalization and nursing personnel utilization.

Today's graduate nurses are capable of being more than just technicians who carry out routine tasks assigned to them by decisions from other sources. Graduate nurses possess the highly developed manual, technical, and judgmental skills required to operate intricate mechanical apparatus, recognize symptoms, and initiate nursing care—and sometimes lifesaving action. Additionally, these nurses are able and are more and more often required to plan with the patient and his family for continued nursing and health care after he leaves the hospital.

Nursing practice leaves much to be desired. Seemingly, each school of nursing has its own ideas about what nursing education and practice is and should be. Furthermore, each nurse, each new graduate, and each veteran has her own ideas about what nursing is and should be and about what she can and wants to do. Aggravating all of this, the general public and physicians are confused about "nursing care." These problems converge at the point where nursing care is rendered.

An organization that does not allow a wide latitude of judgment and decision by a nurse rendering care intensifies the problem by not allowing her to adjust adequately to a multiplicity of pressures. Each patient presents a different case and brings with him and/or assembles about him in the hospital a unique set of requirements. Strict dictation of a formal formula for nursing inhibits freedom of nurse-patient adjustment.

There are probably several workable solutions to this situation, but one seems to be particularly interesting: **encourage the graduate nurse to become an independent professional** in much the same sense as the physician. Thus the nurse would be in a position to exercise professional judgment in practice in the sense that nursing care belongs to the nurse but broad programs of care belong to the community and are discerned by the organization.

The role of today's nurse should be redefined. The role of a **professional** nurse should be developed.

Much of the confusion that has arisen in the name of the ward manager system stems from the failure of the registered nurse to return to the patient's bedside. The needs of today's patients, the changing

composition of care, the academic backgrounds and commensurate attitudes and competencies of registered nurses, the shortage of these nurses, and the schooling and ability of auxiliary nursing personnel, all point to the fact that the registered nurse *will not* return to every patient's bedside.

In the very near future the nurse will not be needed at every bedside. Auxiliary nursing personnel, aided by automation, will soon be able to perform all of the routine activities that have been assigned to nurses for so many years. The development of hospital care into an area of professional management will relieve her of this responsibility.

The professional nurse will be needed to develop comprehensive programs of nursing care, to supervise that care, and to render care to the acutely ill patient. In this role, she will perform as a professional specialist and should be placed in an organizational framework such as that described previously.

This framework allows the organization of nursing and nurse staffing to be structured in such a manner that the nurse may work and be worked with as a professional person. It removes from her the responsibilities for routine care and hospital care and places upon her the responsibility for professional nursing care.

When change of this nature is contemplated, it calls for careful assessment of current practice in view of theory and experience and an exploration of anticipated consequences. For these purposes, nursing care, i.e., activity, should be defined in terms of function. Function refers to activities that maintain or further a goal.*

*See Merton, R. K.: Social theory and social structure, ed. 2, New York, 1957, The Free Press. On pp. 19-82 Merton discusses the concept of function in functional analysis. This concept may play an important role in determining quality indicators of nursing care if nursing function is viewed as having contribution to the maintenance of patient organism as its primary objective.

Consequently, activities may be classified as being functional, i.e., maintain or further a goal; as nonfunctional, i.e., irrelevant to a goal; and as dysfunctional, i.e., hinder or lessen maintenance of a goal. Seen from this point of view, nursing activities may be critically analyzed once desired goals are identified.

This type of functional analysis requires that these questions be asked: "Is the primary function of the nurse self-professional maintenance, maintenance of the professional physician, maintenance of the patient, or maintenance of the hospital organization?" "When these are in conflict, which should and which will she choose?" Since standards are based upon functions, they cannot be established until the preceding question about the nurses' functions and similar questions concerning departmental and organizational functions have been answered.

Proceeding to research the area, *quantity* of function may be recorded, measured, and evaluated through several approaches already in use in many hospitals, i.e., work sampling studies. Means need to be developed, however, that allow *quality* of function to be recorded, measured, and evaluated.

To measure quantity, a work sampling study that identifies nursing hours of specific activity by various nursing personnel at identified levels of skill to patients with identified medical problems in identified stages of progressive care can be developed. Such a study will produce facts and measurements that may be used to establish quantitative standards of nursing care. These standards will become the base of how much of what type of work will be expected under different work loads and staffing conditions. In the future, random work sampling will produce new figures that can be compared to the established base and new facts that can be used in reevaluating the base.

Work sampling studies of this type do not, however, produce any information about how well nursing personnel perform their work or what its effect is on the patient. These questions open the way into the measurement of quality.

One method of exploratory investigation into this area involves the use of written nursing care plans, incorporating an evaluation of the patient and his needs, an evaluation of function required to meet these needs, a record of patient reaction to this function, a record of patient progress, and an evaluation of function in terms of goals, patient reaction, and progress. From such an investigation should come a study that will produce facts and measurements of the quality of nursing function. These results may be used to establish standards of quality for nursing care. Another, quite different approach has been developed by the Commission for Administrative Services in Hospitals; this is discussed in Chapter 10.

Having moved through these considerations, a hospital might choose to undertake experiments in nursing, using an outline similar to the one that follows.

Nursing utilization and manpower development

I. Establish an advisory group

The assistant administrator for patient care will assume responsibility for directing the project; she will be responsible for all policy decisions. Her assistant will assume responsibility for the overall coordination of the project. The advisory group should consist of representatives from appropriate systems and programs, including the medical staff, and representatives from outside institutions and agencies who might be of assistance.

This advisory group should work with the assistant administrator for patient care and her staff in an advisory capacity in establishing and conducting the project. It should be extensively involved in establishing and implementing alternative systems.

II. **Select a study site**

Select two similar nursing units for study purposes; one unit will be used as the control unit and the other as the test unit. The units chosen should

A. Be similar in size to the future size of our existing and future units

B. Have a high occupancy rate, resulting in a high rates of space and personnel utilization and commensurate cost demonstration and pressures of operation

C. Have a mixture of patients to represent appropriate specialty services and acuity of illness

III. **Conduct an initial study to establish base information**

Conduct a study of activities *and* quality of care on the two study units to produce factual base information establishing the similarity of the two units and to show the current activities, quality of care, and dollar cost on the units.

A. Study the activities and quality of care under the current system

B. Study the personnel aptitudes, attitudes, and performance under the current system

C. Study costs of the current system

IV. **Consider alternative systems of personnel utilization and facility design**

Once the base information has been established, alternative systems of personnel utilization and facility design may be considered. In the course of considering alternatives

A. Define proposed philosophy

The formulation of a basic philosophy about management and care on the nursing unit is an imperative step. The philosophy must embody the basic concepts upon which a new program of patient care will be built.

B. Define proposed organization structure

Once the basic philosophy has been established, a new organizational structure that will facilitate the philosophy must be formulated. It is possible that a new organizational structure for the department of nursing and the department of hospital administration will be created. Other departments such as housekeeping, dietary, and the storeroom might be involved.

C. Define proposed activity and responsibility boundaries for the professional nurse, auxillary nursing personnel, and other personnel on the nursing unit

When the proposed philosophy and organizational structure have been formulated, ranges of responsibility and activity must be specified.

D. Define proposed job descriptions

The ranges of responsibility and activity must be assigned to specific job classifications and comprehensive job descriptions must then be written.

E. Define desired results in terms of

1. Activities
2. Quality
3. Cost

The purpose of following the preceding steps (A, B, C, and D) is to design a new, more efficient, and more effective program of care. This program of care must be identified with ultimate points of achievement in terms of activities, quality, and cost. For purposes of phase II (i.e., selecting a study site), these points of achievement may be general; they must be defined in detail, however, before further study is undertaken.

V. **Conduct a research-demonstration study of the selected alternatives**

The selected alternatives may be implemented and studied on the test unit. They should be grouped into categories representing chronologic steps for study. Three categories to be studied in chronologic order might be

A. Personnel abilities and utilization, with corresponding quality of care and dollar cost factors, relating to the use of a ward management system

B. Personnel abilities and utilization, with corresponding quality of care and dollar cost factors, relating to better utilization of nursing personnel not directly involved in ward management (if ward management is not to be studied, this category should become the first phase of study)

C. Personnel abilities and utilization, with corresponding quality of care and dollar cost factors, relating to new facility design and equipment (if categories A and B produce a new, desirable system, then both the new systems on the test unit and the old system on the control unit can be studied as parts of category C)

The steps in each phase should

A. Implement the alternative system on the test unit

B. Study the activities and quality of care under the alternative system on the test unit

C. Study the personnel aptitudes, attitudes, and performance under the alternative system on the test unit

D. Study costs under the alternative system on the test unit

E. Compare results to the old system on the control unit; if desired results are not obtained

1. Determine why
2. Make adjustments
3. Reimplement
4. Restudy

(Repeat unit project until it is brought to a satisfactory conclusion)

NOTE: If extensive personnel retraining is required, create a formal in-service training program for this purpose. Document the training program in detail.

REFERENCES

1. Dennison, A. J.: Pavilion manager, Mod. Hosp. 80:79, June 1953.
2. Vincent, Sister Mary: Floor managers, Mod. Hosp. 78:62, June 1962.
3. Gladstein, S., Prasated, G., and Thorne, M. N.: A floor-manager pattern for the nursing unit, Baltimore, 1959, Sinai Hospital, p. 10.
4. Taylor, C.: How unit manager system works for us, Mod. Hosp. 99:69, Aug. 1962.
5. Mercadante, L. T.: Unit manager plan gives nurses time to care for the patients, Mod. Hosp. 99:73, Aug. 1962.
6. Houtz, D. T.: The unit manager plan provides administrative control of wards, Mod. Hosp. 99:75, Aug. 1962.
7. Martin, S. P.: Medical staff agrees: unit plan is good for patients, Mod. Hosp. 99:76, Aug. 1962.
8. Houtz, D. T.: The unit manager pattern, New England Hospital Assembly, Boston, Mar. 28, 1962.
9. Houtz, D. T.: The nursing unit becomes the patient unit, Ontario Hospital Association, Ontario, Canada, Oct. 31, 1962.
10. Mercadante, L. T.: The effect of unit management on nursing, New England Hospital Assembly, Boston, Mar. 28, 1962.
11. Mercadante, L. T.: An organizational plan for nursing service, Nurs. Outlook 10:305, May 1962.
12. Goffman, I.: Encounters—two studies in the sociology of interaction, Indianapolis, 1961. The Bobbs-Merrill Co., Inc., p. 38.

chapter ten
QUALITY CONTROL

Once personal and group goals are established, the participants want to know how well they are doing. The basis for measuring "how well" is the expectations that they, as participants, help set for themselves. How close they come to meeting expectations may be determined by systematically and objectively collecting quantitative facts and then calculating the difference between what was expected (ideally) and what actually occurred.

The assistant administrator for quality control is available to everyone to help establish expectations and measurements. An accurate evaluation of expectations by means of observations in this manner depends on reliable methods of observing and of recording quantitative, qualitative, and cost factors. Additionally, correlations between these factors must be established.

In the area of quantity, work measurement and standards of the industrial engineering type may be used. These standards form the basis of how much of what type of work is expected from whom under different work loads and staffing conditions. Brief follow-up studies render new figures for periodic checks on how well standards

and expectations are being met. Studies of this type do not, however, produce information about the quality of the work done or the end product unless quality indicators are identified, measured, and then correlated with quantity.

Adequate measures and standards of quality, particularly where patient services are involved, remain to be developed. Already, third-party payers are showing great concern for and curiosity about health services. As third-party reimbursement increases and becomes localized in two or three payers, one can expect more influence on control of health organization operations by allocation of funds. In such a situation it will be imperative to define quality. Only by providing a differential in quality and by substantiating it quantitatively can an institution justify a differential in reimbursement above that of institutions providing less quality.

The Commission for Administrative Services in Hospitals has experimented with a technique that has had considerable success. Using statistical quality control methods, *a quality control plan for nursing service* establishes the relative level of the quality of care and service on a continuing basis.

A QUALITY CONTROL PLAN FOR NURSING SERVICE*
Introduction

The nursing profession has long expressed the need for a quality control plan that would establish, on a continuing basis, the relative level of the quality of care and service. Developing a plan for reporting on the quality of care given is a key step in the ultimate achievement of a high level of quality care. The plan presented here is an opening wedge in this direction. It is the result of considerable research and pilot study by the nursing professionals in a number of major hospitals in Southern California, working in a cooperative effort with the consulting engineers with the CASH program.

The underlying hypothesis for the development of the plan is as follows:

Trained professional personnel may be one of the most effective means of detecting *gross* nursing deficiencies by direct inspection of both the patient and his immediate environs.

Careful and critical review of patient records on the nursing unit can form a valuable supplementary source of information regarding nursing proficiency.†

Testing this hypothesis required the development of a list of meaningful attributes in each of the areas named. This task was undertaken by members of the nursing profession. The means employed to carry out the tests were designed by engineering professionals. The technique is based upon the use of statistical quality control methods.

The plan has shown promise, based on the tests to date. There is no question in the judgment of the participating nurses that it provides a reasonable indicator of the level

of care and service within the parameters of the plan itself. CASH will update this report as further material is adequately tested and introduced.

Objectives of the plan

The primary objectives of the quality control plan for nursing services are stated as follows:

1. To provide a *measure* that will indicate the *level of* the quality of care and service; the *degree* of nursing proficiency
2. To provide such measures on a *continuing* basis as a vital ongoing management *control*
3. To provide *feedback* in order to allow the necessary *corrective action*
4. To provide a means of establishing staffing patterns based upon *optimum* personnel *utilization* and *assured quality* of care and service

Principles of statistical quality control

The statistical quality control method for determining the quality level of the proficiency of people performing work, as reflected in the quality of the end product, has been widely used for roughly 30 years. The primary advantages of this method are that (1) it provides *valid* results, (2) it requires a *minimum* amount of *time* to establish results, and (3) it is universal in its application so that complete coverage of all personnel is possible.

Statistical quality control is based upon the laws of probability, that is, a large enough sample taken at random from a total situation tends to have the same pattern of characteristics as the total situation. Three primary rules must be followed:

1. Samples (in this case, patients, rooms, and charts) must be selected *at random*.
2. A sufficient number of samples (observations) must be taken (made).
3. An affirmative or negative decision regarding the attribute being observed

---

*Pages 200 to 209 (with modification) from Commission for Administrative Services in Hospitals: A quality control plan for nursing service, Los Angeles, 1965, The Commission.

†From Blumberg, M. S., and Drew, J.: Methods for assessing nursing care quality, Hospitals **37**:72, Nov. 1963.

QUALITY CONTROL CHECK SHEET

Medical/Surgical

Floor _2_ Unit _NORTH_ Room _207_ Date _APRIL 19_ Time _9:00 A.M._

Patient _SEWELL_ By _R. NICHOLS_

Diagnosis _APPENDECTOMY_ Age _14_ Date Admitted _APRIL 16_

A. PATIENT WELFARE AND SAFETY

	Yes	No
1. Patient does not appear to require immediate attention?	X	
2. Patient's mental attitude appears satisfactory?	X	
3. Side rails up if required?		X
4. Call lite within easy reach and working?		X
5. Patient's skin condition satisfactory?	X	
6. Dressing clean and comfortable?		
7. Equipment, tube, etc. functioning?	X	
8. Nursing performing procedure correctly and efficiently?		
Total	4	2

B. PATIENT COMFORT AND ACCESSIBILITY OF IMMEDIATE NEEDS

	Yes	No
1. Patient appear to be comfortable?	X	
2. Bed neatly made and comfortably positioned?		X
3. Urinal empty, rinsed, cover on and positioned?		X
4. Bed pan empty, rinsed and positioned?	X	
5. Bedside table and personal effects within easy reach?	X	
6. Before meal – patient prepared?		
7. After meal – finished tray removed?		
Total	3	2

C. PATIENT ROOM

	Yes	No
1. Room appearance satisfactory?	X	
2. Closet orderly and stocked?	X	
3. Lavatory orderly, clean, stocked?	X	
4. Noise level satisfactory?		X
5. Lighting satisfactory to patient?		
6. Temperature and ventilation satisfactory to patient?		
Total	3	1

Observer Comments (Reference Number)

A-3	ONE SIDE UNLATCHED
A-4	CORD TWISTED – CAN'T REACH
B-2	HEAD UP TOO LONG – PAT. TIRED
B-3	NOT COVERED
C-4	CHATTER IN HALL

Fig. 10-1. Quality control check sheet for observing and rating the patient environment. (From Commission for Administrative Services in Hospitals: A quality control plan for nursing service, Los Angeles, 1965, The Commission.)

QUALITY CONTROL CHECK SHEET

All Services

Floor __2__   Unit _SOUTH_   Room __241__   Date _APRIL 7_   Time _3:00 P.M._

Patient   _AVERY_   By   _R. NICHOLS_

Diagnosis   _CARDIAC_   Date Admitted _APR. 6_   Date Discharged _____

D.   PATIENT CHARTS

	Yes	No
1. Is chart assembled in correct order?	x	
2. Are routine activities correctly recorded and position of siderails noted?	x	
3. Have doctor's visits been noted?		
4. Are medicines properly charted with time, method, dosage, initials and signatures indicated? (Sites of injections to be charted in nurse's notes.)		x
5. Are pre-op medicines charted with pertinent comments noted in nursing notes?		
6. Are reasons for PRN medications noted?		x
7. Has effect of PRN medications been noted?	x	
8. Are nurse's notes informative and printed in black or blue ink?	x	
9. Are acceptable abbreviations being used?	x	
10. Are treatments properly charted with time and signature indicated?	x	
11. Is intake and output properly recorded?		
12. Is laboratory work properly recorded?		
13. Are recording persons' signatures, initials and professional status properly noted?	x	
14. Are orders properly transcribed with notation of time and signature of nurse in correct place?	x	
15. Have physician's orders been carried out and charted?	x	
16. If orders are not completed, are pertinent comments acceptable?		
17. Have all orders been signed by physician?	x	
18. Is history and physical completed?	x	
19. Is TPR graphic sheet complete?		x
20. Are admission notes complete?	x	
21. Are discharge notes complete?		
22. Is nursing care plan informative and current?	x	
Totals	13	3

Observer Comments (Reference Number)

4	SOME TITLES NOT INDICATED
6	REASON NOT ALWAYS INDICATED
19	GRAPHIC TIMES NOT CONTINUOUS

Fig. 10-2. Quality control check sheet for inspecting and rating the patient chart. (From Commission for Administrative Services in Hospitals: A quality control plan for nursing service, Los Angeles, 1965, The Commission.)

must truly represent the immediate condition.

Outline of the plan

The plan is named the Unit Quality Index Plan (UQI) since it is based on sampling within a nursing unit, measuring indicators of nursing quality and yielding a single weekly control index.

Three quality control check sheets are provided, covering:

1. The patient and his immediate environs (Fig. 10-1)
2. The patient chart (Fig. 10-2)

3. The nursing unit (Fig. 10-3)

The plan requires a minimum of five of each of the three check sheets to be filled in during each control period (1 or 2 weeks). The times for making these observations should be governed by a random schedule (Fig. 10-4).

Near the end of the control period, additional check sheets may be required based upon the percent acceptable (see p. 216).

At the end of the control period, the control index is calculated for each nursing unit. Separate indices will be computed for each category of control as well as a single

---

QUALITY CONTROL CHECK SHEET

Medical/Surgical

Floor __3__   Unit __EAST__   Date __MARCH 7__   Time __10:30 A.M.__

By __A. JOHNSON__

E.   NURSING UNIT

	Yes	No
1. Are the shelves in the linen room labeled and the linen placed neatly on the appropriate shelf?	X	
2. Are the medicines to be refrigerated on the bottom shelf of the refrigerator?	X	
3. Is the emergency tray accessible, complete and the drugs not outdated?	X	
4. Is the medicine area tidy and clean?		X
5. Have the discontinued drugs been sent to Pharmacy?		
6. Is the kitchen area clean and in order?	X	
7. Is the utility area clean and in order?	X	
8. Are wheel chairs folded, in good repair and in a safe place?		X
9. Are the linen bags prepared properly for laundry pickup?		
10. No unnecessary equipment in the corridor?	X	
11. Are the fire doors and fire escapes readily accessible?	X	
12. Nurses station appear to be organized?	X	
Totals	8	2

Observer Comments (Reference Number)

4	TOWELS SCATTERED ON COUNTER
8	WHEEL CHAIR IN CORRIDOR

Fig. 10-3. Quality control check sheet for observing and rating the nursing unit. (From Commission for Administrative Services in Hospitals: A quality control plan for nursing service: Los Angeles, 1965, The Commission.)

RANDOM SCHEDULE CHART

Patient Environment Check Sheet

Unit   3 S

Week	1		2		3		4	
Time	Day	Rm.No.	Day	Rm.No.	Day	Rm.No.	Day	Rm.No.
7–10	M	321	Tu	322	W	323	Th	324
10– 1	M	325	Tu	326	W	327	Th	328
1– 4	W	329	Th	330	F	331	M	332
4– 7	W	333	Th	334	F	335	M	334
7–11	F	337	Sa	338	Su	340	W	336

Notes:

1. Obtain a minimum of five check sheets per week.

2. If patient is not in scheduled room, go to next occupied room, i.e., 325 N.P., go to 326, etc.

Fig. 10-4. Random schedule chart. (From Commission for Administrative Services in Hospitals: A quality control plan for nursing service, Los Angeles, 1965, The Commission.)

index for the overall control (Fig. 10-5).

All check sheets should be returned to the nursing unit involved for necessary review and corrective action.

Control indices for all units should be recorded and posted as illustrated in Fig. 10-6. Additionally, the indices should be graphed to illustrate trends from period to period (Fig. 10-7).

Observing and rating the patient environment

Observing and rating represents the most important single function in the quality control plan. It is essential to eliminate the possibility of personal bias, which can distort the validity of the results. The nursing committee therefore recommends that the observing and rating be performed by members of nursing administration and/or supervisory nurses.

We strongly recommend that all persons performing the observing and rating function be adequately trained in order to achieve consistency and validity.

The following general procedure is recommended for observing and rating the patient and his immediate environs:

1. Select the time for the observation and the rooms/patients to be observed

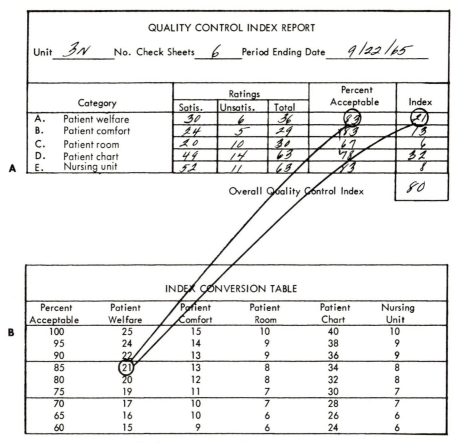

Fig. 10-5. **A,** Quality control index report. **B,** Index conversion table. (From Commission for Administrative Services in Hospitals: A quality control plan for nursing service, Los Angeles, 1965, The Commission.)

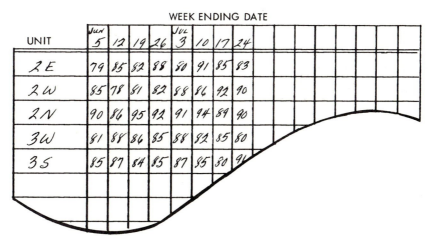

Fig. 10-6. Quality control record. (From Commission for Administrative Services in Hospitals: A quality control plan for nursing service, Los Angeles, 1965, The Commission.)

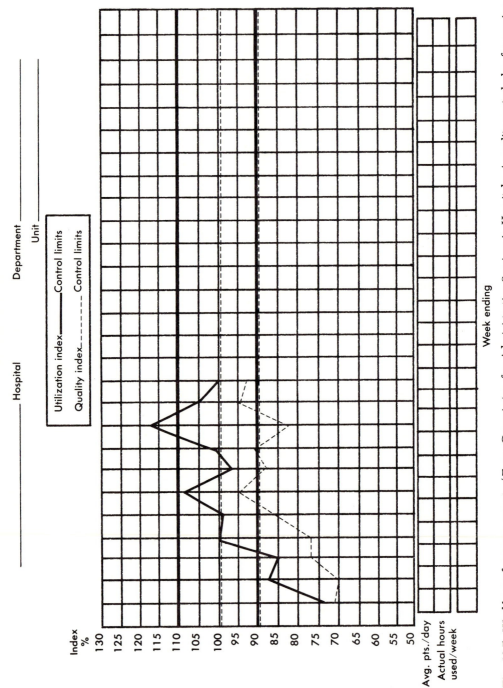

Fig. 10-7. Weekly performance report. (From Commission for Administrative Services in Hospitals: A quality control plan for nursing service, Los Angeles, 1965, The Commission.)

from the random schedule of observations chart (Fig. 10-4).

2. Select the appropriate quality control check sheet for the service involved.
3. Notify the head nurse for the unit. Request the head nurse to accompany, if possible.
4. Observe and rate each factor on check sheet. Rate the *immediate prevailing condition*. (Steps 4 through 8 are illustrated in Fig. 10-1.)
5. Rate only those factors that are present at the time of observation.
6. Consult the nurse in charge if a yes/no rating cannot be made without consultation.
7. Support all negative ratings with appropriate comments.
8. Obtain a minimum of 14 total ratings for each check sheet. If this is not possible, select another room/patient.
9. Obtain a minimum of five check sheets for each unit for each control period.

Inspecting and rating the patient chart

Because of the greater objectivity involved in the inspection and rating of the patient chart, the nursing committee recommends the selection and rotation of staff nurses to perform this function.

It is imperative that the staff nurses receive adequate training in order to achieve consistency and validity.

The following general procedure is outlined:

1. Notify the head nurse for the unit involved.
2. Select the charts at random from chart storage at the unit. (No random schedule is required.)
3. Select the appropriate quality control check sheets for the service involved.
4. Inspect and rate the last 2 complete days only. Refer to Kardex and medication cards, etc. as required. (Steps 4 through 8 are illustrated in Fig. 10-2.)

5. Rate only those factors that apply.
6. Consult the head nurse if a yes/no rating cannot be made without consultation.
7. Support all negative ratings with appropriate comments.
8. Obtain a minimum of 12 total ratings for each check sheet. If this is not possible, select another chart.
9. Obtain a minimum of five check sheets for each nursing unit for each control period.
10. If, in the opinion of the inspector, certain *immediate* corrective actions should be taken, consult the head nurse of the unit involved.

Observing and rating the nursing unit

It is recommended that the observing and rating of the nursing unit be performed by members of nursing administration or supervisory nurses or both.

Adequate training of the observers will ensure consistency and validity.

The following general procedure is outlined:

1. Notify the head nurse for the unit. Request the head nurse to accompany, if possible.
2. Observe and rate each factor on the check sheet. Rate the *immediate* prevailing *condition*. (Steps 2 to 4 are illustrated in Fig. 10-3.)
3. Consult the head nurse in charge if a yes/no rating cannot be made without consultation.
4. Support all negative ratings with appropriate comments.
5. Obtain a minimum of 10 ratings for each check sheet.
6. Obtain a minimum of five check sheets for each unit for each control period.

Calculating the quality control index

1. To ensure validity of the UQI for each nursing unit for the control period, it is essential to check to be sure that a sufficient number of samples (check

sheets) have been made. This procedure follows:

After the first *five* check sheets have been filled in:

A. Determine the percentage of total *acceptable* (yes) ratings in relation to the *total* number of ratings made. Do *not* include unrated factors.

> EXAMPLE: Patient environment check sheet
> Acceptable ratings   62
> Total ratings   75
> $\frac{62}{75} = 83\%$ acceptable

B. Refer to the number of check sheets required chart (see the following) and determine the *additional* number of check sheets required.

> EXAMPLE: (from above)
>   83% acceptable requires 1 additional check sheet

NUMBER OF CHECK SHEETS REQUIRED TO ENSURE VALIDITY TO ±10%*

Percent acceptable	Number of additional check sheets required
100	0
95	0
90	1
85	1
80	2
75	3
70	5
65	8
60	11
55	15
50	20

*From Commission for Administrative Services in Hospitals: A quality control plan for nursing service, Los Angeles, 1965, The Commission.

2. After obtaining a sufficient number of check sheets, the next step involves the calculation of the UQI for the control period.

3. After calculating the percent acceptable for each category, refer to the index conversion table (see Fig. 10-5, *B*) and record each index. The total indices will represent the overall quality control index (see Fig. 10-5, *A*) for the nursing unit.

4. Upon completion, the quality control index report should be sent to the supervisory nurse, together with all check sheets.

5. Supervisory nurse should review results and problem areas with the respective head nurses.

Recording the results

It is recommended that the composite list of all quality indices be recorded on a quality control record (see Fig. 10-6) to indicate the results for the control period involved.

This record may then be posted on the nurses' lounge bulletin board or simply distributed to the supervisory and head nurses involved.

Charting the trends

It is highly recommended that the quality control indices be plotted on a nursing performance report for each nursing unit (Fig. 10-7).

Since each nursing unit is already plotting *utilization indices* for each control period, it is a logical extension to plot the *quality indices* for the same control period on the *same* chart. This provides a quick graphic picture of trends for both utilization and quality control, and further illustrates whether the indices are within the established control limits. Control limits for utilization are indicated by dashed lines. The lower control limit for the quality index is indicated by a double line at "90%."

• • •

It is entirely possible that the CASH approach, which now uses nurses to inspect the patient, his immediate environs, and patient records, can be extended to include the use of written nursing care plans. This would extend quality considerations to an evaluation of patient need for care, the service required to meet that need, and the adequacy with which need was determined and met.

chapter eleven

CASE HOSPITAL INFORMATION SYSTEM

Organization around systems and programs provides flexibility for a high degree of coordination through the use of information upon which to base courses of action. It provides the potential, but the potential is realized only if and when reliable information flows in usable form and is interpretable by those who need it.

Descriptive information must be gathered from all sources. It is correlated with information for and about planning, coordinating, and controlling activities related to resources, programs, and patients in the broad areas of service, research, and teaching. This potential can be realized through a common computer data base (Fig. 11-1) that provides identification, classification, storage, and retrieval of information necessary to the user. As envisioned, the Case Hospital information system would be far more complete than any computer-based system thus far applied to the use of health care information.

Information systems theory and computer applications have evolved from hard sciences such as electrical engineering and are dependent on reliable, consistent information and predictable variables. To the extent that these criteria are met by an organization, hard science and applications

are valid. To the extent that information is not always reliable and not always consistent and that variables are not always predictable, the information system will become less reliable.

Health care organizations are dependent on human beings. Human beings are never completely consistent, reliable, or predictable. They are not completely rational.* Yet these inconsistent, unreliable, unpredictable people will remain the hard core of health care for the foreseeable future. Because of this, health organizations must be particularly aware of the fact that, in developing information systems, it is altogether too easy to develop the system and proceed to build or change the organization to fit it. When this happens the organization may become restricted to the boundaries of the information system. To the extent that the organization stays within these boundaries, it may become incapable of relating to nonroutine situations.

In a health care organization nonroutine situations often arise around patient needs. If the organization is not flexible enough to meet these needs, then the information

---

*That is, rational in terms of hard science or in terms of more general organizational values.

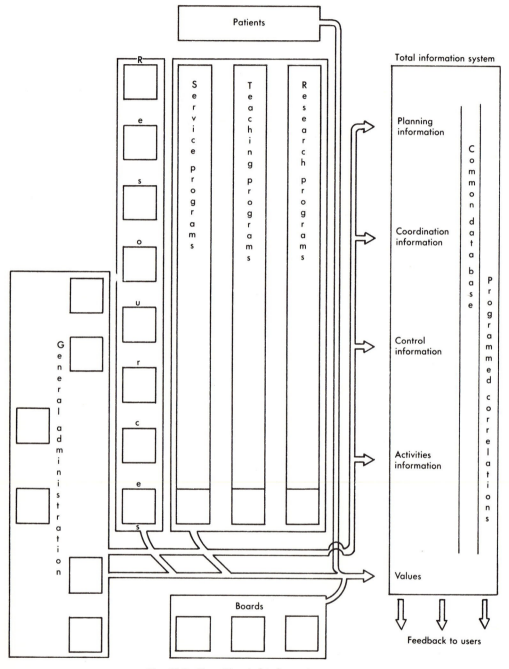

Fig. 11-1. Case Hospital information system.

system may be detrimental to the patient and to the program of care.* As long as patients can create nonroutine situations, the hospital must maintain adequate programs of care and must not be boxed in by an information system.

Added to the complications presented by patients is the fact that the organization encompasses several professional and technical groups that operate with different sets of values. Also contributing to the unpredictability of variables is the fact that the values of these groups may change momentarily as they are pressured by a variety of interrelationships, including relationships with the external environment.

The effect of the external environment is of great importance. It represents the larger social system of which the health care system is a part and to which it should be sensitive. The external environment includes a number of professional and other organizations to which people who work in health organizations belong and from which they bring values into the work place. And not the least important is the fact that, as patients come from the "external" to the "internal" environment, they are confronted with different values of the organization and its professional and technical groups.

Viewing the health care organization as a system in which services are rendered in the form of programs, one can regard an information system as a subsystem. The object of this subsystem is to provide pertinent, accurate information to the proper person at the appropriate time so that the potential for the right decision is maximized. It is imperative that health care information systems be developed to accommodate the full spectrum of health

care, including those areas that need to remain flexible as well as those that may be routinized, and that health care organizations not be required to conform to predetermined parameters established for ease of design.

A comprehensive theory of computerized health information has been slow to focus. Case Hospital seeks this focus. In a major health sciences center the lag between potential information flow and actual flow is gargantuan when it is dependent on manual manipulation. Accuracy too may be nowhere near as reliable as it could be if subjected to computerized screening. The potential advantage for financial affairs, operations, patient care, teaching, and research held by rapid flow and correlation of all information available in the complex is sufficient to warrant a computerized information system. Add to this the information available among other facilities in the region, and the benefits are multiplied many times.

The broad concept of the information system presents the evolution of a computer-based information system that can serve all levels of health care organization. Figs. 6-1, 12-1, and 12-2 depict a hospital organization, a health university, and a regional health authority. The pattern of organization and of information flow are similar in all three so that a Case Hospital information system may be paraphrased "total health information system" on a regional basis.

Case Hospital has been working toward improving present operations to make them more efficient in order to bring them to a point where new, experimental approaches may be tried. An information concept is being developed that, in the future, will involve a data base with input and output mechanisms throughout the health sciences center which can be linked with the entire region, or even beyond. Such a linkup will provide the communication ties between health resources and programs

---

*It is wholly conceivable that a computerized system could make information harder to obtain than a manual system. Under nonroutine conditions this information might be more needed than at any other time, yet may be harder to obtain because it is being sought under nonroutine circumstances.

that must inevitably work together in order to (1) route patients through a gamut of health care, regardless of their location or the location of the services, (2) plan on a regional (or extended) basis how best to use health resources, and (3) determine on a regional basis the need for new resources and programs.

In light of current legislation, enacted and pending, it is evident that regional programs are inevitable, if not by invitation, then by direction. Case Hospital has moved in a number of areas toward diffusing its delivery of care methods, as witnessed by its neighborhood health centers. It has at the same time begun to look toward coordinating with other programs in its region through its teaching affiliations and participation with its health affiliates.

The current information methodology employed in the region, and indeed in most health facilities and regions in the United States, is not adequate to provide the best functioning of individual facilities, much less multiple facility undertakings. The increased ability to ensure adequate care and to manage all resources in an effective and efficient manner within one facility or on a multifacility basis requires an information catalyst for the entire health community.

Obviously, such an ambitious undertaking is a long-term program involving the expenditure of millions of dollars. It ranges from a broad blueprint to the design and implemenation of highly sophisticated and complex data management systems. The initial phase would involve a description of an overall plan. This phase should be a broad-brush blueprint for an automated information-handling system to support the best possible regional health care program. The broad blueprint is a necessary first step that has been overlooked in a number of attempts. Without the blueprint, fragmented programs and operations result that cannot be interfaced into or with a total overall system.

The final result of this phase should be an outline of an implementation plan to make the entire system operational. It should include estimates of personnel, cost, and time requirements for each additional phase. The design should be such that increments may be added as financing is available. Each increment should fit into the master plan. Three major needs will be served: (1) it will assist in improving current operations and in building sound systems and programs for the future, (2) it will handle information necessary for remote health facilities, and (3) it will provide support for a regional health care program.

chapter twelve
EVALUATION

The philosophy of reorganization was basically formulated to integrate resources and programs with institutional missions and objectives by involving appropriate personnel, including physicians, in decentralized decision making related to all types of activity and to blend it all through a participative management environment and process. It was to provide a well-coordinated and economical clinical setting that met the clinical needs of care, teaching, and research with appropriate emphasis on each at the same time that the care activities fit well into the basic health care delivery system. Most of the difficulties encountered with implementation arose from lack of planning. As industry has shown, modern organizations must plan alternatives, decide on courses of action, and obtain commitment and coordination among decentralized decision centers for implementation.

Although considerable effort went into planning organization and operations in the resource systems, the programs were not well thought through and even less consideration was given the coordinating, synergistic mechanism required at the health sciences center level. As a result, reorganization was begun without adequate understanding of the objectives sought or the participative process required to blend activities and direct them toward overall center missions. In short, there was virtually no overall organization or management matrix.

Among the greatest challenges were eight factors presented throughout this chapter.

INADEQUATE SEPARATION OF CARE, TEACHING, AND RESEARCH

Adequate separation of care, teaching, and research interests, with ultimate responsibility for the first retained by the hospital medical staff and for the remaining two reverting to other appropriate decision centers, was not effected. Conflict between care, teaching, and research interests remained because the program directors appointed were also medical school departmental chairmen and often, in addition, chief of the corresponding hospital clinical service.

A basic factor in the clinical setting is how to improve utilization (both in quality and quantity) through organization and delivery of the products of medical science and technology. A second factor is how to secure and maximize financial resources for delivery. The program provides the locus of clinical activity where knowledge may be utilized and new forms of utilization, both professional and administrative, may be devised and experimented with. It is the point where models of care may be developed and where the organization meets the public. This is particularly important to physicians since it provides a platform for exchange of views and services between the profession and the public, but the typical teaching hospital has not maximized this potential.

If these problems are to be correctly managed, the appropriate individuals within the organization must engage in goal implementation with equitable emphasis on each of the missions. Although it is clear that if staff are to conduct clinical teaching and research successfully, they cannot be unreasonably burdened with patient care; it is equally clear that the hospital bears social responsibility for providing excellent care and models for its delivery. Teaching and research activities cannot be substituted for comprehensive care or vice versa. There must be a complete understanding and fulfillment of each as a social instrument, and an understanding of the social, economic, and political environment surrounding each as a link in the larger spectrum of health. The program should become mature to achieve a clinical balance among these interests.

INADEQUATE MANAGERS SELECTED

Managers were selected in both resource systems and programs with too little consideration of management training and ability and, in the case of program directors, their interests and time available for the job were not given adequate attention.

Management is essentially getting optimum results in an assigned area of responsibility. A manager carries the burden of achieving results through the people he is assigned to manage. To do this, he must not only have a firm knowledge of the basics of management such as planning, organizing, staffing, directing, and controlling but must also be adept at using these tools in a situation that involves coordinating the efforts of other people who produce the results. In the modern health complex a manager must be aware that traditional ways of organizing and managing are passing from the scene and new forms are evolving that require the coordination of functional authority through influence as well as command.

Additionally, incentives sufficient to promote innovation, effectiveness, and efficiency were not provided. This is important to people with all levels of ability and need, but especially in relation to professionals if their meaningful participation is to be secured.

AMBULATORY CARE ONLY IN HOSPITAL

Until recent years ambulatory care at the health sciences center in the form of doctors' office visits, other physician services and ancillary service was almost exclusively hospital based and professionally supported by the hospital house staff and voluntary staff physicians. However, two relatively recent changes, full-time medical faculty and reorganization of the hospital outpatient clinics, caused important changes.

Before the medical school recruited its full-time faculty there were few private physicians' offices at the center. Most office visits occurred in hospital outpatient clinics that were staffed by hospital interns and residents rather randomly supervised by voluntary staff physicians. When most medical faculty became full time, many of them established private offices at the center and continued seeing their private patients there. This made more staff physician time available to the outpatient clinics, thus improving the potential for consultation and house staff supervision.

Social and political pressures coupled with the implementation of Medicare and Medicade necessitated an improvement in the professional service available in the clinics and abandonment, in image at least, of a dual-service system that segregated between "private" and "clinic" patients. Thus, the center reorganized the hospital clinics in an effort to cope with these pressures and a poor financial situation. The physical, administrative, and professional changes resulting from this reorganization created a situation in which the new group practice type of operation was more like, but often physically separate from and not quite equal to, private practice. Comprehensive delivery was partially lost sight of and the pattern became fragmented, retaining remnants of two levels of care between private and nonprivate patients, resisting coordination between inpatient and outpatient activities, and confronting patients with multiple registration, appointment, billing, and referral systems. Multidisciplinary activities did not materialize and an interface between the various disciplines within each program was incomplete. Adequate triage was not provided from the emergency department and referrals between programs and neighborhood health centers presented many mechanical difficulties.

The center must move into a system in which all ambulatory doctor's office visits, other physicians' services and ancillary services conducted under its auspices are organized as an integral part of the center's health services delivery system managed by an associate vice-president. This office should be held accountable for effective and efficient operation of the entire system, but must delegate appropriate responsibility and authority to operating units such as programs and resource systems. The administrative and professional management of ambulatory office visits, other physicians' service, and inpatient service related to each program should be managed on a combined basis by each program with program managers reporting directly to the office of the associate vice-president.

At least the following professional and administrative characteristics should be present for the ambulatory portion of the system, but should function for all parts of the system whenever possible.

Organization and management

The original concept of clinic reorganization was visualized as a gradual wedding of clinics and private practice that would achieve ambulatory care goals in an organizational and management structure where ambulatory and inpatient responsibilities were combined in the management of each program. Accountability for the management of the collective programs would rest with an overall administrative office, with considerable authority and decision-making responsibility delegated to program managers.

As a step toward this ultimate organization and management structure, a group practice administrative unit was formed and given responsibility for planning and implementing the transition from hospital clinics. It was to gradually transfer management to each group, retaining those functions necessary for overall coordination. This unit originally reported to an associate vice-president for clinical services. When he left, responsibility was transferred first to a temporary replacement and finally to the medical school dean.

Coordinating mechanisms for inpatient and outpatient areas switched to separate management centers and the organizational arrangement of the center, hospital services, and ambulatory services, along with the process for their management became extremely unclear. In fact, they were frequently referred to as "nonorganization," "nonmanagement," and "nonsystem." This must be rectified before policy or operational improvements or changes can be undertaken with any assurance of success.

Accountability

A process of accountability must be established in which:
1. There is a definite chain of command from the vice-president of the health

sciences center to every individual and operating unit in the center.

2. The chain of command is reflected in an organizational chart.
3. The chain of command is backed by a management process, which enumerates the following:
   a. Job and performance descriptions for each person.
   b. What authority and responsibility is assigned to each person.
   c. Who each person is responsible to for his performance.

Overall management accountability of health services must rest with an associate vice-president. This office should establish a clear-cut administrative process that:

1. Provides a clear chain of command from each person and operational unit in the system to the associate vice-president.
2. Manages the center's entire health delivery system.
3. Coordinates ambulatory doctors' office visits and other physicians' services with hospital-based ancillary service, inpatient care, and other hospital and center activities.
4. Establishes a method of health services audit and review that will enforce policies of nondiscrimination in facilities, administration, and professional care and will assure a high standard of care. This should be part of the institution's overall program of peer review and quality assurance.
5. Provides centrally managed planning and policy development, implementation, and maintenance.
6. Provides central accountability for uniformity of services and tightening of audit and control.
   a. Creating uniformity of ambulatory facilities, reception and portal of entry, financial screening and registration, appointments, medical records, billing-collections-accounting, and professional care.

(1) *Facilities.* Despite the considerable progress that has been made toward consolidating ambulatory care space, the goal of providing equal and contiguous space and functions for all ambulatory patients has not been achieved, largely because of a lack of enough contiguous space to handle the entire load and a diversity of poorly coordinated management practices. The following steps should be taken:

(a) Evaluate space utilization in the outpatient building in an effort to devise recommendations for using the building entirely for ambulatory care. It is conceivable that if the identification of geographic service boundaries reduces the number of ambulatory patients treated and if the space is used to capacity with a different operating schedule, all or nearly all ambulatory patients could be treated in the outpatient building. Every effort should be made to eliminate all dual offices and facilities that are used by a single program.

(b) If all ambulatory practices cannot be consolidated in the outpatient building, facilities must be upgraded to provide functional and esthetic equality among all ambulatory service areas.

(c) Seek out situations where programs or individual practitioners have or believe they have informal agreements that allow circumvention of institutional policy, and take remedial action.

(d) Seek out and correct physical appearances that suggest discrimination.

(2) *Reception and portal of entry.* There should be one, centralized portal of entry for all ambulatory patients making initial entry into the system unless they are referred directly to a specific service by their private physician.

(3) *Financial screening and registration.* There should be one, centrally managed financial screening and registration system for all patients making initial entry into the system, including those referred by a private physician.

(4) *Appointments.* There should be one, centrally managed appointment system for all patients seen in the ambulatory care system, including patients referred by a private physician. Appointments for new patients to various office locations must be on a random basis.

(5) *Medical records.* Medical records for all patients seen in the ambulatory care system should be incorporated into the hospital-unit record system, including the records of patients referred by private physicians.

(6) *Billing-collections-accounting.* There should be one, centrally managed billing-collections-accounting system for all patients seen in the ambulatory care system, including patients referred by a private physician.

(7) *Professional care.* Continual

use of the terms "private practice" and "group practice" tends to perpetuate an image of a two-class system of care. The lack of contiguous physical space also supports this image. In addition to the measures suggested above, it would also be helpful to:

(a) Establish an episodic care unit that is a forerunner of the larger, comprehensive community care practice. This unit should provide triage and episodic care for many patients now treated in the emergency department, thus diverting nonemergency cases from that area and providing a single portal of entry to the ambulatory care system.

(b) Eliminate the terms "private practice," "group practice," and "clinics" from the institution's vocabulary and use instead, a term such as "professional care" or "ambulatory care."

(c) Insist on uniform involvement of house staff in ambulatory care, with the extent of their involvement determined only by disease complexity and patient need.

b. Tightening audit and control mechanisms. An audit and control system for both professional and nonprofessional activities must be created that does the following:

(1) Sets measurable standards reflective of the single standard of care goals and objectives sought. The goals and objec-

tives must be stated in policy form and the policy, in turn, must provide the basis for beginning to enumerate tangible standards against which success or failure in satisfying policy can be obtained.

(2) Obtains feedback about performance through systematized appraisal.

(3) Evaluates feedback to see if performance is meeting standards.

(4) Makes evaluation available for decisions on corrective or change action when indicated.

The result of such a process as auditing and control must be intimately linked with the administrative and professional organizational structures for delivery of care throughout the center and, in the end, must related resources-use evaluation as well as provide comparative evaluations of program management and performance. The process should also project ways of maintaining standards that surpass accreditation and reimbursement requirements and provide models for community health organizations and affiliated institutions. For purposes of establishing and maintaining a high standard of care, the associate vice-president should evaluate existing policies and recommend new policies that would collectively describe the single standard of care sought for all patients and enable a control system for the policies that meets the criterion outlined above.

The problems inherent in a good ambulatory system that fits comprehensively with inpatient care are many, of course, and call for a broad administrative perspective. First of all, ambulatory care, like inpatient care, should reflect the community

it serves. To be truly representative, there must be continual communication between the community and the health institution. This is usually accomplished by including interested, intelligent members of the community on the board of trustees.* Physicians' advice and participation are often overlooked at the board level too, despite the fact that these professionals are the most highly trained and informally influential participants in the delivery of care. Thus a platform of broad administrative perspective should be created at the board of trustees level and should include input from community members and physicians.

The intricate organizational and administrative complex required to implement the system must be headed by a capable administrator of all health services at the associate vice-president level. He must be assisted by people who are expert in the management of both inpatient and outpatient services and be advised by a medical advisory board linked to the executive committee.

The people who the associate vice-president assigns to coordinate ambulatory services must work as smoothly as possible with all departments since there will be overlapping of decision on every level. But their primary responsibility is ambulatory service and they must be willing and able to promote decisions in support of the prevailing philosophy of the institution. They must be involved in a central appointment system, work closely with all specialties and the physicians who are apprised of bed availability in the inpatient facility, and coordinate all the activities of ambulatory service with inpatient service.

The social service department will need to move freely between the inpatient and ambulatory facilities just as patients should,

*Residents of low-income areas have never really been a part of policy making in agencies serving them, however, and they are now asking for "a piece of the action." The inclusion of their advice at the board level makes good sense.

and a strong medical-record committee that has a sincere belief that good patient care can be identified though good record keeping will be needed. To avoid as much duplication of equipment and personnel as possible, services such as laboratories, radiology, medical records, and the emergency room should be located as close to both inpatient and ambulatory services as possible. The business office is another important connecting link, since one office can do all the accounts receivable and payable. However, before building a large staff to provide these services one should take an inventory to see if outside firms more economically provide these functions.

All these efforts must add up to an easy flow of materials, services, records, personnel, and patient back and forth between inpatient and ambulatory services. To achieve this, there must be continuing communication, cooperation, and dedication to a common objective—the dispensing of the best quality of medical care. Barriers must be removed and everyone must participate in a vital, vigorous organization where each individual has the freedom to function to the limit of his ability. It can be a dynamic and engrossing experience, with the patient reaping the benefits.

HOPED-FOR CENTERWIDE FINANCIAL MANAGEMENT SYSTEM NOT COMPLETED

The overriding reason for attempting a complete reorganization at one time was the financial deficit. A new method of handling income and expenses that many felt would substantially reduce the deficit was devised. The program budgeting system was to parallel the new management design, identifying costs specifically related to care, teaching, and research activities, and analyzing income sources to support each. Each cost center, corresponding to a management-decision center, was to have a program budget and be heavily involved in its construction and management. Program financial management for resource

systems and programs was to be tied into an overall centerwide financial and accounting framework. Although individual pieces of the system have been started, the overall framework has not materialized, resulting in inadequate information for multiple decision centers and little institutional review of expenditures and commitments.

IMPROPERLY DESIGNATED SYSTEMS

With implementation, a number of departments originally designated as "resource systems" became "programs." This reflected interplay by a number of factors, including a poor planning and implementation process as well as concession to political interplay.

The original goal and policy statements provided for the following programs:

1. Neurosurgery (neurosurgery, neurology, otorhinology, and ophthalmology).
2. Human growth and development (obstetrics, pediatrics, and gynecology).
3. Musculoskeletal (orthopedics, rheumatology, and physical medicine and rehabilitation).
4. Cardiopulmonary (thoracic and cardiovascular surgery, cardiology, chest disease and inhalation therapy, and bronchoesophagology).
5. General surgery.
6. Internal medicine.

As discussion progressed, *psychiatry, orthopedics* (originally in *musculoskeletal*), *dermatology,* and *community health* were added to the list, and by the time implementation was affected it included all of the above except *cardiopulmonary*, in addition to *physical medicine and rehabilitation* (originally in *musculoskeletal*), *laboratories and pathology, radiology,* and *anesthesiology.* Some specialties with a "loose" fit such as urology, head and neck tumor, bronchoesophagology, oral surgery, and proctology remained ostensibly outside of the management system although their professional responsibilities seemed to be adequately monitored. The situation created a concept breakdown and considerable organizational confusion, allowing political, status, and emotional considerations to prevail over any objective rationale that selectively included some areas of activity as programs and excluded others.

IMPROPER REMOVAL OF MANAGEMENT OF PROGRAMS

Management of programs was removed from the hospital organization and the terms "systems," "programs," "clinical management divisions," and "program budgeting" became ill defined and confusing. As discussed earlier, the first significant organizational changes took place when the hospital was reorganized into systems that later became known as "resource systems." Hospital departments were examined from a systems point of view where inputs to a system are processed for purposes of changing them into outputs usable in programs. Where processing similarities were found among several departments they were grouped together in a resource system.

Goals and objectives for the hospital, resource systems, and departments were established and a management process that complemented the new organization with greater decentralization of responsibility, authority, and decision making to assistant administrators and department heads was begun. Since the implementation of resource systems a number of organizational shifts within the hospital have occurred, and some systems and departments have moved from a hospital to a centerwide base of operations. Nevertheless, the concept of service departments as systems providing resources for the primary institutional programs of research, education, and care remains intact.

As these hospital changes took place, it became increasingly apparent that the focus of management and operations was centered predominantly on hospital service departments and that the coordination of departmental outputs for patient service was still suffering from traditional neglect. It was at this point that interest expanded to include comprehensive management of inpatient and outpatient service in a manner that would be compatible with the program floor concept of the new hospital and thus the term "programs" was brought into common use. Unfortunately this term was not clarified by the center with a sense of official meaning and became the source of considerable confusion. Among the multiple meanings frequently associated with "programs" were the following:

1. A program based in the medical school or health sciences center including all of the department's teaching, research, and care activities.
2. A major health sciences center program of activities focusing on either research, teaching, or care.
3. A group of activities based on a hospital program floor, related to a medical body system and including clinical research, teaching, and care interests.

From the hospital's point of view "programs" related to the third meaning and were described along the lines presented on pages 97 to 117.

Later the dean of the medical school gave up his post to become a deputy vice-president of the health sciences center with the purpose of implementing the systems and programs idea on a wider basis than originally conceived by the hospital. His new emphasis retained a partial focus within the original context of the hospital and program floor but extended to many other management functions in the medical school and health sciences center. In addition, his plan would add a potentially sophisticated planning-programming-budgeting system type of budgeting and accounting mechanism to the scheme that was patterned on the hospital cost-finding studies of the late Dr. Augustus J. Caroll and affected financial management throughout the center.

In the same year, conversion of the hospital outpatient clinics to a group-practice operation began. The term "clinical management division" (C.M.D.) was coined to highlight the organizational position of group practice within hospital-based clinical management divisions and to distinguish the original meaning of the term "programs" (within the hospital) from its newer configuration of activities extending beyond the hospital organization. This crystallized the idea that clinical activities could be grouped into hospital management units concentrating on centerwide missions where these multiple interests (research, teaching, and care) must respond to patient need. During the same time period a document detailing the organization, management, and financial implications of the changes underway was prepared. The following statement provides a picture of what was happening at that time:

The health sciences center has three basic objectives:
1. The education of health personnel (in this document physician education will be used as the example).
2. Research in health (both basic biologic research and research into the methods of organizing and delivering health care).
3. The actual delivery of health care to some defined population.

The latter objective is the one that is most difficult to rationalize for an educational institution and deserves some comment. Education in medicine differs from other educational programs in one major respect. It is not possible to utilize simulated models for learning. An engineering student can design a bridge, but the bridge need not be constructed. In medical education, the patient is the model for learning and it is necessary to conduct patient care in the highest quality fashion both to utilize the patient for a teaching model and to assure that the care received meets all appropriate expectations of the patient. Thus, the objective of patient care is necessary to provide the laboratory experience for the medical student as well as for the other health professional students.

In pursuing its objectives the health science center produces three different products that are purchased by three different beneficiary groups. The cost of patient care is appropriately chargeable to the patient or the third-party agency responsible for financing his care. Research is purchased by the national community through federal granting agencies and private foundations. The costs of education are supported by state subsidy and tuition charged to the student. Two of these beneficiary groups, research and patient care, are now demanding more accurate cost definition and are relating their purchasing price to audited costs. One can envision that the same type of accountability will ultimately be required by the agencies of the public that support the educational function.

The health sciences center is an industry that produces three separate products purchased by three different markets. One major difference from other industries, however, is the fact that the center must engage in the production of all three simultaneously, since the conduct of each is dependent on the others. Teaching can occur only in an environment of research and patient care. Although it is difficult to describe the exact amount of each of these activities needed, one needs to make judgments on the size of each program. This can best be illustrated by examining the most specific and simple example—that of one teacher, one student, and one patient.

Neglecting research activity for the moment, the functions of the center can be visualized by examining the way in which one physician-teacher conducts patient care and utilizes this activity to teach a student. If one represents each of these activities in Fig. 12-1, *A*, as a circle, then the

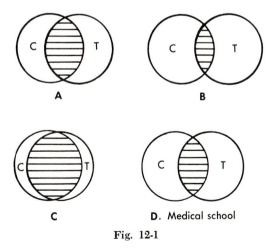

Fig. 12-1

area contained within the circle represents the amount of activity expended for the purpose. The overlapping of the two circles denotes that some of the care activity is utilized for teaching. The teacher may also expend effort beyond that which he would ordinarily expend in pure patient care if the student were not present. Obviously the degree of overlap will vary from one situation to another and depends on the status of the particular student. The involvement in care in Fig. 12-1, B, by an undergraduate medical student may be relatively slight. The involvement of an advanced student in a residency may be extensive, as in Fig. 12-1, C.

One can use this diagram to gain some understanding of the problem of accountability. The area in Fig. 12-1, C, included within circle C (care) is that which would be expended even though no teaching were being conducted and is appropriately (under existing laws and ethics) allocated as a cost to the patient. Generally speaking, we have not done so, at least in reference to that part of the cost directly attributable to the cost of the faculty member. Rather, we have allocated his cost for the entire circle T to the teaching budgets. In the past this was entirely appropriate since it was possible to charge for the entire circle C even though costs were not allocated there. With the change to cost reimbursement based on actual allocated costs, this is no longer possible. Immediately one can see that there is a potential double charging for that activity contained within the shaded overlap area.

One must understand that this diagrammatic presentation is accurate only in relationship to those costs related to part A of Medicare. The mechanism of billing the direct physician fee to the patient (part B) is quite confusing and must be treated separately. It is not related to a cost basis and the only way to anticipate amount of income is related to the number of people who are capable of paying a physician bill in addition to a hospital bill.

At this point of time it is still necessary to utilize double billing if the institution is to achieve fiscal solvency. This situation occurs because of incomplete implementation of Medicare and other governmental programs. Although most inpatient care will be reimbursed at cost (Medicare, Blue Cross, Medicade), there will still remain some patients who are not eligible for Medicade but do not have adequate financial resources to pay their full costs. If these patients are to be continued at all, it will be necessary to find some source of revenue other than from basic hospital income. Further, ambulatory care is supported at cost only by Medicare.

The mechanism that must be used is obvious. The total resources available to the combined teaching-care activity must be treated in a unified fashion. Whenever possible, those costs of teaching that overlap with patient care must be charged as patient care in order that they can be collected from those able to pay (this is entirely legal). When this is done, the resources that previously were expended from teaching budgets for this portion will be freed and become available to support the care for those patients who do not pay.

Continuing to use the microelement of the center (one physician, one patient, one student) as the model, one can envision certain management changes that would be required and the elements of program budgeting and accountability can be illustrated. The effort of the faculty can be divided into several distinct program categories (teaching of medical students, teaching of residents, care of the patient and research). Includable under hospital part A costs are the activities expended for teaching the resident and that portion of patient care included in hospital costs (supervision of laboratories, interpretation of electrograms, etc.). Chargeable to the patient directly or to part B of Medicare is that effort expended in direct professional diagnosis and treatment of the patient. This latter activity is not limited to reimbursement on cost basis and represents potential allowable profit. That attributable to part A currently allocated to the teaching budgets will represent new income available if transferred and will simultaneously release an equivalent number of dollars from the teaching budgets. Thus the multiple program activities will yield a profit from those patients who pay that can be used to compensate for losses on those who do not pay.

Perhaps some of the existing confusion related to current administrative structure can be realized. One individual faculty member accomplishes both program activities simultaneously, but he currently conducts these under two different management systems. His teaching function is administered by the medical school and his care function by the hospital. It is not surprising that some confusion should occur referable to the overlap area in Fig. 12-1, D. It would appear more appropriate if the management system could be unified at a level closer to the individual teacher, thus allowing for more accurate cost identification and optimal allocation of fiscal and other resources in the interest of better integration of the program activities, which are occurring simultaneously.

Obviously each individual faculty member cannot relate to central administration directly. Rather there must be aggregates of faculty identified and defined in order that collections represent coherent functional entities. The individual faculty members of such a unit should have comparable or complementary abilities, knowledge, and skills that are appropriate to specific categories of patient illness and teaching needs, e.g., a group of surgeons have comparable skills and treat comparable patient ills.

There are many ways in which one could define units. For the purposes of this institution the programs that have been tentatively identified are in many instances identical to other existing departments. In other instances, the program represents a collection of disciplines that work together in a unified fashion; e.g., the neurosensory program contains neurologists, neurosurgeons, otorhinologists, and ophthalmologists. All of these persons treat diseases of the nervous system and teach the students in a coordinated fashion.

The program is a functional entity that contains a group of professional persons (faculty) who have common specialized expertise (e.g., internists) together with all of the activities that they undertake within the geographic limits of the health sciences center. The teaching, research, and patient care functions of the unit are conducted simultaneously and all would be coordinated and managed by the program director (who would ordinarily be the academic department chairman). Each of the functions undertaken can be identified and costed, and this cost can be utilized to develop a program budget that, by allocation of costs to appropriate activities, can assure the maximum opportunity for cost reimbursement from the proper beneficiary or resource category. All the services provided by departments of the institution (housekeeping, dietary, nursing, etc.) to the program would be viewed as inputs to the program and costed to the program. Patients admitted for care within the program would be selected by the professional members and it would be their responsibility to aid in assuring payment for the patient's care.

If a patient were unable to pay, it would be the responsibility of the program manager to allocate available budgetary resources of the program to underwrite this payment (somewhat in the form of a patient scholarship). The resources available to meet this cost would come from one of three possible sources:

1. The profit that the hospital can derive on some services paid for at a level above cost.
2. Teaching resources that may currently be expended for salaries that can be freed by appropriate reallocation to patient care and

residency teaching and that can be collected from most patients.
3. Any of the income to the program derived from professional fees the collective professional personnel are willing to expend for this purpose.

This program concept would place the authority and responsibility on the persons who make the decisions on patient care and teaching. It is necessary to create the units rather than do this in a more generalized fashion for one very obvious reason. Some of the resources that would be utilized to meet currently unreimbursed costs would be those derived by the professional activities of the faculty. They are usually willing to divert these if it is done in the interest of their own program but are unwilling to do so if they see such diversion as working to the benefit of others and not to their own interests.

There are a number of implications that the institution of this policy might have. Among them are the following:

1. Administrative support would be needed in relationship to each program. To some extent there would be a decentralization of many administrative functions.
2. Since the program director would be responsible for all the activities conducted within his program, he would have to be directly responsible to the office of the vice-president for the ultimate coordination of all of the functions within his program.
3. Certain service systems that are currently hospital departments would need to function at the level of the health sciences center.
4. A unified fiscal office would be essential.

The proposed management system would not create a series of autonomous units. Basic budgetary allocations would be the responsibility of the administration of the health sciences center. The dean of a school would have the budgetary authority for applying teaching-budget inputs into each program. It would, however, produce incentives for the program director to identify all costs and to allocate them most appropriately in the interest of maximizing his financial resources. Judgment made on the amount of patient care cost accumulating on patients who do not pay would also be subject to fiscal incentives. If such costs could be reduced, the available resources could be utilized for program improvements.

One interesting facet of this approach is that of envisioning the way in which it might lead to a better mechanism of cost control and efficiency of operation. If it is possible to establish a balanced budget in the face of some existing unreimbursed costs and then when the time arrives when all patient care costs are covered, it should be possible to consider reducing costs to patients or reducing costs allocated to the teaching budgets. If successful, the program concept would ultimately allow the institution to request less from the state for teaching support than it would in the absence of such system with equivalent program quality.

From this discussion one may see that the term "programs" assumed a new meaning and that the peg that would hold the scheme together was program budgeting.

Evolving situation

A period of confusion and maneuvering for advantage followed during which the center underwent considerable instability. Recent administrative and attitudinal changes have reestablished a forward-looking momentum however, and it appears as if programs will be developed as management units within the hospital clinical setting only, an adequate program budgeting system will be developed, and the phrase "clinical management division" will be dropped. In the evolving scheme program organization and management are much more adequately defined along the following lines.

Organization of the professional medical component of Case Hospital. Those duly recognized academic departments of the Case School of Medicine and Dentistry that have major responsibilities centered around the hospital's functions in patient care, teaching, and research serve as the professional medical resource system of the hospital. These will be referred to hereafter as "university departments." The guidelines and principles under which the university departments operate are covered by the bylaws of their respective schools. Those members of the university departments who are professionally active in the hospital comprise the professional medical staff of the hospital. They remain primarily based in the academic department of their interest. However, for carrying out their professional clinical care they function as the professional medical staff of the hospital

and are governed by the principles set forth in the bylaws of Case University and the hospital and the bylaws of the professional medical staff. In the hospital they will be organized and function by the principles set forth in those bylaws.

Programs. The programs serve as the operationally active clinical units of the hospital through which the patient care, teaching, and research functions of the university departments and hospital are carried out. They are based in specifically designated physical facilities, guided and administered by a program director, and provided with appropriate professional and nonprofessional personnel as well as the necessary fiscal resources. The professional medical component for each of these programs will be active professional medical staff members from the staff of one or more of the university departments.

Appointment of the director for each of the programs is made by the associate vice-president in consultation with the various university department chairmen whose staff work within each particular program and subject to the approval of the vice-president for health sciences.

Interrelationship between the program concept at Case Hospital and the Case School of Medicine and the health sciences center

1. The program concept represents a hospital organizational mechanism designed to provide a more effective means for discharging the patient care, teaching, and research activities conducted by the schools of the health sciences center and Case Hospital. It is to be recognized that this organizational mechanism is for operational purposes in Case Hospital only and that the program director has a role separable and distinct from the role of the heads of university departments in the schools of the health sciences center.

   a. The programs do not contain all of the educational and research activities of the schools in which the university departments participate or are responsible for. Since only a portion of the teaching and research activities assigned to the heads of the university departments are implemented through programs, the program director need not be the head of a university department.

b. The programs have educational responsibilities that are not limited to the medical school but include those of the other health professional schools of the health sciences center that provide part of their education at Case Hospital.

c. The programs facilitate other teaching, research, and care responsibilities unique to the hospital, its medical staff, and its personnel and are separate from those of the schools and university departments.

2. Considering the differences between the programs and the university departments (composition and nature of their personnel, the schools to which they relate, kinds and nature of their facilities, budgetary sources, etc.), the programs, for their successful operation, must derive their authority from and be directly responsible to the office of the vice-president of the health science center. For the vice-president of the health science center to assume this role, he will require an associate vice-president. The associate vice-president will organize and administer the activities of the multiple programs and will be responsible to the office of the vice-president of the health sciences center for this as well as for the operation of the hospital as a whole.

Responsibility and authority of the program director

1. The program director is responsible for providing the hospital clinical environment for educational programs for medical students and other students of the health sciences center that take place in the facilities of his program. In this regard, he must be responsive to the respective chairmen of the university departments in the medical or other professional schools (or, when appropriate, to the chairman of interdisciplinary teaching committees) for that segment of the teaching program assigned to his facility.

2. The program director is responsible for providing the hospital clinical environment in which research activities take place within the facilities of his program. This must be carried out within the guidelines established for human research at the health sciences center.

3. The program director is responsible for the operational aspects of the patient care activities conducted within the facilities of his program. In this regard, he must be responsive to the respective university departmental chairmen.

4. The program director participates with the appropriate university departments or appropriate segments of these departments or both in planning the operations to be conducted in his facilities, and he participates in the budgeting for each of them. After this, he assumes the management responsibility for the operation of his program and its budget.

5. The program director has the authority to utilize the total resources made available to him in whatever way seems most appropriate to fulfill his various commitments. However, any major deviations from previous operational and budgetary planning requires appropriate consultation with the administrative officers, department heads, or specialty unit heads, who provide these resources.

6. The program director is responsible

for remaining within the total budgetary constraints that have been established for his program. He may alter budgetary categories and has the opportunity to seek additional income resources that, if obtained, may be made available for further program alteration or amplification. However, all professional fees generated by the full-time professional personnel within his program are the property of the university department in which these personnel have their primary academic appointment but with the understanding that the department will be responsive to the needs of the program.

7. The program director, in accomplishing his operational management responsibilities, must be provided with the multiple services and support he requires from the hospital resource systems, the university departments, the health science center and the university at large. Essential to the efficient conduct of his management responsibilities is the availability of timely and accurate fiscal and statistical information.

8. The program director's policy-making responsibilities are limited to the function of his operational unit. Also, as a faculty member, he may participate in academic policy formulation. In addition, as a program director, he may contribute to the formulation of hospital policy. In his role as program director, he is responsible for implementing all policies pertaining to his program.

9. Each program director recognizes that he does not function in isolation but participates with the other directors in assuring optimal institutional unity.

10. The collective program directors recognize that the number of programs and the scope contained within each

is flexible and that there is need, from time to time, to review and consider modifications in each program or alterations in the total number of such programs.

Shifts in power and authority

With the program as locus for decision-making two shifts in using power and authority in a participative environment must take place simultaneously. First, managers in resource systems must accept decision-making responsibility that has usually been held under the command authority of top management, and exercise this responsibility in a participative manner to support the needs of programs through decisions made at that level. Second, professionals who have usually made decisions at the program level outside the influence of top management's command authority must begin to share responsibility by making decisions in a participative manner. To accomplish this, missions and objectives must be delineated in advance and there must be one ultimate source of authority by balanced command and influence that meshes all systems into a synergostructure supporting the missions of the center.

A number of organizational arrangements have been suggested, several of which are pictured in Figs. 12-2 to 12-7. If resource system and program management is to remain almost exclusively a hospital responsibility, with program directors representing care, teaching, and research interests, variations of model A may be used. Model B is similar to the structure originally implemented and removes program management from the usual hospital structure and places it in broader perspective for balancing clinical interests. Model C is, in a sense, dynamically qualified, since it considers where the organization has been, where it is now, and where it may want to go in the future. There are, of course, many variations of each model that might be tried.

Text continued on p. 243.

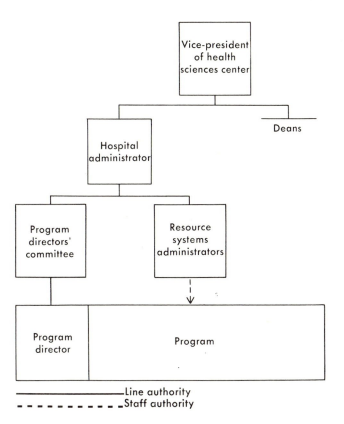

VICE-PRESIDENT OF HEALTH SCIENCES CENTER—responsible to president of the university for all operations of the health sciences center and its entities.

DEANS—responsible to vice-president of health sciences center for respective educational programs; clinical interests represented in program management by program directors.

HOSPITAL ADMINISTRATOR—responsible to vice-president of health sciences center for all patient care and resource activities in the hospital; care interests represented in program management by program directors.

PROGRAM DIRECTORS' COMMITTEE—responsible to hospital administrator for coordinating program operations; incorporates hospital medical staff organization and medical director.

PROGRAM DIRECTOR—responsible to hospital administrator for overall program management and patient care, and to deans for respective clinical interests; director's personal orientation may have substantial influence on the way care, teaching, and research are emphasized.

RESOURCE SYSTEMS ASSISTANT ADMINISTRATORS—responsible to hospital administrator for management of resource systems and providing resource outputs to programs; incorporates professional service departments as a resource system under a director of professional services.

Fig. 12-2

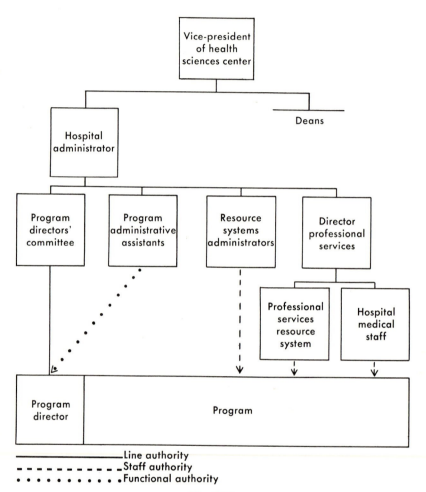

Fig. 12-3

VICE-PRESIDENT OF HEALTH SCIENCES CENTER—responsible to president of the university for all operations of the health sciences center and its entities.

DEANS—responsible to vice-president of health sciences center for respective educational programs; clinical interests represented in program management by program directors.

HOSPITAL ADMINISTRATOR—responsible to vice-president of health sciences center for all patient care and resource activities in the hospital; care interests represented in program management by program directors and program administrative assistants.

PROGRAM DIRECTORS' COMMITTEE—responsible to hospital administrator for coordinating program operations.

PROGRAM DIRECTOR—responsible to hospital administrator for overall program management and patient care, and to deans for respective clinical interests; director's personal orientation may be balanced by that of the program administrative assistant.

PROGRAM ADMINISTRATIVE ASSISTANTS—responsible to hospital administrator and program director as a person working for the program director with functional authority assigned by the hospital administrator; responsible for representing the hospital's interests in patient care and for day-to-day program operations.

RESOURCE SYSTEMS ASSISTANT ADMINISTRATORS—responsible to hospital administrator for management of resource systems and providing resource outputs to programs.

DIRECTOR OF PROFESSIONAL SERVICES—responsible to hospital administrator for management of the professional services resource system and for the professional service and organization of the hospital medical staff.

Fig. 12-3—cont'd

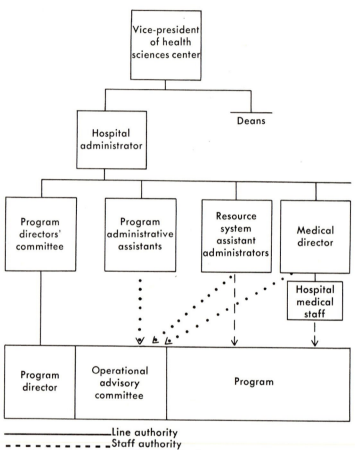

Fig. 12-4

VICE-PRESIDENT OF HEALTH SCIENCES CENTER—responsible to president of the university for all operations of the health sciences center and its entities.

DEANS—responsible to vice-president of health sciences center for respective educational programs; clinical interests represented in program management by program directors.

HOSPITAL ADMINISTRATOR—responsible to vice-president of health sciences center for all patient care and resource activities in the hospital; care interests represented in program management by persons serving on the operational advisory committee including the program director, the program administrative assistant, a nurse, and a member of the hospital medical staff; other persons with functional authority might also be assigned to the committee.

PROGRAM DIRECTORS' COMMITTEE—responsible to hospital administrator for coordinating program operations.

PROGRAM DIRECTOR—responsible to hospital administrator for overall program management and patient care and to deans for respective clinical interests; director's personal orientation may be balanced by the operational advisory committee.

PROGRAM ADMINISTRATIVE ASSISTANTS—responsible to hospital administrator and program director as a person working for the program director with functional authority assigned by the hospital administrator; responsible for representing the hospital's interests in patient care and for day-to-day program operations; other persons assigned to the operational advisory committee would fulfill a similar role related to care and resource systems integration.

RESOURCE SYSTEMS ASSISTANT ADMINISTRATORS—responsible to hospital administrator for management of resource systems and for providing resource outputs for programs; may provide resource personnel with functional authority to operational advisory committees; incorporates professional service departments as a resource system under a director of professional services.

MEDICAL DIRECTOR—responsible to hospital administrator for the hospital medical staff organization.

Fig. 12-4—cont'd

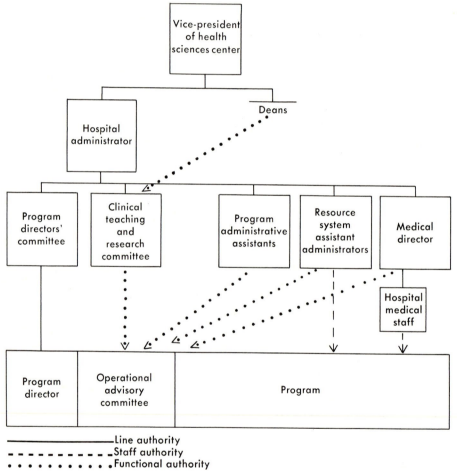

Fig. 12-5

VICE-PRESIDENT OF HEALTH SCIENCES CENTER—responsible to president of the university for all operations of the health sciences center and its entities.

DEANS—responsible to vice-president of health sciences center for respective educational programs; clinical interests represented in program management by program directors and appointed teaching and research representative on the clinical teaching committee.

HOSPITAL ADMINISTRATOR—responsible to vice-president of health sciences center for all patient care and resource activities in the hospital; care interest represented in management by persons serving on the operational advisory committee including the program director, the administrative assistant, a nurse, and a member of the hospital medical staff; other persons with functional authority might also be assigned to the committee.

PROGRAM DIRECTORS' COMMITTEE—responsible to hospital administrator for coordinating program operations.

CLINICAL TEACHING AND RESEARCH COMMITTEE—responsible to hospital administrator for coordinating the overlay of teaching and research interests on patient care; the committee would be composed of the program directors, hospital administrator, medical director, and a representative of each school with clinical teaching and/or research concerns; representatives of this committee should be assigned to work with operational advisory committees.

PROGRAM DIRECTOR—responsible to hospital administrator for overall program management and patient care and to deans for respective clinical interests; director's personal orientation may be balanced by the operational advisory committee.

PROGRAM ADMINISTRATIVE ASSISTANTS—responsible to hospital administrator and program director as a person working for the program director with functional authority assigned by the hospital administrator; responsible for representing the hospital's interests in patient care and for day-to-day program operations; other persons assigned to the operational advisory committee would fulfill a similar role related to care and resource systems integration.

RESOURCE SYSTEMS ASSISTANT ADMINISTRATORS—responsible to hospital administrator for management of resource systems and for providing resource outputs for programs; may provide resource personnel with functional authority to operational advisory committees; incorporates professional service departments as a resource system under a director of professional services.

MEDICAL DIRECTOR—responsible to hospital administrator for the hospital medical staff organization.

Fig. 12-5—cont'd

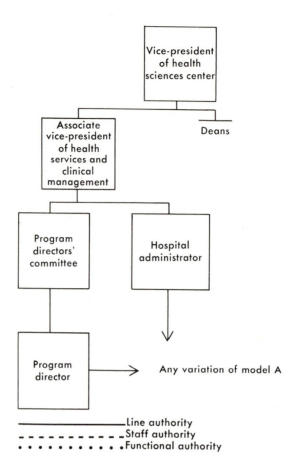

VICE-PRESIDENT OF HEALTH SCIENCES CENTER—responsible to president of the university for all operations of the health sciences center and its entities.

ASSOCIATE VICE-PRESIDENT FOR HEALTH SERVICES AND CLINICAL MANAGEMENT—responsible to vice-president of health sciences center for all center-sponsored health services and clinical management.

DEANS—responsible to vice-president of health sciences center; responsibilities approximately like those outlined in model A or model B.

HOSPITAL ADMINISTRATOR—responsible to associate vice-president for health services and clinical management; responsibilities approximately like those outlined in model A or model B.

PROGRAM DIRECTORS' COMMITTEE—responsible to associate vice-president for health services and clinical management; responsibilities approximately like those outlined in model A or model B.

Fig. 12-6

Operational advisory committees are shown for models A to C. Committees of this type have not been implemented and, as a result, there has been general failure to achieve hard-hitting management within programs. An operational advisory committee will lend balance and coordination in any overall structure from models A to C, with effectiveness increasing in proportion to the caliber and functional authority of the participants.

A variation of the committee might be for the superiors of persons on the committee to collectively write composite job-description/management expectations for the committee as if it were a person and to collectively supervise its performance as a single superior. In this role it would become a functional operating group, possibly replacing the program director and reporting to a group of superiors, which would report to the associate vice-president. This, of course, demands management ability to gain a vibrant in-depth group process working toward shared missions.

Unfortunately, it is virtually impossible to design a useful structure before missions and objectives are determined in a working planning and management process.

LACK OF AGREEMENT

There was a lack of agreement on missions and goals of the institution and no common *will* to achieve institutional purposes.

The center's goal and policy statements were substantial and futuristic. Problems arose not so much from the statements themselves as from the facts that (1) they were not created through meaningful participation by organizational members, (2) they were not internalized within the center and its entities because of the lack of well-coordinated planning and management processes that could reduce them to operating objectives and communicate and coordinate them throughout the organization,

and (3) they were not systematically re-evaluated and changed or updated over time.

The hospital's goals were stated separate from the center's and, although they were derived with knowledge of some of the points eventually stated in the center goals and policies, they were not thoroughly incorporated. To the extent of broad resource system objectives the hospital experienced a degree of success, but overall directions were not specifically reconciled with the center's objectives, and as the center gradually failed to achieve operational emphasis, progressively larger gaps developed between the center and the hospital.

These gaps are exemplified by the following three points.

Need for planning and implementing systems for the public

It did not seem that the best interest of social and political necessity or of developing and demonstrating new knowledge in the area of health care delivery could be met without participating in planning and implementing systems that help make service available to the general public. Social and political pressures have made it clear that the center and the hospital cannot practice disinterest or passive tolerance where their immediate geographic community's total health needs are concerned. Furthermore, regional and national trends look to major health institutions for new concepts for health care delivery as demonstrated by federal health maintenance organization legislation, Ameriplan, state insurance commissioner's statements on Blue Cross and hospitals, and regional comprehensive health planning recommendations. The position of providing service that emphasizes teaching and research is defensible, but it does not absolve the center of the responsibilities arising from its commitment to create and demonstrate new knowledge, its state-relatedness, or its position in an urban university. There has been

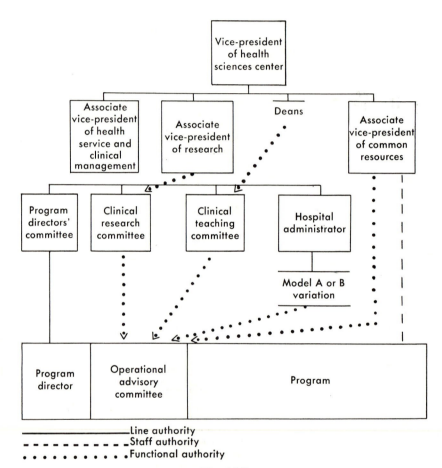

Fig. 12-7

VICE-PRESIDENT OF HEALTH SCIENCES CENTER—responsible to president of the university for all operations of the health sciences center and its entities.

ASSOCIATE VICE-PRESIDENT FOR HEALTH SERVICES AND CLINICAL MANAGEMENT— responsible to the vice-president of health sciences center for all center-sponsored health services and clinical management.

ASSOCIATE VICE-PRESIDENT FOR RESEARCH—responsible to the vice-president of health sciences center for coordination of all research conducted in the center, including clinical research.

DEANS—responsible to vice-president of health sciences center for respective educational programs; clinical interests represented in program management by research and teaching representatives on the clinical research and clinical teaching committees.

ASSOCIATE VICE-PRESIDENT FOR COMMON RESOURCES—responsible to vice-president of health sciences center for resources commonly used throughout the center as maintenance and personnel services.

PROGRAM DIRECTORS' COMMITTEE—responsible to the associate vice-president for health services and clinical management for coordinating program operation.

CLINICAL RESEARCH COMMITTEE—responsible to the associate vice-president for health services and clinical management for coordinating the overlay of clinical research interests on patient care. The committee would be composed of representatives from each school, the offices of the associate vice-president for health services and clinical managment and hospital administrator and from the program directors' and clinical teaching committees; representatives of this committee should be assigned to work with operational advisory committees.

CLINICAL TEACHING COMMITTEE—responsible to the associate vice-president for health services and clinical management, for health services for coordinating the overlay of clinical teaching interests on patient care; the committee would be composed of representatives from each school, the offices of the associate vice-president for health services and clinical management and hospital administration and from the program directors' and clinical research committees; representatives of this committee should be assigned to work with operational advisory committees.

HOSPITAL ADMINISTRATOR—responsible to the associate vice-president for health services and clinical management; responsibilities should approximate those outlined in model A or model B.

PROGRAM DIRECTOR—responsible to the associate vice-president for health services and clinical management; responsibilities should approximate those outlined in model A or model B.

Fig. 12-7—cont'd

little indication as to whether hospital or center will bear prime responsibility for this area.

Exceeds hospital parameters

Original center goals called for the hospital to demonstrate ideal and practicable forms of organizing and applying new knowledge to clinical science. Original hospital goals assumed this responsibility and included in it new forms of organization and management.

Subsequent development of programs (originally identified in a very general sense) raised organizational questions that exceed the parameters of the "hospital," as the term is often used to identify a provider of hotel services to a doctors' workshop, and left unidentified the seat of responsibility and decision making that will accomplish the stated objectives.

Organization and management insufficient for complexities

Center objectives such as "single standard of care," "eradication of the distinction between social classes of patient," "treating the whole patient," "formation of teams of mutually reinforcing health care personnel," "extending appointment hours," and "making the most rational use of scarce and qualified health personnel" are matters of significant consequence that focus on the hospital (whether inclusive or exclusive of program management) but are closely interrelated with other activities throughout the center. Centerwide organization and management was not developed sufficiently to handle the complex interplay involved and consequently specific responsibilities for meeting these objectives are left unassigned.

With these and a host of other areas, goals and responsibilities are not clear and the hospital, other entities, and the center have often gone in different directions with diverging interpretations of the requirements and different, often conflicting, meth-

ods of satisfying them. In some instances *no* action has been taken.

Each of these problem areas reflects inadequate planning and management. At the same time many similar but broader problems related to the overall organization of the center and its relationship to central university administration antagonized the situation and intensified the void at those critical junctures where intense communication and close interface should have occurred.

FUTURE NECESSITIES

The future of the center will depend on its adaptness at clarifying relationships with the main university, defining and internalizing missions and objectives, and organizing and creating viable planning and management processes. Thus the center must move with special emphasis on the following eight points:

Placing itself in perspective with the total management of the university. This should be accomplished through a strong office of the vice-president that is vested with full authority and accountability for the management of a flexible center operating within university-wide policies and procedures.

Providing in-depth statements of missions and objectives that update original goal statements and guide the center's operational components toward them.

Creating a meaningful management development and training program that promotes realization of management responsibility for producing optimum results in assigned areas and acknowledges that many organizational participants cannot be managed through command authority but may be constructively influenced through communication and motivation in a participative process (a primary means of integrating individual aspirations with the needs and missions of the center). The center must have vigorous managers who set a personal example of the will to work and innovate for energetic employees who are self-motivated to achieve.

Implementing a planning process that ensures a sense of direction of where the center is going, by deliberate choice, and provides for reaching and revising agreement in a decentralized, participative management decision-making process where influence is as important as command authority.

Establishing a flexible but unified organizational structure with decentralized decision centers integrated in a well-coordinated pattern of health sciences center management. Emphasis must be placed on an assignment of specific responsibilities.

Effectively integrating with the social, economic, and political environment that supports the Center. This integration, of course, introduces the possibility of changing present modes of operation to bring them more in line with the realities of environment and must stress relationships with (1) outside agencies and groups such as community-negotiating teams, local and regional hospital planning committees, the regional health planning council (Public Law 89-749), and the regional health affiliates, (2) teaching and research affiliations with other institutions, and (3) institutions that may organizationally integrate with the center in the future.

Realistically evaluating resources, with a special eye to the future, and maximizing their use to achieve evaluated consumer needs. The center should develop program budgeting with precise cost identification so that future operations may be predicated on ability to find adequate financing. This requires setting forward-looking missions and objectives (operating in the interest of society and seeking outside funding for public interest programs), undertaking only such programs as can be funded, and restricting *all* activities to those having priority and adequate fiscal support. Prepayment arrangements and operat-

ing or participating in health maintenance organizations must also be explored.

Developing a comprehensive, automated information system incorporating control feedback measured against established production, cost, and quality standards for care, teaching, and research.

• • •

The resource systems and programs concept departs from traditional approaches. It places the question of organizational missions squarely in controversial focus and recommends that organizational structure and management process be arranged to provide for optimal achievement. The basic building blocks of the organization become resource systems and programs. A program might be a unit that devotes its energies to any of a number of missions, including care, teaching, or research, or a unit where these are brought into clinical perspective such as clinical programs.

Resource system organization discourages isolationism and reduces the cumbersome process of responding in a large hierarchy. It is more flexible, and, with the use of functional authority, places decision making at points of timely response and appropriate coordination. Programs offer units concentrating on missions where multiple clinical interests must respond to patient need. Each participant can concentrate on his particular expertise within a management process that provides coordination, collaboration, and balance. Again, as in resource systems, there is a decision center where the action is promoting quick response among appropriate participants and greater, more in-depth group process and motivation.

Programs introduce new management possibilities into the usual medical-center complex. Here practitioners, professors, and scientists can meet in a matrix of collaborative endeavor to determine directions mutually beneficial to their vested but interdependent roles. Much depends, of course, on quantification and integration of center goals, since even mature men may not act rationally when values are in conflict and goals are ambiguous. As a decentralized unit well-coordinated within the framework of the center, the program offers an opportunity to involve the professional directly in an organizational and administrative network in a way that gives him assigned accountability in a specific decision center that has a uniqueness all its own. Where growing concern centers on delivery of care, the program, developed to its full potential, holds a key to new models. It is a decision center that can experiment under a director accountable for a wide range of decisions within latitude provided by overall center guidelines.

In other complexes, program goal emphasis might be different, but its organizational and management principles would remain constant. Since any number of programs might exist in one center and since the manner in which they are collectively coordinated may be arranged to fit a variety of grand designs influenced by available resources, environment, mission, and a host of other factors, the program is an appropriate candidate for pilot development and applied research study.

Despite some discouraging overtones, the experiment has been productive. Many conditions that remain unchallenged in other institutions have surfaced and been dealt with at the center. Predictably, most progress has been in the areas of minimum stress, but other more difficult areas have yielded too, sometimes by design, often by compromise. But compromise should be expected and welcomed as a sign of change; original thinking will seldom emerge unchanged although it is desirable to achieve a systematic process for changing it.

Other organizations considering similar endeavors should proceed with well-stated and -understood purposes and with planning and management strengths sufficient for the task, lest they experience a *free-floating apex*, which, according to Dr. Laurence J. Peter, is the "rare phenomenon of a hierarchical pyramid consisting solely of the capstone, suspended aloft without a base to support it."*

---

*Peter, L. J., and Hull, R.: The Peter principle, New York, 1969, William Morrow & Co., Inc., p. 22.

PART FIVE
PROJECTION

Perhaps the greatest need in health care
is the need to project organization beyond
the traditional patterns.

chapter thirteen

BEYOND TRADITIONAL PATTERNS

HEALTH UNIVERSITY

There remains in this country a considerable gap between health theory and health practice. A partnership between the academician and the practitioner should be created to bridge this gap. A health university that assumes responsibility for developing new knowledge, teaching it to students, and experimenting with ways of applying it through a partnership with practitioners can accomplish this. It will become the home of theory. The synergistic framework, with its systems and programs, may be extended to this level with the specific objective of reducing human suffering and bettering the health of the individual.

From the university platform, resources are assimilated for teaching, research, and service. Fig. 13-1 provides the framework. The use of boards, as shown in the illustration, is significant since they are a major influence on the university in determining what programs are most advantageous to the total community. Such an undertaking will be only as successful as its leadership and its ability to provide the input into the action-oriented programs that provide a product or service.

Health university systems

Systems for the university will follow the criteria outlined in Fig. 13-2, with the ex-

ception of the medical staff system, which becomes the professional system, embracing all faculty including physicians. This system is the pivotal point of the university. It forms the backbone of service, education, and research. In this area will be found the practicing physicians and possibly also a number of doctors of veterinary medicine, Ph.D.s, physiologists, and biochemists. The main consumers are the various programs providing direct service, including clinical teaching programs, community mental health programs, neighborhood health center programs, outpatient or ambulatory programs, extended care facilities, and home care programs.

At the university level the professional system director will view this system as one that can provide inputs into any program in a fashion that will be functional to the program's purpose. Organization within the program may range from group or institutional practice to solo practice. The system must be flexible enough to allow input of professionals who can adapt themselves and must not be so inflexible that they will feel compelled to conform to existing philosophies of the area from which they came. This flexibility will be paramount in the area of community service, where new patterns of health care and its delivery are evolving.

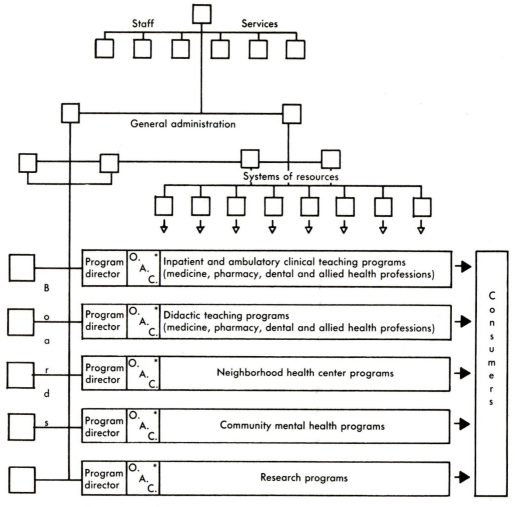

*Operational advisory committee

Fig. 13-1. Health university.

Linking the university professional system with the program medical staff system will probably be accomplished through group practice, with departments providing inputs to program floors. Program floor physicians will be members of line operational committees working in harmony with other providers of health care. This means that physicians will participate as members of a committee responsible for planning and initiating action decided upon by the committee. This committee will report to its specialty committee within the medical staff and also to an overall executive committee (see Fig. 5-2, p. 94). The same type of organization could apply to any program of the total operation and would allow for the continuity and quality factors of the practice of medicine being enforced on a standard basis throughout all programs.

The organization of the professional system should also allow for a broad spectrum of organization, from a heirarchy to a flat

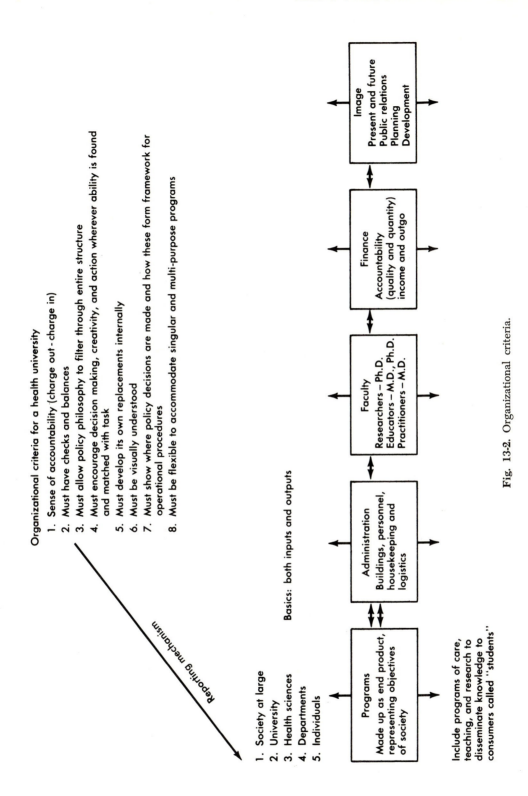

Organizational criteria for a health university

1. Sense of accountability (charge out - charge in)
2. Must have checks and balances
3. Must allow policy philosophy to filter through entire structure
4. Must encourage decision making, creativity, and action wherever ability is found and matched with task
5. Must develop its own replacements internally
6. Must be visually understood
7. Must show where policy decisions are made and how these form framework for operational procedures
8. Must be flexible to accommodate singular and multi-purpose programs

Reporting mechanism

Basics: both inputs and outputs

1. Society at large
2. University
3. Health sciences
4. Departments
5. Individuals

Include programs of care, teaching, and research to disseminate knowledge to consumers called "students"

Programs
Made up as end product, representing objectives of society

Administration
Buildings, personnel, housekeeping and logistics

Faculty
Researchers – Ph.D.
Educators – M.D., Ph.D.
Practitioners – M.D.

Finance
Accountability (quality and quantity) income and outgo

Image
Present and future
Public relations
Planning
Development

Fig. 13-2. Organizational criteria.

line. The use of committees and consultants is recommended and encouraged at every level. The organization is built so that abilities are recognized and decision making occurs at the level where the ability is found to make responsible decisions.

Health university programs

The health university will be organized around programs of service, teaching, and research carried out by the schools of medicine, pharmacy, and dentistry, the college of allied health professions, and the clinical teaching programs.

Major emphasis on education will occur in the schools of medicine, dentistry, and pharmacy and the college of allied health professions. The college of allied health professions will be concerned with the development of professionals for other medical professional areas such as nursing, medical records, medical record science technicians, laboratory technicians, x-ray technicians, pharmacy technicians, and registered nurses at the 2-year, baccalaureate, and master's degree levels. It will have in its curriculum means for developing programs lasting 6 weeks, 6 months, or even longer for employee training and retraining. In addition, it will add new specialists such as cardiac and intensive care specialists, electronic nursing specialists, and medical technologists as they are needed.

The organization of these educational programs will be under the direction of a dean in each program, with advisors to gear the teaching to the needs of the community. These include community leaders, program directors, and experts from the main university. Clinical teaching programs provide the clinical environment for these educational programs.

Policy for the broad, educational programs will be decided at the level of the health university in collaboration with its community-oriented board and the requests of the individual programs. The curriculum will be designed in a manner compatible with the basic objectives of the health university. It will provide for participation by those involved in the practice of health care and for the introduction of new members to the health university. It will change continually, based on needs of society, not on those of individual faculty members alone.

Research programs will emanate primarily from a research section in the professional system and will be supported largely by outside grants administered through a provost and his subdirector for research. This section will consist of Ph.D.s and other professional groups devoted to seeking out and solving problems relating to the relief of human suffering and betterment of the individual, both in the theory and in application. Researchers will be coordinated in a flexible organization in order to encourage the creativity and initiative necessary to research. This will create an environment that allows freedom of thought and action according to ability. The size and scope of the research section will be determined by the demand for its services, their social and economic* implications, and the objectives of the health university.

Service, research, and education must be incorporated in a setting that will encourage a bridging of the gap from the ivory tower to the workshop. Since the service programs are community as well as teaching oriented, they will be one of the university's major vehicles for practical application of these areas to modes of practice and operation.

The health university must integrate with the rest of the university in developing a viable philosophy that is based on the needs of man and not on the needs of a mechanized society per se. This is the

---

*Performance and program budgeting, as discussed in Chapter 7, are applicable throughout the university as the means of weighing competing demands upon resources in light of total objectives and the social and economic implications of those objectives.

evolution of the **human sector:** the merging of the private sector with the public sector, which results in the creation of a new sector. Here the needs of many may be better met through private enterprise and government's forming a partnership where both will contribute toward reaching the total objective.

In the human sector, historic movement has followed the lines of vested interests in a free-enterprise system oriented toward the industrial approach. The current demand is for coordinated achievement in a planned system oriented toward human need. The implications here are many. There is much potential. There is also danger. If the human sector works for the causes of success in a partnership with the government, we will build creative service organizations. If, on the other hand, a partnership does not materialize, broader public authority will become predominant, and creative potential in individual service organizations may be lost. The workability of such a partnership rests solely on the extent of mutual philosophic understanding. The health university will use the resources of the private sector and the public sector to evolve the human sector. Once the health university has done this, the human university will naturally follow.

HOSPITAL SERVICE CORPORATION

Hospitals have been harassed since their beginning by having to engage in too many businesses. They are collection agencies, laundries, bakeries, cafeterias, carpenter shops, personnel experts, teaching institutions, research centers, and much more. There was a time when the services of bakeries, laundries, and the like were not available to hospitals (at least these commercial enterprises were not interested in hospitals—the mystique scared them away). Furthermore, hospitals considered themselves to be charity institutions and wanted to be served at less than cost. Hospitals are now recognizing the fact that they are businesses and that they must be aware of the necessity of reducing costs whenever possible. Though their primary role may be patient care, certain ancillary services are unavoidable. These lend themselves to modern, imaginative business techniques such as the hospital service corporation.

The corporation should be organized as a nonprofit organization. Since no profits will accrue, the tax structure of the hospitals will not be altered. One administrative member and one board member from each participating hospital will comprise the governing board. A director will not be named, but the board will act as the directing force and as the arbitrator of conflict.

The appointment of personnel to the corporation will be by board appointment for the board representative and by position in the hospital for the administrative members. The chairmanship will be determined by the action of the governing board of the corporation, and no salaries will be paid. All business will be conducted during working hours at hospital expense.

Space and facilities can be acquired either from space in the existing hospitals or rented from some outside source. Ownership of these facilities by the corporation is not felt to be advisable at this time.

Computer services

Participating hospitals that have reached the stage in their growth that requires the services of a computer might obtain this service from the corporation, in conjunction with a large computer-manufacturing company, on a time-shared basis. The hospitals would be the initial users, and the service would eventually extend to nursing homes, clinics, and individual doctor's offices.

Many aspects of this type of computer operation are attractive to the service corporation. The hospitals would have consoles and other peripheral equipment in their offices and would be able to use the computer simultaneously. They would be connected through telephone lines to the computer center. What is envisioned is a kind of keyboard in each hospital by which information can be fed into the central computer. This will not be the same as the system whereby several companies go together to buy a computer and then must take turns using it. All participants will be able to use the computer concurrently. It can also be used by many individuals within the same hospital, with no waiting in line.

Within any given hospital the most likely users of the computer are the business office, medical records, purchasing, and dietary, but other departments will find at least limited uses for it, e.g., storing information, staffing, quality control, and pricing of service.

For billing, budgeting, payroll, maintaining and aging accounts receivable, cost accounting, etc. the computer will be invaluable. A central collection agency can be set up for the hospitals; or, if they do not want to actually operate the collection agency, the volume of their combined business will make it possible for them to negotiate with an outside agency at more favorable terms than at present because of the volume.

In fact, the bargaining status with the number of employees of the combined hospitals is very favorable when it comes to dealing with the third-party payers or government agencies or for negotiating for insurance, pension plans, and health insurance for the group.

Credit ratings can be maintained for the convenience of all the hospitals, a service that could easily be extended to physicians and to other related health agencies. It could become a central referral point, and appointment systems could be centrally maintained.

There are some individuals with unlimited imaginations who feel that, with this setup, hospitals would be in a position to formulate actuaries and thus determine their ability to underwrite the cost of care, thereby becoming the providers and financiers of health care. However, Sumner Marcus, writing in the January 1965 issue of the *Harvard Business Review*, cautioned that no "two companies which are major competitive factors in a given market can merge with each other under any circumstances."[1] Whether this would apply in any of the situations mentioned is a point that must be clarified as the plan unfolds.

Medical records

The feasibility of two or more hospitals' using a joint computer center to serve all hospitals has been proved. Vast amounts of medical information are gathered, stored, and partially retrieved. Why not share this information with each hospital or institution on a need basis? Custom says, "No, do not release information from one hospital to another, and certainly not 'privileged' information such as is contained in a medical record." But the information cannot be used to the fullest unless it is used wherever it will benefit the patient.

Let all medical data be available wherever the patient is currently receiving care or treatment. If progressive care from home environment to hospital to nursing home is to work to full advantage, then medical data must flow freely as the patient moves. A central computer would simplify this procedure.

Medical research would certainly be speeded by this process and would include area studies with a broad base. There need be no loss of individual identity of the participating hospitals. This would not remove control from the hospitals but would expand their resources and capabilities.

Dietary

Dietary will use the computer for maintaining inventories, for ordering, and for tallying selective menus as well as for dealing with problems involving portion control, quality control, and preference.

Dietary, one of the more cumbersome supportive services, desperately needs a real expert to manage it. A centralized kitchen for the hospitals, where food can be prepared and frozen (to be later reconstituted with electronic ovens), will use the computer to calculate the number of portions needed at projected future dates. In the volume that the combined hospitals will use this service, it is a worthwhile challenge to any large food concern.

Purchasing

The advantage of using the computer in maintaining inventories for purchasing, in calculating maximum and minimum limits in inventory, and in ordering requires no further elaboration. The convenience will be keenly felt, however, by everyone involved.

The same is true of the bargaining power when purchasing for three hospitals instead of one. Each hospital will be able to maintain its own individuality and autonomy, however, while taking advantage of the volume leverage when convenient.

Education

Hospitals have in the past maintained their own schools of nursing and other specialties when it became apparent that there were shortages in the fields. Education, however, is community business. No one hospital should have to support any school by taxing the sick, paying patient. This is everybody's business and is best supported by using everybody's tax dollars. Besides, who is better equipped to do the educating if not the educator? State schools of higher education are very willing to assume this task when they become aware that a need exists. Cooperation between the hospitals in the hospital service corporation could lead to cooperative educational innovations.

One group of hospitals in the Southwest has formed a program of this type. These hospitals are actively supporting a junior college in an adjoining community in starting a school of nursing that offers an associate degree. The hospitals provide the

clinical experience and housing facilities for the students during this period and augment the college staff by providing the clinical instructors.

For a number of years in the same community an intern and resident program has been combined, with three hospitals participating. The quality of the program was greatly improved when this merger was agreed upon and started, but the cost to each hospital has been reduced. Administrative detail need not be repeated in each hospital, and, although the quantity of teaching material has been increased, the cost has been spread over a broader base and therefore costs each individual hospital less. Medical staff members who are interested in teaching have been used to good advantage, with compensations made to everyone concerned. It is helpful that all physicians in the program have staff appointments at all three hospitals. A fully approved internship and residency in medicine and surgery are functioning, and, for the first time, the results of the matching program were successful. A notable increase in the quality of the program and in the quality of its interns and residents is apparent.

There is a possibility that a housing project for the use of the interns and residents will be shared by all three participating hospitals.

Personnel

A central personnel office for all hospitals brings a consistency in standards of all hospitals. This is something that could be done by a professional or by an outside agency such as an employment agency. Records could be kept centrally so that one hospital's misery does not become another's sorrow.

Laundry

One well-equipped laundry could presumably do the laundry for all hospitals. Commercial laundries can do the laundry for 18 cents per pound, whereas the nonprofit hospital laundry can do it for 12 cents per pound. Whether more volume could bring this still lower is worth investigating, for the profit margin does not have to be reckoned with, and it is unlikely that using a commercial laundry in the near future will be considered worthwhile.

• • •

Before such a hospital service corporation can be undertaken it is necessary to break down some of the barriers that separate health institutions. The establishment of a hospital planning council and a regional hospital council can do much to open up avenues of communication. This concept will be rejected by the empire-builders who have frantically added as many enterprises as possible in order to make themselves big and ostensibly invulnerable. The rising costs of medical care, however, are forcing hospitals to take a realistic look at their practices and to make some attempts at eliminating unnecessary duplication and fringe activities that add little but a superficial aura.

REGIONAL HEALTH AUTHORITY

As the healthy university will become the home of health theory, so the health care industry will become the home of health practice. In meeting America's new health demands, every health resource and program must be exploited for its maximum potential. Institutions and leaders must collaborate on a regional basis to produce a mature industry. The Comprehensive Health Planning and Public Health Service Amendments of 1966 provide a mechanism through which this may be done.

It would be reassuring to feel that voluntary efforts could bring about the needed change at an acceptable rate. However, history has shown and present experience continues to support the fact that, where change is needed in the human sector for human good, a more representative spokesman for the public must exert considerable pressure. This point is borne out by the recent position of many hospitals that the government's insistence that government reimbursement to hospitals under Titles XVIII and XIX of amounts representing depreciation and interest attributable to capital items must be used in accordance with a state's overall planning under the Partnership for Health Act (Public Law 89-749) is unwarranted control over a normal cost item of the hospital and results in interference with the *inherent rights* of hospital trustees to control finances of individual hospitals. It is also reflected in the feeling of hospital associations that hospitals are so complex, with responsibilities extending in so many charitable endeavors, that they cannot be subject to the management guidelines for other fields.

A more realistic approach is one of proper perspective and change in attitude. Only at a regional level can sufficient perspective be gained to effectively organize and apply the varied resources of the community. But perspective alone is not enough; it cannot be useful unless it is applied. Traditional attitude defends the sacredness of individuality and of differing ideologies. These are necessary to a dynamic and creative world, for it is through individual curiosity and contention between ideologies that we advance to new discoveries. However, the full potential of these advances is continually hindered at the point of application for the common good because of the lack of coordination and collaboration. The regional health authority is visualized as bringing this necessary element into the picture. The regional health authority is visualized as an organization at the regional level to create administrative mechanisms necessary to maximize efforts. The authority should be designed to combine the interests of government with the creativity and flexibility of private enterprise. It must be free from detailed governmental regulations for personnel and financial administration and have flexibility

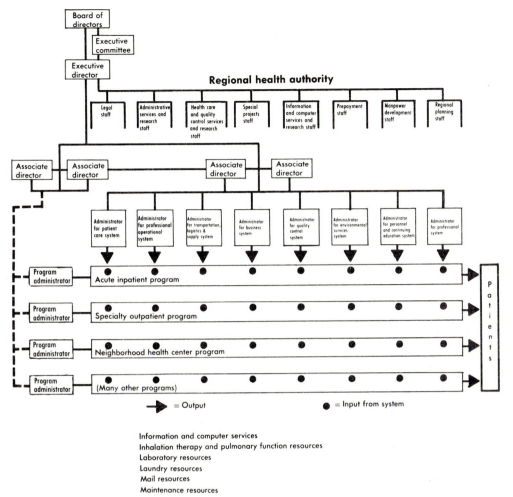

Fig. 13-3. Regional health authority.

to work within broad governmental policy.

The board of directors (Fig. 13-3) is appointed by the chief governmental official subject to established checks and balances. It must be representative of the resources and of the programs that draw from them. It must be a body that is competent to receive and use broad powers in a fair and equitable way. An executive director should be appointed by the board as its principal administrative officer. He will be responsible for implementing board policy and for conducting the financial and ad-

ministrative activities of the authority. Associate directors will assist him in fulfilling his duties.

Success in realizing the full potential of available resources and services will depend to a great extent on developing capable staff activities. At the staff level, projects will be undertaken to meet existing needs for improvement and to experiment and develop new innovations. As a minimum, the staff activities should include legal work, administrative services and research, health care and quality control services and research, special projects, information and computer services research, prepayment, and regional planning.

These staff activities should pursue ways of encouraging independent, efficient resource utilization and effective programs, incentives aimed at increasing productivity and cutting employees costs per unit produced, and comprehensive long-range planning with adequate financing. Thus an administrative framework is established through which resources and programs of service may be coordinated.

Resources

An inventory of the health resources in a region might include:

Referral and admitting resources
Anesthesiology resources
Blood bank resources
Business and financial resources
Communications resources
Construction resources
EEG resources
EKG resources
Food service resources
Housekeeping resources
Personnel resources
Pharmacy resources

These resources can be arranged into systems in much the same order as they are for the medical center and health university. They can be applied in a similar manner to regional programs, which might include:

Acute inpatient care programs
Convalescent inpatient care programs
Dental care programs
Domiciliary inpatient programs
Emergency care programs
General outpatient care programs
Home care programs
Medical research programs
Mental health programs
Neighborhood health center programs
Preventive medicine programs
Public health education programs
Public health service programs
Regional hospital council programs
Regional planning council programs
Rehabilitation programs
Specialty outpatient care programs
State, county, and city welfare programs

A collaborative relationship between the program administrator and the associate directors for the authority gives the program access to higher authority administration and staff function support. Thus collaboration is established to undertake the cooperative administration of many experts in a situation where a single boss has been outmoded.

There are currently in action a number of activities that could move in the direction of an authority. These are geographically isolated and sometimes limited in scope, but the possibility of grouping and coordinating the concepts in a single region is real.

Witness:

The growing success of regional planning associations in coordinating the planning and allocation of physical facilities, notably in the states of New York and California

The effect of Hill-Harris legislation and state governments on the geographic location of facilities coupled with the allocation of public monies

The success of the Hospital Councils of Southern and Northern California and the Commission for Administrative Services in Hospitals in soliciting the cooperation of a large number of leading citizens and hospitals to jointly undertake a common exploration of

1. Legal matters
2. Computer utilization
3. Efficient manpower utilization
4. Quality of patient care

The success of growing numbers of physician group practices and their efforts to provide services for identifiable groups of patients

The sudden interest of management, planning, and information systems consultants in the health care industry

The success of prepaid health insurance plans

The insistent interest of the federal government in supporting the exploration of the nation's health care needs and in experimenting with new ways of packaging and delivering care to meet those needs

The proposed federal legislation that would

give control of monies reimbursable under government sponsorship to an authority

The coordination of such activities toward efficient and effective utilization could occur as an entirely voluntary, collaborative effort.

POSTSCRIPT

As an industry, American health care is in its infancy. Like its big brothers in the profit sector, it will grow hard and fast. Because it is an industry, it must establish a committed objective and move toward it with objective intelligence. Unlike the profit sector, its impetus will be social pressure for change.

The American public is demanding change in health care. The nature, means, and direction of that change is still very general. But simple and cursory scanning of "the handwriting on the wall" can reach no other conclusion than that of inevitable change.

Change requires cause, hope, and direction. Resistance to change indicates that the greatest cause, hope, and direction lies in the status quo. Social change is largely evolutionary because a common cause sufficient to spawn revolutionary action does not often occur among the masses. In administrative organizations, however, specific boundaries are identifiable and organizational environments may be deliberately generated and worked with. Revolutionary change may be created and molded in predetermined directions.

Voluntary health care institutions and practitioners, and the system that they constitute, will be brought to response by the public and their governments. The question begging for an answer is: "Who will take the initiative and who will call the shots?"

In this book, health care is presented as a system, both from the perspective of a single organization and from that of a larger geographic base. An interlinking between individual entities and the larger whole of which they are a part and between the larger whole and the general social, economic, and political forces is achieved through a model that views resources pooled in **systems** and channeled into **programs** of service. This is the type of overview in which voluntary health care can find sufficient cause, hope, and direction to move to change under its own initiative. It is a frame of reference that establishes rights on the basis of ability, creates organizational structures that release human energy, and meshes the private and public sectors to produce meaningful payoffs through choices among representative courses of action.

As a system of organizations and individuals deliberately committed to promoting and maintaining health, the voluntary system has a wealth of experience. It is, at the moment, America's expert. Will it remain so?

As academicians and practitioners, we find ourselves squarely in the middle of a highly complex setting. We are faced with the responsibility for ongoing operations of a large health care organization while hypothesizing about the conduct of such organizations in our changing society. We are often reminded of the words of Thoreau:

> If a man does not
>   Keep pace
> With his companions,
>   Perhaps it is because
> He hears
>   A different drummer.
>   Let him step
> To the music which
>   He hears,
> However measured
>   Or far away.

This has been our philosophy in exploring the **organization and administration of health care.**

REFERENCE

1. Marcus, S.: New weapons against bigness, Harvard Bus. Rev. 43:104, Jan.-Feb. 1965.

SELECTED READINGS

BOOKS

American Hospital Association: Budgeting procedures for hospitals, Chicago, 1971, The Association.

American Hospital Association: Internal control and internal auditing for hospitals, Chicago, 1969, The Association.

Anthony, R. N.: Planning and control systems: a framework for analysis, Boston, 1965, Harvard University Press.

Argyris, C.: Personality and organization, New York, 1957, Harper & Row, Publishers.

Batten, J. D.: Tough minded management, New York, 1963, American Management Association.

Blau, P. M.: Bureaucracy in modern society, New York, 1956, Random House, Inc.

Blau, P. M., and Scott, W. R.: Formal organizations: a comparative approach, San Francisco, 1962, Chandler Publishing Co.

Brim, O. G., Jr., Glass, D. C., Lavin, D. E., and Goodman, N.: Personality and decision process: studies in the social psychology of thinking, Stanford, 1962, Stanford University Press.

Brown, R. E.: Judgement in administration, New York, 1966, McGraw-Hill Book Co.

Burkhead, J.: Government budgeting, New York, 1956, John Wiley & Sons, Inc.

Clark, J. M.: Competition as a dynamic process, Washington, D. C., 1961, The Brookings Institution.

Coe, R. M., editor: Planned change in the hospital, New York, 1970, Praeger Publishers, Inc.

Corson, J. J., and Paul, R. S.: Men near the top, Baltimore, 1966, The Johns Hopkins Press.

Dale, E.: Management: theory and practice, New York, 1965, McGraw-Hill Book Co.

Drucker, P. F.: The practice of management, New York, 1954, Harper & Row, Publishers.

Drucker, P. F.: The age of discontinuity: guidelines to our changing society New York, 1969, Harper & Row, Publishers.

Eells, R.: The government of corporations, New York, 1962, The Free Press.

Etzioni, A.: Modern organizations, Englewood Cliffs, N. J., 1964. Prentice-Hall, Inc.

Fayol, H.: General and industrial management, London, 1949, Sir Isaac Pitman & Sons, Ltd.

Fellner, W.: Competition among the few, New York, 1965, Augustus M. Kelly, Publishers.

Galbraith, J. K.: The new industrial state, Boston, 1967, Houghton Mifflin Co.

George, C. S., Jr.: The history of management thought, Englewood Cliffs, N. J., 1968, Prentice-Hall, Inc.

Georgopoulos, B. S., and Mann, F. C.: The community general hospital, New York, 1962, The Macmillan Co.

Gerth, H. H., and Mills, C. W.: From Max Weber: essays in sociology, New York, 1958, Oxford University Press, Inc.

Gouldner, A. W.: Organizational analysis. In Merton, R. K., et al., editors: Sociology today: problems and perspective, New York, 1959, Basic Books, Inc., Publishers.

Greenwalt, C. H.: The uncommon man, New York, 1959, McGraw-Hill Book Co., Inc.

Gulick, L., and Urwick, L., editors: Papers on the science of administration, New York, 1937, Institute of Public Administration, Columbia University Press.

Henderson, A. M., and Parsons, T.: Max Weber: the theory of social and economic organization, New York, 1947, The Free Press.

Hughes, E. C.: Professions. In Lynn, K. S., editor: The professions in America, Boston, 1965, Houghton Mifflin Co.

262

Kornlauser, W.: The interdependence of professions and organizations. In Vollmer, H. M., and Mills, D. L., editors: Professionalization, Engelwood Cliffs, N. J., 1966, Prentice-Hall, Inc.

Levinson, H.: The exceptional executive, Cambridge, 1968, Harvard University Press.

Lindberg, R. A., and Cohn, T.: Operations Auditing, New York, 1972, American Management Associations, Inc.

Likert, R.: The human organization: its management and value, New York, 1967, McGraw-Hill Book Co.

March, J. G., and Simon, H. A.: Organizations, New York, 1958, John Wiley & Sons, Inc.

McGregor, D.: The human side of enterprise, New York, 1960, McGraw-Hill Book Co.

Mortin, J. A.: Organizing for innovation, New York, 1971, McGraw-Hill Book Co.

Odiorne, G. S.: Management by objectives, New York, 1965, Pitman Publishing Corp.

Olsson, D. E.: Management by objectives, Palo Alto, Calif., 1968, Pacific Books, Publishers.

Peter, L. J., and Hull, R.: The Peter principle, New York, 1969, William Morrow Co., Inc.

Selznick, P.: Leadership in administration, New York, 1957, Row, Peterson & Co.

Selznick, P.: T.V.A. and the grass roots, Berkeley, 1949, University of California Press.

Simon, H. A.: Administrative behavior, New York, 1961, The Macmillan Co.

Simon, H. A.: The shape of automation: for men and management, New York, 1965, Harper & Row, Publishers.

Simon, H. A., Smithburg, D. W., and Thompson, V. A.: Public administration, New York, 1950, Alfred A. Knopf, Inc.

Sloan, A. P.: My years with General Motors, New York, 1964, Doubleday & Co., Inc.

Sloane, R. M., and Sloane, B. LeBov: A guide to health facilities personnel and management, St. Louis, 1971, The C. V. Mosby Co.

Somers, A. R.: Health care in transition: directions for the future, Chicago, 1971, Hospital Research and Educational Trust.

Soule, G.: Planning U.S.A., New York, 1967, The Viking Press, Inc.

Taylor, C.: In horizontal orbit: hospitals and the cost of efficiency, New York, 1970, Holt, Rinehart & Winston, Inc.

Taylor, F. W.: Scientific management, New York, 1947, Harper & Row, Publishers.

Thompson, V. A.: Modern organization, New York, 1965, Alfred A. Knopf, Inc.

Townsend, R. C.: Up the organization, New York, 1970, Alfred A. Knopf, Inc.

Toynbee, A. J.: Change and habit: the challenge of our time, New York, 1966, Oxford University Press.

Whyte, W. F.: Industry and society, New York, 1946, McGraw-Hill Book Co.

Whyte, W. H., Jr.: The organization man, New York, 1956, Simon & Schuster, Inc.

Wilcox, C.: Public policies toward business, Homewood, Ill., 1966, Richard D. Irwin, Inc.

ARTICLES AND PAPERS

Livermore, S.: The management of science: future guidance and leadership in science and technology, Program of Policy Studies in Science and Technology, Paper Number 8, George Washington University, Apr. 1965.

Peltz, D. C.: Creative tensions in the research and development climate, Science **157**:160, July 14, 1967.

Planning-programming-budgeting system: A symposium, Pub. Admin. Rev. **26**:243, Dec. 1966.

INDEX

265